Attention and Vision in Language Processing

Ramesh Kumar Mishra · Narayanan Srinivasan
Falk Huettig

Editors

Attention and Vision
in Language Processing

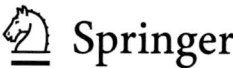 Springer

Editors
Ramesh Kumar Mishra
Center for Neural and Cognitive Sciences
University of Hyderabad
Hyderabad
Andhra Pradesh
India

Falk Huettig
Max Planck Institute for Psycholinguistics
Nijmegen
The Netherlands

Narayanan Srinivasan
Centre of Behavioural and Cognitive
    Sciences
University of Allahabad
Allahabad
Uttar Pradesh
India

ISBN 978-81-322-2442-6   ISBN 978-81-322-2443-3   (eBook)
DOI 10.1007/978-81-322-2443-3

Library of Congress Control Number: 2015940985

Springer New Delhi Heidelberg New York Dordrecht London

Printed on acid-free paper

Springer (India) Pvt. Ltd. is part of Springer Science+Business Media
(www.springer.com)

Preface

It is perhaps obvious that language interacts with vision and attention. In many everyday situations people give or receive directions or instructions for action or talk about things in their surroundings, say, a photo or a painting, the state of the kitchen sink, or an unfolding sports event. Moreover, our shifts in eye gaze are often (consciously or subconsciously) directed by spoken language input. A parent may tell a child to look at the beautiful leaf or a visitor may ask about a new gadget he has spotted in our living room. In short, the ability to integrate visual and auditory input with stored linguistic and nonlinguistic mental representations is a hallmark of human cognition. It follows from these observations that it is very likely to be a mistake to study language, vision, and attention independently of one another. It is surprising therefore that many of the cognitive processes occurring under such circumstances traditionally have been investigated in isolation although they are all involved when language is used.

The traditional approach to investigate language separately from other cognitive systems is a consequence of the theoretical development in the language sciences. Hockett, for instance, developed his list of features of human language (Hockett and Altmann 1968) and displacement (the fact that concepts need not refer to an object that is physically present) was considered a (or the) key feature of human language. Recent eye-tracking research however suggests that when the object of spoken language is actually physically present individuals express a strong tendency to refer to it. The cognitive system does this by orienting its visual sensory apparatus toward the object thereby linking a linguistically activated type representation to a specific perceptual token in the outside world. Cooper (1974), for instance, simultaneously presented participants with spoken fictional stories such as a safari in Africa and a visual display containing nine line drawings of concrete objects (e.g., a lion, a zebra, a tree, a camera, etc.). Participants in the study were asked to just listen to the stories. Cooper found that listeners' fixations of the objects were very closely time-locked to the unfolding speech input. Whenever a spoken word referred to an object participants rapidly shifted their overt attention to the object or similar objects even though this was not required

Mishra and Singh (Chap. 10) present evidence for language nonselective activation in Hindi–English bilinguals using an oculomotor task. They show that bilinguals suffer interference during a simple visual task suggesting that they activate translations of spoken words unintentionally. Mishra and Singh discuss the detrimental influence such nonselective activation may have on cognitive processing.

Finally, Part IV focuses on language processing in a social context. Lev-Ari (Chap. 11) discusses how the identity of interlocutors influences which cues we attend to during language processing. She points out that adjustments in the allocation of attention can have cascading linguistic and social consequences. Lev-Ari argues that it is indispensable for our understanding of language processing to study cognitive processes in different social contexts.

Vinson, Dale, Tabatabaeian, and Duran (Chap. 12) further take up the issue of language processing and social context. They review the literature suggesting that social cues (including low-level perceptual variables, perception of another's gaze, knowledge of another's belief states) influence language processes. They make the case for a systematic research agenda to uncover how various processes work together to bring about multimodal coordination between two or more interacting persons.

This volume emanates from the first "Attentive Listener in the Visual World" workshop held in 2012 at the Centre of Behavioural and Cognitive Sciences at the University of Allahabad, India. Studies of language, vision, and attention are intrinsically related. We hope that this volume will encourage further workshops and research on this crucial topic for the language sciences.

Hyderabad, India   Ramesh Kumar Mishra
Allahabad, India   Narayanan Srinivasan
Nijmegen, The Netherlands   Falk Huettig

References

Allopenna, P. D., Magnuson, J. S., & Tanenhaus, M. K. (1998). Tracking the time course of spoken word recognition using eye movements: Evidence for continuous mapping models. *Journal of Memory and Language, 38*, 419–439.

Cooper, R. M. (1974). The control of eye fixation by the meaning of spoken language: A new methodology for the real-time investigation of speech perception, memory, and language processing. *Cognitive Psychology, 6*, 84–107.

Dahan, D., & Tanenhaus, M. K. (2005). Looking at the rope when looking for the snake: Conceptually mediated eye movements during spoken-word recognition. *Psychonomic Bulletin and Review, 12*, 453–459.

Ferreira, F., & Tanenhaus, M. K. (2007). Introduction to the special issue on language–vision interactions. *Journal of Memory and Language, 57*(4), 455–459.

Fodor, J. A. (1983). *The modularity of mind: An essay on faculty psychology.* Cambridge: MIT Press.

Hartsuiker, R. J., Huettig, F., & Olivers, C. N. (2011). Visual search and visual world: Interactions among visual attention, language, and working memory (introduction to the special issue). *Acta Psychologica*, *137*(2), 135–137.

Hockett, C. F., & Altman, S. (1968). A note on designfeatures. In TASebeok (Ed.), *Animalcommunication: Techniques of study and results of research* (pp. 61–72). Bloomington: Indiana University Press.

Huettig, F., & Altmann, G. T. (2004). The on-line processing of ambiguous and unambiguous words in context: Evidence from head-mounted eyetracking. In M. Carreiras, & C. Clifton (Eds.), *The online study of sentence comprehension: Eyetracking, ERPs and beyond* (pp. 187–207). New York: Psychology Press.

Huettig, F., & Altmann, G. T. M. (2005). Word meaning and the control of eye fixation: semantic competitor effects and the visual world paradigm. *Cognition*, *96*, B23–B32.

Huettig, F., & Altmann, G. T. M. (2007). Visual-shape competition during language-mediated attention is based on lexical input and not modulated by contextual appropriateness. *Visual Cognition*, *15*, 985–1018.

Huettig, F., Rommers, J., & Meyer, A. S. (2011). Using the visual world paradigm to study language processing: A review and critical evaluation. *Acta Psychologica*, *137*, 151–171.

Huettig, F., Olivers, C. N., & Hartsuiker, R. J. (2011). Looking, language, and memory: Bridging research from the visual world and visual search paradigms. *Acta psychologica*, *137*(2), 138–150.

Logan, G. D. (1988). Toward an instance theory of automatization. *Psychological Review*, *95*, 492–527.

Mishra, R. K., Olivers, C. N. L., & Huettig, F. (2013). Spoken language and the decision to move the eyes: To what extent are language-mediated eye movements automatic? In V. S. C. Pammi, & N. Srinivasan (Eds.), *Progress in Brain Research: Decision making: Neural and behavioural approaches* (pp. 135–149). New York: Elsevier.

Tanenhaus, M. K., Spivey-Knowlton, M. J., Eberhard, K. M., & Sedivy, J. C. (1995). Integration of visual and linguistic information in spoken language comprehension. *Science*, *268*, 1632–1634.

Yee, E., & Sedivy, J. C. (2006). Eye movements to pictures reveal transient semantic activation during spoken word recognition. *Journal of Experimental Psychology: Learning, Memory, and Cognition*, *32*, 1–14.

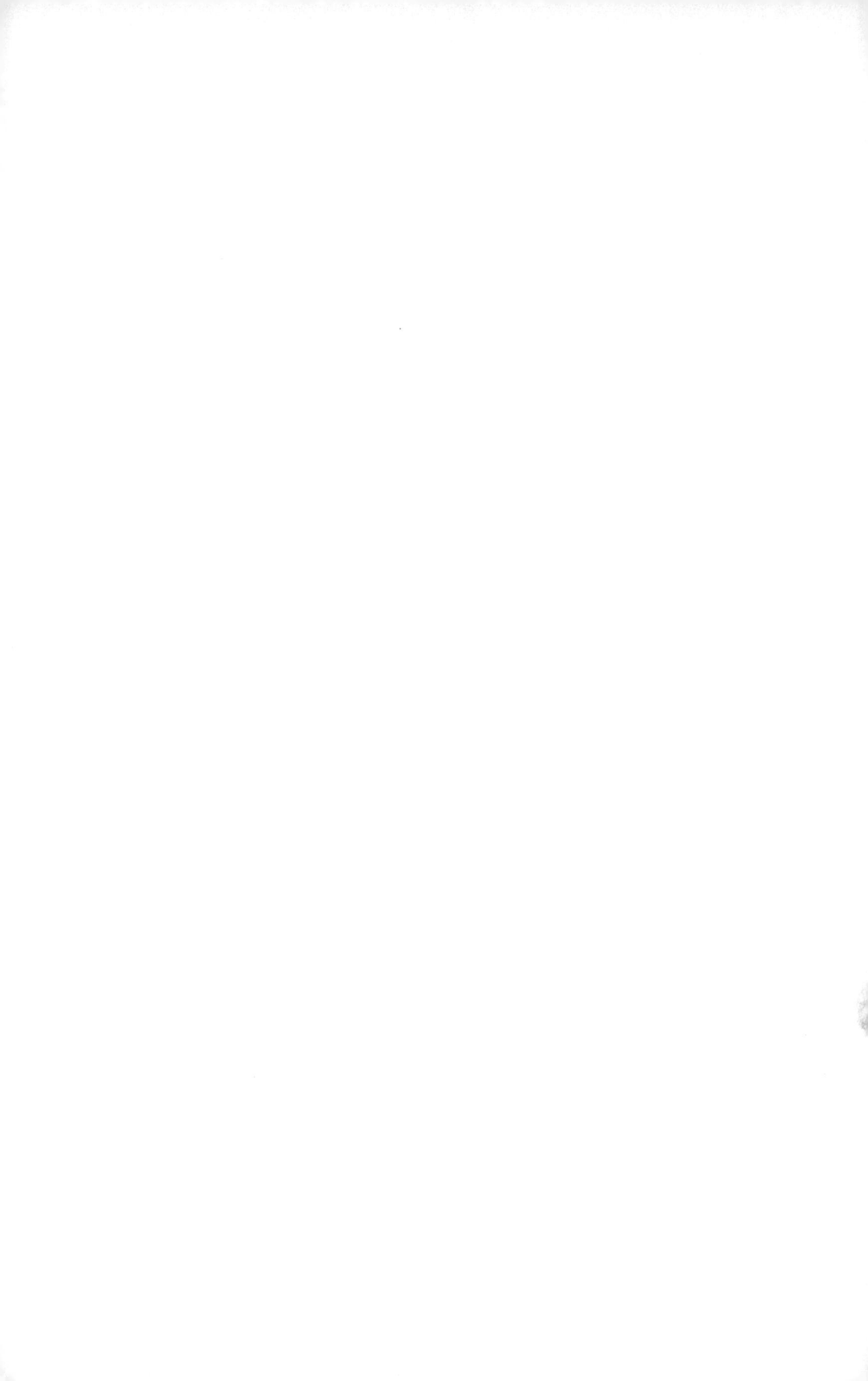

Contents

Editors and Contributors

About the Editors

Ramesh Kumar Mishra has a Ph.D. from the University of Delhi and is currently associate professor and Head at the Center for Neural and Cognitive Sciences, University of Hyderabad. He earlier taught at the Centre of Behavioural and Cognitive Sciences, University of Allahabad, India. Dr. Mishra has published widely in the area of psycholinguistics and cognitive science of language and has edited books in the area of language and cognition. His current research focuses on how language and other important cognitive processes like attention and vision interact during cognitive processing. Dr. Ramesh Mishra is on the editorial board of journals like Journal of Theoretical and Artificial Intelligence, Frontiers in Cognition. He also co-edits the International Journal of Brain, Culture and Cognition.

Narayanan Srinivasan is currently Professor and Head at the Centre of Behavioural and Cognitive Sciences, University of Allahabad, India. Professor Srinivasan was a visiting scientist at the Riken Brain Science Institute (2006–2012). He has a master's degree in Electrical Engineering from the Indian Institute of Science and subsequently earned his Ph.D. in Psychology from the University of Georgia, USA in 1996. He has been working at the Centre for more than a decade. His primary research interests are attention, perception, emotions, and consciousness. He employs multiple methodologies to study cognitive processes. Professor Srinivasan has edited six books and a special issue and has published more than a hundred journal articles, book chapters, and conference proceedings papers. He was the editor-in-chief of the International Journal of Mind, Brain, and Cognition and the associate editor of the journals, Frontiers in Cognitive Science, Cognitive Processing, Neuroscience of Consciousness, Royal Society Open Science, and Psychological Studies.

Falk Huettig is a Senior Investigator at the Max Planck Institute for Psycholinguistics in Nijmegen, Netherlands and a Visiting Professor at the University of Hyderabad, India. He received a B.Sc. and an M.Sc. from the University of Edinburgh and a Ph.D. in Psychology from the University of York, UK. His main research interest is in multimodal cognition. Other main interests include the effect of cultural inventions such as reading on general cognition in children, illiterate adults, and individuals with reading impairments; and predictive language processing. Falk Huettig is an editorial board member of the Journal of Memory and Language and editor-in-chief of Brain, Cognition, and Culture.

Contributors

Nicole Altvater-Mackensen Max Planck Institute for Human Cognitive and Brain Sciences, Leipzig, Germany

Sarah Chabal Department of Communication Sciences and Disorders, Northwestern University, Evanston, IL, USA

Rick Dale Cognitive and Information Sciences, University of California, Merced, CA, USA

Nicholas D. Duran Arizona State University, Tempe, USA

Robert J. Hartsuiker Department of Experimental Psychology, Ghent University, Henri Dunantlaan 2, Ghent, Belgium

Florian Hintz Max Planck Institute for Psycholinguistics, Nijmegen, The Netherlands

Falk Huettig Max Planck Institute for Psycholinguistics, Nijmegen, The Netherlands; Donders Institute for Brain, Cognition, and Behavior, Radboud University, Radboud University, The Netherlands

Raymond M. Klein Dalhousie University, Halifax, Canada

Pia Knoeferle Research Group "Language and Cognition", CITEC, Cognitive Interaction Technology Excellence Center, Bielefeld University, Bielefeld, Germany

Agnieszka E. Konopka Max Planck Institute for Psycholinguistics, Nijmegen, The Netherlands

Shiri Lev-Ari Nijmegen, Netherlands

Nivedita Mani University of Göttingen, Göttingen, Germany

Viorica Marian Department of Communication Sciences and Disorders, Northwestern University, Evanston, IL, USA

Ramesh Kumar Mishra Center for Behavioural and Cognitive Sciences, University of Allahabad, Allahabad, India; Center for Neural and Cognitive Sciences, University of Hyderabad, Hyderabad, India

Elisabeth Norcliffe Max Planck Institute for Psycholinguistics, Nijmegen, The Netherlands

Lillian Rigoli Cognitive and Information Sciences, University of California, Merced, CA, USA

Jean Saint-Aubin Université de Moncton, Moncton, Canada

Niharika Singh Center for Behavioural and Cognitive Sciences, University of Allahabad, Allahabad, India

Michael J. Spivey Cognitive and Information Sciences, University of California, Merced, CA, USA

Maryam Tabatabaeian Cognitive and Information Sciences, University of California, Merced, CA, USA

David W. Vinson Cognitive and Information Sciences, University of California, Merced, CA, USA

Heather Winskel Psychology, School of Health and Human Sciences, Southern Cross University, Coffs Harbour, NSW, Australia

Part I
Attention and Vision in Spoken Language Comprehension and Production

Chapter 1
Real-Time Language Processing as Embodied and Embedded in Joint Action

Lillian Rigoli and Michael J. Spivey

1.1 Introduction

The take-home message of this chapter is that language processing happens not only *inside* people's brains but also *outside* people's brains. From the perspective of the cultural evolution of language, this would not be a surprising message. For example, diachronic language change—over the course of decades and centuries—is clearly a process of information transmission that involves computational operations that are gradually performed on words and grammatical structures to change how the language is used (Christiansen and Kirby 2003; Tabor 1995). These gradual transitions in the content and form of a language constitute computational operations that are taking place in between individuals (not solely inside their brains) and across generations of the population. On a somewhat shorter timescale of months and years, groups of children have been observed to create their own communication systems that evolve into full-fledged languages (Senghas and Coppola 2001). On the shorter-still timescale of hours and days, undergraduate participants in a non-linguistic communication game will gradually settle on depictions of compact and distinctive symbols that become remarkably standardised over time (Bergmann et al. 2013; Galantucci 2005). Again, these kinds of cultural change in the content and form of a communication system are perhaps sensibly described as a form of information processing that is happening in the environment, not solely in the brains of the language users themselves.

However, moving down to the timescale of seconds and minutes, it may seem rather surprising to a cognitive scientist to conceive of the real-time language processing that takes place during a natural everyday conversation as involving

L. Rigoli · M.J. Spivey (✉)
Cognitive and Information Sciences, University of California,
Merced, CA 95343, USA
e-mail: spivey@ucmerced.edu

© Springer India 2015
R.K. Mishra et al. (eds.), *Attention and Vision
in Language Processing*, DOI 10.1007/978-81-322-2443-3_1

computational operations that happen in the environment, *in between* the brains of the language users. In much of the cognitive and neural sciences, we are accustomed to focusing our analyses on the mind and brain of an individual person. The sciences of language tend not to embrace the fact that a large proportion of the natural occurring situations that exhibit language exchange involve people co-creating their dialogue by contributing incomplete utterances, ungrammatical sentences, interruptions and completions of each other's sentence fragments (Clark 1996). Instead, much of linguistics and psycholinguistics has approached their science using individual carefully constructed complete sentences that are either delivered to a comprehender or elicited from a speaker. As such, the vast majority of our studies of real-time language processing have been devoted to identifying the computational operations that take place *inside* a single listener, or reader, or speaker.

In this chapter, we will briefly recount a series of experimental findings that are intended to stretch the reader's conception of language processing, step-by-step, further and further out of the realm of the traditional "language module" and into the realm of joint action. In the next section, a handful of laboratory results will be described that point to language processing in the brain as being richly interactive, perhaps even coextensive, with other perceptual and cognitive processes. This first step pulls real-time language processing out of its putative module and places it amid a vast network of brain areas that process a variety of mental faculties in a distributed fashion. The section after that describes a series of experiments showing that perceptual and cognitive representations in general (which, by then, the reader may see as also including language processing) are richly interactive, perhaps even coextensive, with action representations. Thus, how we interpret and think about our sensory input is shaped by what kinds of potential actions (affordances) we have at our disposal. This "embodiment of cognition" leads to the next section in this chapter, where we describe some experiments showing that motor action is itself interactive with real-time language processing. Importantly, motor action (with its linguistic information embedded in it) rarely takes place in a vacuum. The environment often contains other language users performing actions as well. Thus, the chapter concludes with a treatment of the joint action literature—where coordination between people produces shared behaviour—as a potential home for situating some of the information processing that constitutes real-time language use. Like joint action, joint language use may be best described as a process in which many of the important computational operations are happening in the environment, not solely in the brains of the participants.

1.2 Language Processing Is Coextensive with Perception and Cognition

Decades ago, George Lakoff argued for treating language not as a domain-specific module in the mind (Fodor 1983), but instead as part and parcel of the rest of cognition (Lakoff and Johnson 1980). The way we use everyday language reveals that our linguistic idioms and metaphors are tightly coupled with our general conceptual structure about how the world works. Moreover, recent work shows that a graph-theoretical analysis of the results from more than 30 neuroimaging studies reveals that several different mental faculties, including language, are subserved not by individual brain areas but instead by networks of brain regions, with most regions participating in multiple different networks (Anderson et al. 2010). Thus, the differences between mental faculties are better attributed to differences in patterns of cooperation between brain regions, rather than to differences in which brain region is used for each faculty.

A great many laboratory behavioural experiments have convincingly shown that, rather than being solely the function of a domain-specific communication mechanism, real-time language processing is tightly coupled with other cognitive and perceptual processes. One of the most convincing findings of interaction between language processing and another cognitive faculty is the McGurk Effect. McGurk and MacDonald (1976) audio-dubbed the spoken syllable "bah" over a video of a person saying "gah", and found that the resulting stimulus is compellingly perceived as the syllable "dah." Essentially, the visible mouth shape for "gah" is inconsistent with a bilabial place of articulation for the sound "bah", so the next closest syllable for that acoustic input is the alveolar place of articulation for the sound "dah," which is also consistent with the mouth shape being viewed. But rather than a long drawn out problem solving process of considering these alternatives, the listener usually experiences an instantaneous percept of hearing "dah." When the listener closes her eyes, the auditory percept instantly changes to the veridical "bah." Importantly, electroencephalography (EEG) measures indicate that this audiovisual integration takes place early on in perception (Colin et al. 2002).

More recently, headband-mounted eyetracking has provided a variety of findings showing how spoken language processing is quickly influenced by visual context (for a review of this methodology, see Richardson et al. 2007b). For example, at the timescale of dozens of milliseconds, phoneme perception is influenced by the set of visual objects available in the scene (McMurray et al. 2003). Likewise, as a spoken word unfolds over the course of a few hundred milliseconds, lexical representations of words that share those first couple phonemes become partially active (Marslen-Wilson 1987), and this pattern of lexical activations can be modulated by the set of objects that are visible in the environment (Eberhard et al. 1995). When instructed to "pick up the candy," listeners will often look briefly at a *candle* in the display before finally settling their attention on the candy. Not only does this effect work for cohorts such as candy/candle, tower/towel and penny/pencil, but it also works for rhymes such as candle/handle and beaker/speaker (Allopenna et al. 1998). Interestingly, it is not only phonetic similarity between the names of objects that causes these eye movements to competitor objects. Competitor objects that are visually similar and semantically related also draw brief eye movements, such as fixating a rope when instructed to "click the snake" or fixating a trumpet when instructed to "click the piano" (Dahan and Tanenhaus 2005; Huettig et al. 2006; Yee and Sedivy 2006).

Now, we move up from the timescale of dozens of milliseconds from one phoneme to the next, and focus on the timescale of hundreds of milliseconds from one word to the next. In much the same way that each incoming phoneme is being processed in the context of the visual environment, each incoming word is being interpreted in that visual context as well. For example, when instructed to "pick up the starred yellow rectangle," listeners are already fixating on the starred objects in the display before the noun is even spoken (Eberhard et al. 1995). If a single adjective is being immediately interpreted with respect to the visual context, what consequences does this have for complex visual search scenarios? Traditional visual search paradigms assume that when searching for a target object that conjoins two features (e.g., a red vertical bar), the search process is effortful, inefficient and substantially slowed down by distractor objects, but searching for a target object defined by a single feature (a red bar) is effortless, efficient and largely unaffected by the number of distractors. Thus, if listeners can start identifying the starred objects in a display before hearing the rest of "...the starred yellow square...," one might expect that they can also begin a visual search process for red objects before hearing the rest of "...red vertical bar." That initial visual search process would be guided by a single feature, not a conjunction of features, and should thereby proceed effortlessly and efficiently. Indeed, when participants hear "red" and then "vertical" while concurrently viewing the visual search display, their reaction times are largely unaffected by the number of distractors (Chiu and Spivey 2012; Reali et al. 2006; Spivey et al. 2001). This tells us that as the language system in the brain is engaging in its uptake of spoken lexical items, and the visual system in the brain is engaging in its visual search process, the two are interacting with each other and resolving each other's uncertainties within a fraction of a second.

When we move further up the timescale, from the hundreds of milliseconds for each word to whole seconds across the delivery of an entire spoken sentence, we can examine the effects of syntactic parsing in a visual context. Compared to word recognition, syntactic parsing is often treated as a qualitatively different kind of system. Whereas word recognition is typically assumed to involve the accessing of a pre-existing representation in something equivalent to a lookup table, syntactic parsing is typically assumed to involve each representation (or piece of syntactic structure) being produced anew using generative rules (Frazier 1995). As a result, syntax is often thought of as the more "truly linguistic" component of the language system, whereas word recognition can be seen as rather similar in style to other perceptual and cognitive processes, such as visual object recognition and memory retrieval. Therefore, for some linguists and psycholinguists, it may not be surprising that word recognition is so tightly coupled with visual context, but syntactic parsing can be expected to operate in a more context-free manner than that. After all, if syntax does not use pre-existing representations, then how could they receive spreading activation from the pre-existing representations used by another cognitive modality, such as visual object representations?

Irrespective of what format of representation is used by vision or by syntax, the evidence has nonetheless come to the fore that real-time syntactic processing is indeed immediately influenced by visual context. Based on eye-tracking experiments by Tanenhaus and colleagues (Spivey et al. 2002; Tanenhaus et al. 1995), when listeners are confronted with a classic temporary ambiguity in the syntax of an unfolding spoken sentence, referential properties of the visual context to which the sentence refers can bias the syntactic parsing process towards one structure or the alternative structure. When instructed to "Put the apple on the towel in the box," in a context where there is one apple already on a towel, an extra irrelevant towel, and a box, listeners often look briefly at the irrelevant towel shortly after hearing "Put the apple on the towel…". By contrast, if the visual context has multiple apples, then the prepositional phrase "on the towel" is instead parsed as part of the noun phrase "the apple on the towel", and looks to the irrelevant towel are rare. Thus, the exact same spoken instruction is syntactically parsed differently depending on the visual context.

Even without tracking people's eye movements during the course of their real-time comprehension of language, but instead simply recording reaction times long after the entire sentence has been processed, one can still observe evidence for visuospatial information playing an important role in language comprehension. When presenting visual probes after a sentence, the spatial orientation properties of that visual probe (e.g., vertical or horizontal) elicit faster or slower reaction times when they are consistent or inconsistent with the spatial orientation properties of the event described in the sentence (Richardson et al. 2003; Stanfield and Zwaan 2001). This suggests that the comprehension of the sentence may generate a kind of internal "perceptual simulation" of the event described by the sentence (Barsalou 1999). Likewise, when eliciting reaching movements after a sentence, the spatial orientation properties of that movement (away from the body or towards the body) exhibit faster or slower reaction times when they are consistent or inconsistent with the implied direction of the event bring described (Glenberg and Kaschak 2002; Kaschak and Borreggine 2008). In addition to static spatial properties, spatiotemporal properties of language (e.g., verbs of motion and metaphors of motion) also appear to recruit visuospatial information in carrying out the process of linguistic comprehension (Huette et al. 2012; Meteyard et al. 2008; Spivey and Geng 2001; Zwaan et al. 2004).

As can be seen from this short review, over the past couple of decades, a substantial amount of evidence has been accumulated that suggests that language in the brain is no longer productively seen as an independent cognitive module that uses its own domain-specific rules to conduct its internal information processing in a context-free manner. Rather, language in the brain is richly interactive with other cognitive and perceptual processes in the brain. However, as the progression through this chapter attempts to argue, this is only the first step in widening the scope of defining what language is. All the while that a handful of psycholinguists were re-interpreting language as part and parcel of the rest of perception-and-cognition, a handful of perceptual and cognitive psychologists were busy re-interpreting perception-and-cognition as part and parcel of action!

1.3 Perceptual and Cognitive Processes Are Coextensive with Action

Decades ago, Gibson (1979) encouraged the field to think of the job of perception not as a producer of internal object representations, but instead as crucially linked to motor movement contingencies. On a millisecond timescale, every bodily movement changes the sensory input in law-governed ways, and every change in sensory input alters the propensities for the next body movements. This perception-action loop (Neisser 1976) generates mathematical invariants in the information stream that can directly guide adaptive behaviour, without requiring intermediate stages of categorised information being presented to a central executive. Gibson's ecological perception treats sensory input as describable in terms of the associated actions it affords (Gibson 1977; Turvey 1992), and it treats motor output as describable in terms of the expected perceptual results of such actions (Jordan and Hunsinger 2008; Kawato 1999). In this account, perception and action are not discretely separable; and recently, cognition has been included in this superposition. For example, passively estimating the steepness of a hill or the distance to an object is influenced by the anticipated effort that would be expended in traversing them, thus inflating those judgments when one is wearing a heavy backpack (Proffitt 2006).

The actions we are able to perform on our environment immediately alter the way we perceive and cognize about it. By acting on our environment in ways that essentially perform some of our cognition for us, we enhance efficiency and accuracy in many cognitive tasks while lowering cognitive demand. This reliance upon the world keeps us from wasting energy that could be used elsewhere, and also provides tools for us to use when certain tasks are too complex.

For example, it seems as though the stable spatial interactions between our attention and our actions in the environment act as a fundamental asset to mental processes and to what we call "cognition". Deubel and Schneider (1996) investigated the spatial interaction of visual attention and saccadic eye movements, by having subjects make saccades to locations within horizontal strings of letters on the left and right of a central fixation cross. They then proceeded to make discriminatory judgments on a capital "E" presented tachistoscopically both upright and upside down within the distractor letters. The discriminatory performance by the participants was taken as a measure of visual attention. Results show that visual discrimination is best when both the discrimination stimulus and the upcoming saccade target are the same; discrimination of neighbouring items is near chance level. Furthermore, it seems to be impossible to direct attention to the discrimination target while making a saccade to a spatially close target, despite prior knowledge of the discrimination target position. The data clearly speak for a coupling of saccades and visual attention to one target object, thus favouring a system in which one attentional mechanism is responsible both for the selection of objects for perceptual processing and for providing the information required for motor action. The existence of substantial overlap in the processes of the visual attentional mechanism and the oculomotor mechanism (see also Corbetta 1998) implies that saccade programming and attentional focus on a target are not easily dissociated or decoupled, and points to a coextension and codependence between cognitive processes and action processes.

The relationship between neural activation patterns that are involved in motor movement and those that are involved perception is especially clear in electro-physiology research with monkeys. The accumulation of sensory information favouring one interpretation over others can be seen in the neural circuits corre-lated with the behavioural response. Gold and Shadlen (2000) trained monkeys to use their saccadic eye movements towards visual targets to indicate direction judgments about dynamic random-dot motion. Motion viewing was interrupted with electrical microstimulation of the frontal eye fields, and the evoked eye movements were analysed for continued activity associated with the oculomotor response. Gold and Shadlen found that the evoked eye movements actually devi-ated in the direction of the monkey's evolving perceptual decision, and that the magnitude of the deviation depended on motion strength of the random-dot stim-ulus and viewing time. While the perceptual information about motion direction gradually accumulated over hundreds of milliseconds in visual and parietal corti-cal areas, this information was continuously cascading into oculomotor processes in the frontal eye fields, such that when the microstimulation evoked a saccade, the resulting eye movement was a weighted average of the evoked direction and the partially-evolved perceptual decision direction. Thus, motor planning and decision formation appear to share much of their neural organisation, strongly suggesting another necessary coupling of cognitive processes with motoric action.

Taking advantage of eye movements as an index of visual attention, Ballard et al. (1995) used a block-copying task with humans to show how constant reli-ance on the environment is a natural tendency that facilitates task solving by serving as a form of external memory. Participants were presented with a dis-play divided into three sections: one section containing the block arrangement to be copied, a second consisting of the resource of blocks used to recreate the arrangement, and a third serving as the workspace in which the copy was assem-bled. Although it was entirely within visual memory limitations to individually memorise four sub-patterns consisting of two blocks each and copy the pattern with only four total fixations on the model block arrangement, participants often times made as many as 18 fixations on the model itself during the course of the task. In fact, it was common for participants to make more than one fixation of the model even while copying only a single block. Despite the instructions being sim-ply "copy the pattern as quickly as possible," participants employed a task-solving strategy which made constant use of the environment for memory storage, allow-ing participants to postpone accumulation of task-relevant information until just before it was needed to continue on with the task. These results display our nat-ural tendency to reduce mental workloads through motoric interaction with the environment.

As another example, Kirsh and Maglio (1994) used the game of Tetris as an experimental tool to compare the strategies of highly skilled Tetris players to the strategies of novice players. One might intuitively guess that skilled players are perhaps more competent in the art of quick mental rotation and pattern solving. Instead, the data showed that skilled players actually exploited the use of quick button presses in order to have the game quickly rotate the objects for them. The rotations and translations made by skilled players were perhaps best described as actions which make use of the environment to offload some internal cognitive processing. These external actions are not the result of an a priori plan; they are simply used by the player to streamline the task at hand. In the same way that a mental rotation of a Tetris shape in the brain (via the visual system) provides new information about whether the shape would fit into the game array, a physical rotation of that shape on the screen (via button press) provides equivalent new information. For this reason, Kirsh and Maglio referred to these motor movements as epistemic actions. Epistemic actions generate knowledge in much the same way as manipulating, turning and prying at a metal puzzle in your hands generates new knowledge about its potential solutions.

Another example of generating new knowledge, or performing cognitive operations, via interaction with the environment comes from problem solving research. Grant and Spivey (2003) tracked participants' eye movements while they attempted to solve Duncker and Lees' radiation problem (1945), which has proven to be an abundant resource for scientists studying insight and human inference making. In the first experiment, 36 % of the participants were successful in solving the problem, while 64 % failed to solve the task and required the use of hints. Analyses of eye-tracking data showed that during the last 30 s before inferring the solution, successful participants spent significantly more time looking at a specific part of the diagram than unsuccessful participants did. To further explore how situated cognition allows for improved problem solving, Grant and Spivey had a group of participants in Experiment 2 view an animated diagram that highlighted the critical feature discovered in Experiment 1, thereby controlling the perceptual properties of the environment to guide visual attention in a way that might assist reasoning skills. Under this manipulation, 67 % of participants successfully solved the problem without hints. How can simply highlighting one of the stimulus features result in twice as many participants able to infer the solution? In this study, Grant and Spivey manipulated the direction of participants' attention towards a critical feature of the diagram, inducing patterns of eye movements that not only revealed to the experimenters that they were approaching the solution but actually assisted cognitive processes towards insightful solving of the problem.

This set of results provides evidence for an intimate coupling between actions in the environment and mental operations. Through this intertwinement, we are better able to solve complex problems and make high-level inferences by using the world as an active part of our cognitive processes. Thus, while Sect. 1.2 of this chapter provided evidence for treating language as coextensive with perception and cognition, Sect. 1.3 here provides evidence for perception and cognition being treated as coextensive with action. This raises the question: Is language processing also coextensive with action?

1.4 Language Processing Is Coextensive with Action

Decades ago, Herbert Clark argued for treating language not as a series of coded messages that senders and receivers transfer to one another (Shannon 1948), but instead as part and parcel of the collective actions we carry out together in our environment (Clark and Schaefer 1989). Spoken utterances are not merely attempts to recreate in the listener's mind an idea that is in the speaker's mind. Spoken utterances have purpose and intent for changing some aspect of the environment. For example, if you are standing by a window and I say, "It's hot in here. Do you mind?" with a pointed gaze and a deictic gesture, all of a sudden, like magic, the window gets opened. My spoken utterance and gesture did not simply transfer a thought from my mind to yours, it caused action in the world. It was a speech act (Austin 1962; Searle 1969).

Since then, a great many laboratory studies have shown powerful evidence in favour of treating human language processing as coextensive with human action. For example, research on gesture during spoken conversation has been showing again and again that a variety of hand movements, arm movements and facial expressions are naturally enacted with precise timing relative to the speech stream, and non-matching or poorly timed gestures can actually impair communication of the linguistic signal (Alibali 2005; Goldin-Meadow 1999; McNeill 2008). There is evidence that gestures are commonly used both for the purpose of assisting the listener in comprehending (Bavelas et al. 2002) and also for the purpose of assisting the speaker in word-finding (Kita 2000).

The tightly coupled relationship between linguistic information and motor processes is especially clear when one examines the real-time temporal dynamics of language comprehension and motor action. For example, Farmer et al. (2007) replicated Tanenhaus et al.'s (1995) results with "Put the apple on the towel in the box" (Sect. 1.2), by recording computer-mouse movements instead of eye movements. Their results showed that on trials where the irrelevant towel attracted attention, while it was briefly mis-parsed as a potential destination for the "put" event, the computer-mouse trajectory curved partially towards the irrelevant towel while dragging the apple across the screen towards the box. Thus, even on individual trials that may or may not have had eye fixations of the irrelevant destination object, the reaching movement nearly always curved slightly towards that irrelevant destination object. Moreover, Chambers et al. (2004, Experiment 2) found that the Gibsonian affordances for action in a given environment could modulate how the visual context influenced syntactic parsing in an instruction like, "Put the whistle on the folder in the box." If there were two graspable whistles in the environment, then an extra irrelevant folder did *not* attract eye movements because "on the folder" was parsed as a noun phrase modifier, not as the destination for the "put" instruction. However, if participants were using a small hook to move objects around, and only one of the whistles had a string attached to it (affording manipulation via the hook), then all of a sudden the very same instruction in the very same visual context caused listeners to ignore the non-graspable whistle, and then briefly parse "on the folder" as a destination for the "put" event (drawing eye fixations to it).

Similar findings can be found by tracking a reaching movement with motion-capture technology. Nazir and colleagues (2008) continuously recorded the 3-D position of joints on the arm while participants made a reach-and grasp movement and performed a lexical decision task. The letter string was presented after initiation of the reaching movement. If the letter string was a word, then they were to continue the reaching movement and complete the grasp, but if the letter string was not a word, they were to cancel the reaching movement mid-flight and return their hand to the start position. They found that when the word was an action verb (e.g., paint, jump, cry), the acceleration profile of the reaching movement was reliably different from the acceleration profile for when the word was a noun denoting a non-graspable concrete object (e.g., star, meadow, cliff). Thus, even after motor movement had been initiated, information from new linguistic input was able to cascade to the motor system in time to influence the dynamics of the movement.

Not only does activation of linguistic representations spread to motor processes on the timescale of dozens of milliseconds, but activation of motor representations also spreads to linguistic processes as well. Pulvermüller et al. (2005) delivered weak pulses of transcranial magnetic stimulation to the leg and arm regions of motor cortex while participants were carrying out a lexical decision task. They found that mild activation of motor cortex influenced reaction times to visual word stimuli. Activating the leg area of motor cortex induced faster reaction times to action verbs that involve the legs (e.g., kick, run, etc.), and activating the arm area of motor cortex induced faster reaction times to action verbs that involve the arms (e.g., throw and catch). Thus, during the few hundred milliseconds that it takes to process a written letter string, neural activation patterns in motor cortex contributed selectively to the process of determining whether that letter string was a word or not a word.

The findings from these various studies clearly point to a substantial amount of overlap between the real-time processing of language and of action. They suggest that there may be overlap between the network of brain areas involved in language and the network of brain areas involved in motor processing. The question that is raised next is: Once language in the brain is seen as coextensive with action in the world, how does one deal with the fact that action in the world frequently involves not just inanimate objects that are passively waiting for us to interact with them, but also other language-using agents who are actively interacting with those same objects?

1.5 When Action Becomes Joint Action, Language Becomes Joint Language

Although we have discussed the ubiquitous use of actions in the environment to assist in cognitive and language processes, we have yet to discuss the role of other human beings as making up a significant portion of our environment and assisting in the actions we perform. Just as we employ the environment to do some of our language and cognition for us, we regularly coordinate with other human beings to assist in our task completion and problem solving. Two people, when working together on a shared-task, can temporarily become one synergistic, functional perception-action system and can share their cognitive workload by sharing their cognition (e.g., Chang et al. 2009; Isenhower et al. 2010; Richardson et al. 2007b). Language is an essential tool in the efficient spreading of cognition; as soon as we formulate an idea in words, it becomes a manipulable and shareable object for both ourselves and for others (Clark 2010). In this final section of the chapter, we explore how linguistic exchange contributes to the emergence of cooperative actions, and suggest that the emergence of such patterns of behaviour is required for robust and flexible joint-action systems.

First, it is pivotal to reconsider the multifaceted cognitive functions provided to us by the environment. Constant reorganisation of our environment efficiently enhances performance by reducing the energy, memory, and time demands required for problem solving and task completion. Intelligent spatial arrangements of the objects in our environment can simplify perception and choice, while the dynamics of our spatial arrangements can greatly simplify internal processing (Kirsh 1995). In the field of artificial intelligence, this manipulation of the environment to simplify problem solving is characteristic of situated reasoning. In one famous example (de la Rocha 1985), an interviewer asked a participant "How much cottage cheese would you have if you served three-fourths of the day's allotment, which is two-thirds of a cup?" The participant measured out two thirds of a cup of cottage cheese which he proceeded to lay out on the counter in the shape of a circle. After dividing the circle into four quadrants, he removed one quadrant and announced his completion of the task. Here, rather than internally multiplying three-fourths by two-thirds to equal half a cup, this participant exploited the world and its resources in order to visualise the problem and therefore externalise a part of his cognition.

In problem solving tasks such as the one described above, individuals act according to their perception of the world, their embedded actions become their next perception, they then act upon their altered environment and so on. The whole of their cognition is realised throughout this interactive channel of bidirectional influence between their actions and environment. Contrary to the popular belief that cognitive faculties are separable modules each with their own delineable seat in the brain (e.g., Fodor 1983; for critique, see Uttal 2001), the embodied embedded cognition perspective emphasises the way that the brain, body and environment interact with one another in a continuous feedback loop. Cognition, then, is not limited to one of the components in this loop, but rather extends beyond the brain and into the body and environment. From the perspective of ecological psychology, humans cannot help but be a continuous part of this feedback loop, as the terms *animal* and *environment* make an inseparable pair. Although it is tempting to consider the environment of each observer as being unique or private, this sort of description works with stationary points of observation rather than moving points of observation. The environment surrounds all observers nearly the same way that it surrounds one observer. The available paths of motion in an environment make up the set of all possible points of observation. Notwithstanding the fact that no two animals can be in the same place at the same time, any animal can stand in all available places, and all animals can stand in the same place at different times (Gibson 1979). As long as the substantial layout of the environment persists, all inhabitants have equal options for exploration. Therefore, it is important to note not only the interdependence of observers with their environment, but also the complementary relationship between a set of observers and their common environment. It is this common environment that provides the arena for social behaviour and cooperative actions.

A fundamental part of human social behaviour is characterised by the interpersonal cooperation that occurs during face-to-face or co-present goal-directed interaction. These complementary actions appear to emerge naturally from the physical and informational constraints inherent in a shared task (Knoblich and Jordan 2003). Research in the field of embodied embedded cognition has challenged the commonly held belief that there is always a clear separation between "me" and "you" (e.g., Goldstone and Gureckis 2009; Marsh et al. 2009; Sebanz et al. 2006). Under the assumption that the environment plays a significant role in shaping one's cognition, it seems to follow that interaction with another person (i.e. interacting with your environment) can make the boundary between two peoples' cognition unclear, if not indeterminate. This research is beginning to provide evidence that perception, action and cognition are not confined within one individual but can be shared across two or more individuals through the dynamic interaction between linguistic exchange, action and the environment. The spreading/sharing of these mechanisms can lead to groups of individuals temporarily constrained to behave together as a single coherent unit, with cognitive operations being performed by the network of individuals in the group (e.g., Roberts and Goldstone 2009; Riley et al. 2011).

Armed with the above theoretical approach, we can begin to take our focus away from internal mental processes that extend no further than the physical material of the brain and instead begin exploring how these information flows are intimately coupled within the interaction between the brain, body and environment (which includes other human beings). Previous research has suggested that the dynamics of perceptual-motor coordination that emerges from interaction between humans serves to embody and reflect the underlying cognitive coordination required to successfully achieve joint actions (Shockley et al. 2009). Given the exceedingly large number of degrees of freedom present at the micro-levels of the perceptual-motor system (e.g. neurons, synapses, muscles, joints, etc.), it can be much more efficient to infer their coordination by focusing on the few collective degrees of freedom observed at the macro-level of behaviour.

By examining cognitive phenomena between people at the macro-level of behaviour, we can start to understand how a schism between the cognition of one person and another is vague and fickle at best. Traditionally, cognitive science has focused experimental practice and theory on individuals in isolation; however, extraordinary insights into the brain's dependency on, and plasticity with, social and cultural influences are providing evidence for the temporary formation of cooperative cognitive systems of human beings (Hutchins 1995). As noted in Sect. 1.4 of this chapter, Herbert Clark popularised the radical idea of language being a process that is realised across social systems rather than being a secluded mental process unique for every individual. In part as a response to this idea, contemporary research has begun heavily concerning itself with ecological validity so as to strengthen the study of situated cognition (e.g. Robbins and Aydede 2009) and interactions among humans (see e.g. Sebanz et al. 2006).

As we begin to explore the endless complex organisation that naturally emerges from groups of interacting individuals, we begin to see how language not only enables information transfer between a pair of human beings; it allows for groups and societies to share information collectively. This type of information transfer makes it so that intelligent behaviour can naturally emerge from the interactive dynamics of the group as a whole. These emergent collective behaviours often exhibit higher levels of intelligence than can be seen in the behaviours coming from a single individual (e.g. Williams and Sternberg 1988; Mataric 1993; Druskat and Wolff 2001). This intelligent collective behaviour that is greater than the sum of its parts may be due to the fact that certain cognitive functions from individual minds can be offloaded onto other brains through the use of language, thereby reducing the cognitive workload placed on one brain and allowing other brains to take up some of this workload. In this sense, language makes it possible for cognition to be spread across multiple minds.

Acknowledgement of the remarkably blurred boundaries between the brain, behaviour and the environment is crucial to understanding the true nature of language, as language is fundamentally rooted in the dynamic interaction between these things. It is impossible to confine language to merely one aspect of this interdependent design; the true nature of linguistic exchange is discovered only through rigorous exploration of the coupled underpinnings of the totality of language. Through the use of language, groups of people are able to form sophisticated social systems whose dynamic qualities can give rise to intelligent behaviour. By examining social systems through the scientific lens of complex systems theory, we are given tools that allow for the explication of intricate networks of dynamical interaction within groups of individuals embedded in certain environmental contexts. Intelligent behaviours arise out of the complex interactions between individuals of the system. This behaviour is self-organised, meaning that the behaviour arises despite there being no a priori plan or controller; the elements, or agents, of the system are simply interacting with local elements, but these interactions spread over time and influence the system as a whole. In turn, the system as a whole influences the interactions between the elements. The collective behaviour of these systems may be difficult if not impossible to anticipate from knowledge of the individual agents making up the system, since even exhaustive knowledge of the intentions and desires behind an agent's actions will fall short of providing any descriptive information about what emergent behaviours will arise from the dynamic interplay within the system.

Often, these emergent behaviours can exhibit coherent patterns or even apparent purposiveness. For example, a person's social group may be a non-obvious consequence of the complex interactions between many group members and environmental constraints (e.g. Read and Miller 2002; Smith 1992; Freeman and Ambady 2011; Arrow 1997). Additionally, a work-team can form a robust collective system, spreading cognitive workload throughout its members until some semi-stable arrangement is found. Allocation of work and sharing of ideas build up over time until eventually the team becomes a highly efficient stable collaborative system whose emergent behaviour transpires through the continuous linguistic and environmental interactions among group members (Arrow 1997). Similarly, task sub-roles and divisions of labour can emerge spontaneously from communication during joint action or social tasks (Eguíluz et al. 2005). Language use can also lead to increased social rapport and therefore lead to better productivity and collaboration. For example, linguistic interactions among individuals demonstrate convergence in dialect (see, e.g. Giles 1973), vocal intensity (see, e.g. Natale 1975), pausing frequency (see, e.g. Cappella and Planalp 1981), and speaking rate (see, e.g. Street 1984). Moreover, during dyadic conversation, two people can also spontaneously exhibit coordinative linguistic behaviour in terms of speaking duration, turn duration, response latency and accent. Bodily postures and gaze patterns can also spontaneously converge, suggesting that these coordinated actions go beyond mere external interactions; they seem to reflect cognitive convergence as well (Shockley et al. 2009). The use of language in these coordinated behaviours is facilitating cooperative and intelligent actions emerging from groups and also makes up an active *part* of these things. Linguistic exchange is thus a tightly integrated part of the conjoint process in which we continuously coordinate our bodies, actions and intentions in order to realise shared perspective and joint goals (Clark 1996). When cooperative behaviours such as these are considered using models in physics, biology and complex systems, internal mental representations may be circumvented on the grounds that the coordinative structure that emerges speaks for the system as a whole and not just the brain.

In one study, researchers explored the possibility that coordinated patterns of postural sway may be mediated by the convergence of speaking patterns over time. Their data demonstrate that shared postural patterns of activity are more robust when conversational partners speak the same words or words with similar stress patterns, but not when compared to a different participant speaking the exact same word sequence (Shockley et al. 2007). These findings suggest that postural coordination between people conversing is mediated by converging speaking patterns. In a study investigating the coupling between a speaker and listener's eye movements, a group of four participants were recorded speaking freely about a television show while viewing the cast members of the show on a display. Afterwards, a large group of participants listened to these monologues while viewing the same display of the cast members. In general, listener's eye movements tended to correlate with those of the speaker, with a lag of about 1.5 s. Essentially, the speaker would look at a cast member on the screen and about 750 ms later refer to that person in their speech, and then the listener would make an eye movement to that cast member another 750 ms after hearing the reference. Moreover, analysis of eye movements revealed that the more closely a listener's eye movements matched a speaker's eye movements, the better the listener performed on a final comprehension test (Richardson and Dale 2005). Interestingly, when the paradigm was modified into a bidirectional dialogue—with two participants co-creating their conversation in real-time in two rooms with two headsets, two microphones and two eyetrackers—that 1.5 s lag in their eye-movement correlation disappeared (Richardson et al. 2007c). When involved in a shared unscripted dialogue, participants were anticipating their shifts in the topic of conversation on a dozens of milliseconds timescale, such that they were typically looking at the same thing at the same time. Experiments such as these strongly argue for a close coupling of actions and cognitive processes across human beings engaging in a shared task.

Recent work in cognitive neuroscience is beginning to extend its focus from the mind of the individual in isolation to two or more individuals interacting and coordinating together. During interpersonal communication—including unidirectional communication—an accumulation of shared mental representations takes place in the minds of the individuals throughout the unfolding of the conversation (Clark and Brennan 1991; Garrod and Pickering 2004). To explore this at a neural level, Kuhlen et al. (2012) investigated the patterned coupling of EEG activation between speakers and listeners and found strong coordination of electrophysiological activity in the processing of communicated content. They had a male speaker and a female speaker tell unrelated stories to a video camera while their EEG patterns were recorded. These two audio–video clips were then overlaid with one another, and participants were instructed to watch and attend only the male speaker or only to the female speaker, while their own EEG patterns were recorded. Even though they were observing the same audio–video stimulus, participants who were attending to the female speaker had greater EEG correlation with the EEG patterns of the female speaker, than those of the male speaker; and vice versa for those participants who were attending the male speaker. These results are in line with previous neuroimaging studies that also discovered neural coordination between communicating individuals (e.g. Schippers et al. 2010; Fuchs and Jirsa 2008). More and more convincing evidence examining neural coordination among individuals is pointing towards a fully integrated, tightly interwoven coupling of individuals in joint action and communication, taking place at many different timescales and spread out over a broad range of frequencies.

The use of language vastly facilitates this coupling by acting as a tool for directing attention as well as aligning perspectives and action. Fusaroli et al. (2012) expanded upon this idea by employing a novel experimental design in which participant dyads cooperated through linguistic exchange to solve a psychophysical perceptual task. Dyads that outperformed their best individual performance on the perceptual task tended to exhibit greater global linguistic convergence than dyads that did not outperform their best individual. As dyads began using recurring and coordinative structures in their linguistic exchange, their joint performance in the perceptual task improved substantially. It seems as though language serves as an efficient tool for coordination, particularly when the linguistic tools are fitted to the affordances of the task and when the tools are successfully shared by interlocutors. Mere creation of linguistic tools for use in a task is insufficient for achieving optimal collective benefit; shared linguistic repertoires evolve and stabilise as a result of selective processing of reciprocative local alignment and constant attentional sensitivity to the task environment.

Upon careful, open-minded consideration of the plethora of powerful evidence in research on linguistic exchange and interpersonal action, we begin to realise that the extended mind hypothesis applies to interpersonal interactions as well as individuals in isolation (e.g. Fusaroli et al. 2013). Through linguistic exchange, we easily manage to radically expand the interaction space in which our actions occur and are constrained (Tylén et al. 2010), and we blur the boundaries between our own cognitive processes and those of others. In a wide range of everyday social interactions and contexts, language plays a key role in allowing for the emergence of many advantages that coordinating minds have over individual cognition. The concept of *collective minds* describes how the dynamic activity of language enables the formation of unified cognitive systems (Tollefsen 2006; Theiner et al. 2010) and emphasises the importance of a fundamental extension of cognition onto the surrounding environment and those within it. Building on these ideas, the growing conglomeration of compelling empirical and conceptual arguments provides strong evidence for treating language as a social coordinative device, constantly undergoing development, maintenance and adaptation to contextual and interpersonal constraints. Consequently, it may be that by defining language and cognition as separate from other individuals and from our actions in the environment, much of the field has been overlooking the powerful capacity realised within these continuous interactions and hence missing the very essence of language itself.

References

Alibali, M. W. (2005). Gesture in spatial cognition: Expressing, communicating, and thinking about spatial information. *Spatial Cognition and Computation, 5*(4), 307–331.

Allopenna, P. D., Magnuson, J. S., & Tanenhaus, M. K. (1998). Tracking the time course of spoken word recognition using eye movements: Evidence for continuous mapping models. *Journal of Memory and Language, 38*(4), 419–439.

Anderson, M. L., Brumbaugh, J., & Şuben, A. (2010). Investigating functional cooperation in the human brain using simple graph-theoretic methods. In *Computational neuroscience* (pp. 31–42). New York: Springer.

Arrow, H. (1997). Stability, bistability, and instability in small group influence patterns. *Journal of Personality and Social Psychology, 72*(1), 75.

Austin, J. L. (1962). *How to do things with words*. Cambridge, MA: Harvard University Press.

Ballard, D., Hayhoe, M., & Pelz, J. (1995). Memory representations in natural tasks. *Journal of Cognitive Neuroscience, 7*(1), 66–80.

Barsalou, L. W. (1999). Perceptions of perceptual symbols. *Behavioral and Brain Sciences, 22*(04), 637–660.

Bavelas, J., Kenwood, C., Johnson, T., & Phillips, B. (2002). An experimental study of when and how speakers use gestures to communicate. *Gesture, 2*(1), 1–17.

Bergmann, T., Dale, R., & Lupyan, G. (2013). The impact of communicative constraints on the emergence of a graphical communication system. In *Proceedings of the Thirty-Fifth Annual Conference of the Cognitive Science Society* (pp. 1887–1892).

Cappella, J. N., & Planalp, S. (1981). Talk and silence sequences in informal conversations III: Interspeaker influence. *Human Communication Research, 7*(2), 117–132.

Chambers, C. G., Tanenhaus, M. K., & Magnuson, J. S. (2004). Actions and affordances in syntactic ambiguity resolution. *Journal of Experimental Psychology. Learning, Memory, and Cognition, 30*(3), 687.

Chang, C. H., Wade, M. G., & Stoffregen, T. A. (2009). Perceiving affordances for aperture passage in an environment–person–person system. *Journal of Motor Behavior, 41*(6), 495–500.

Chiu, E., & Spivey, M. J. (2012). The role of preview and incremental delivery on visual search. In *Proceedings of the 34th Annual Conference of the Cognitive Science Society* (pp. 216–221).

Christiansen, M. H., & Kirby, S. (Eds.). (2003). *Language evolution.* New York: Oxford University Press.

Clark, A. (2010). *Supersizing the mind: Embodiment, action, and cognitive extension.* Oxford University Press.

Clark, H. H. (1996). *Using language.* Cambridge: Cambridge University Press.

Clark, H. H., & Brennan, S. E. (1991). Grounding in communication. *Perspectives on Socially Shared Cognition, 13,* 127–149.

Clark, H. H., & Schaefer, E. F. (1989). Contributing to discourse. *Cognitive Science, 13*(2), 259–294.

Colin, C., Radeau, M., Soquet, A., Demolin, D., Colin, F., & Deltenre, P. (2002). Mismatch negativity evoked by the McGurk–MacDonald effect: A phonetic representation within short-term memory. *Clinical Neurophysiology, 113*(4), 495–506.

Corbetta, M. (1998). Frontoparietal cortical networks for directing attention and the eye to visual locations: identical, independent, or overlapping neural systems? *Proceedings of the National Academy of Sciences, 95*(3), 831–838.

Dahan, D., & Tanenhaus, M. K. (2005). Looking at the rope when looking for the snake: Conceptually mediated eye movements during spoken-word recognition. *Psychonomic Bulletin & Review, 12*(3), 453–459.

de la Rocha, O. (1985). The reorganization of arithmetic practice in the kitchen. *Anthropology & Education Quarterly, 16*(3), 193–198.

Deubel, H., & Schneider, W. X. (1996). Saccade target selection and object recognition: Evidence for a common attentional mechanism. *Vision Research, 36*(12), 1827–1837.

Druskat, V. U., & Wolff, S. B. (2001). Building the emotional intelligence of groups. *Harvard Business Review, 79*(3), 80–91.

Duncker, K., & Lees, L. S. (1945). On problem-solving. *Psychological Monographs, 58*(5), i (Whole No. 270).

Eberhard, K. M., Spivey-Knowlton, M. J., Sedivy, J. C., & Tanenhaus, M. K. (1995). Eye movements as a window into real-time spoken language comprehension in natural contexts. *Journal of Psycholinguistic Research, 24*(6), 409–436.

Eguíluz, V. M., Zimmermann, M. G., Cela-Conde, C. J., & San Miguel, M. (2005). Cooperation and the emergence of role differentiation in the dynamics of social networks1. *American Journal of Sociology, 110*(4), 977–1008.

Farmer, T. A., Anderson, S. E., & Spivey, M. J. (2007). Gradiency and visual context in syntactic garden-paths. *Journal of Memory and Language, 57*(4), 570–595.

Fodor, J. A. (1983). *The modularity of mind: An essay on faculty psychology.* Cambridge: MIT press.

Frazier, L. (1995). Constraint satisfaction as a theory of sentence processing. *Journal of Psycholinguistic Research, 24*(6), 437–468.

Freeman, J. B., & Ambady, N. (2011). A dynamic interactive theory of person construal. *Psychological Review, 118*(2), 247.

Fuchs, A., & Jirsa, V. K. (2008). *Coordination: Neural, behavioral and social dynamics* (Vol. 1). Berlin: Springer.

Fusaroli, R., Bahrami, B., Olsen, K., Roepstorff, A., Rees, G., Frith, C., & Tylén, K. (2012). Coming to terms quantifying the benefits of linguistic coordination. *Psychological Science, 23*, 931–939.

Fusaroli, P., Vallar, R., Togliani, T., Khodadadian, E., & Caletti, G. (2002). Scientific publications in endoscopic ultrasonography: A 20-year global survey of the literature. *Endoscopy, 34*(06), 451–456.

Fusaroli, R., Gangopadhyay, N., & Tylén, K. (2013). The dialogically extended mind: Language as skilful intersubjective engagement. *Cognitive Systems Research, 29*, 31–39.

Galantucci, B. (2005). An experimental study of the emergence of human communication systems. *Cognitive Science, 29*(5), 737–767.

Garrod, S., & Pickering, M. J. (2004). Why is conversation so easy? *Trends in Cognitive Sciences, 8*(1), 8–11.

Gibson, J. J. (1977). The concept of affordances. In *Perceiving, acting, and knowing* (pp. 67–82).

Gibson, J. J. (1979). *The ecological approach to visual perception*. London: Psychology Press.

Giles, H. (1973). Accent mobility: A model and some data. *Anthropological Linguistics, 15*, 87–105.

Glenberg, A. M., & Kaschak, M. P. (2002). Grounding language in action. *Psychonomic Bulletin & Review, 9*(3), 558–565.

Gold, J. I., & Shadlen, M. N. (2000). Representation of a perceptual decision in developing oculomotor commands. *Nature, 404*(6776), 390–394.

Goldin-Meadow, S. (1999). The role of gesture in communication and thinking. *Trends in cognitive sciences, 3*(11), 419–429.

Goldstone, R. L., & Gureckis, T. M. (2009). Collective behavior. *Topics in Cognitive Science, 1*(3), 412–438.

Grant, E. R., & Spivey, M. J. (2003). Eye movements and problem solving guiding attention guides thought. *Psychological Science, 14*(5), 462–466.

Huette, S., Winter, B., Matlock, T., & Spivey, M. (2012). Processing motion implied in language: eye-movement differences during aspect comprehension. *Cognitive Processing, 13*(1), 193–197.

Huettig, F., Quinlan, P. T., McDonald, S. A., & Altmann, G. (2006). Models of high-dimensional semantic space predict language-mediated eye movements in the visual world. *Acta Psychologica, 121*(1), 65–80.

Hutchins, E. (1995). *Cognition in the Wild* (Vol. 262082314). Cambridge, MA: MIT press.

Isenhower, R. W., Richardson, M. J., Carello, C., Baron, R. M., & Marsh, K. L. (2010). Affording cooperation: Embodied constraints, dynamics, and action-scaled invariance in joint lifting. *Psychonomic Bulletin & Review, 17*(3), 342–347.

Jordan, J. S., & Hunsinger, M. (2008). Learned patterns of action-effect anticipation contribute to the spatial displacement of continuously moving stimuli. *Journal of Experimental Psychology: Human Perception and Performance, 34*(1), 113.

Kaschak, M. P., & Borreggine, K. L. (2008). Temporal dynamics of the action–sentence compatibility effect. *The Quarterly Journal of Experimental Psychology, 61*(6), 883–895.

Kawato, M. (1999). Internal models for motor control and trajectory planning. *Current Opinion in Neurobiology, 9*(6), 718–727.

Kirsh, D. (1995). The intelligent use of space. *Artificial Intelligence, 73*(1), 31–68.

Kirsh, D., & Maglio, P. (1994). On distinguishing epistemic from pragmatic action. *Cognitive Science, 18*(4), 513–549.

Kita, S. (2000). How representational gestures help speaking. In *Language and gesture* (pp. 162–185).

Knoblich, G., & Jordan, J. S. (2003). Action coordination in groups and individuals: learning anticipatory control. *Journal of Experimental Psychology: Learning, Memory, and Cognition, 29*(5), 1006–1016.

Kuhlen, A. K., Allefeld, C., & Haynes, J. D. (2012). Content-specific coordination of listeners' to speakers' EEG during communication. *Frontiers in Human Neuroscience, 6*, 266.

Lakoff, G., & Johnson, M. (1980). *Metaphors we live by*. Chicago: University of Chicago Press.

Marsh, K. L., Johnston, L., Richardson, M. J., & Schmidt, R. C. (2009). Toward a radically embodied, embedded social psychology. *European Journal of Social Psychology, 39*(7), 1217–1225.

Marslen-Wilson, W. D. (1987). Functional parallelism in spoken word-recognition. *Cognition, 25*(1), 71–102.

Mataric, M. J. (1993, August). Designing emergent behaviors: From local interactions to collective intelligence. In *Proceedings of the Second International Conference on Simulation of Adaptive Behavior* (pp. 432–441).

McGurk, H., & MacDonald, J. (1976). Hearing lips and seeing voices. *Nature, 264*, 746–748.

McMurray, B., Tanenhaus, M. K., Aslin, R. N., & Spivey, M. J. (2003). Probabilistic constraint satisfaction at the lexical/phonetic interface: Evidence for gradient effects of within-category VOT on lexical access. *Journal of Psycholinguistic Research, 32*(1), 77–97.

McNeill, D. (2008). *Gesture and thought*. Chicago: University of Chicago Press.

Meteyard, L., Zokaei, N., Bahrami, B., & Vigliocco, G. (2008). Visual motion interferes with lexical decision on motion words. *Current Biology, 18*(17), R732–R733.

Natale, M. (1975). Convergence of mean vocal intensity in dyadic communication as a function of social desirability. *Journal of Personality and Social Psychology, 32*(5), 790.

Nazir, T. A., Boulenger, V., Roy, A., Silber, B., Jeannerod, M., & Paulignan, Y. (2008). Language-induced motor perturbations during the execution of a reaching movement. *The Quarterly Journal of Experimental Psychology, 61*(6), 933–943.

Neisser, U. (1976). *Cognition and reality: Principles and implications of cognitive psychology*. WH Freeman/Times Books/Henry Holt & Co.

Proffitt, D. R. (2006). Distance perception. *Current Directions in Psychological Science, 15*(3), 131–135.

Pulvermüller, F., Hauk, O., Nikulin, V. V., & Ilmoniemi, R. J. (2005). Functional links between motor and language systems. *European Journal of Neuroscience, 21*(3), 793–797.

Read, S. J., & Miller, L. C. (2002). Virtual personalities: A neural network model of personality. *Personality and Social Psychology Review, 6*(4), 357–369.

Reali, F., Spivey, M. J., Tyler, M. J., & Terranova, J. (2006). Inefficient conjunction search made efficient by concurrent spoken delivery of target identity. *Perception and Psychophysics, 68*(6), 959–974.

Richardson, D. C., & Dale, R. (2005). Looking to understand: The coupling between speakers' and listeners' eye movements and its relationship to discourse comprehension. *Cognitive Science, 29*(6), 1045–1060.

Richardson, D. C., Spivey, M. J., Barsalou, L. W., & McRae, K. (2003). Spatial representations activated during real-time comprehension of verbs. *Cognitive Science, 27*(5), 767–780.

Richardson, D. C., Dale, R., & Kirkham, N. Z. (2007a). The art of conversation is coordination common ground and the coupling of eye movements during dialogue. *Psychological Science, 18*(5), 407–413.

Richardson, D. C., Dale, R., & Spivey, M. J. (2007b). Eye movements in language and cognition. In *Empirical methods in cognitive linguistics* (pp. 323–344).

Richardson, M. J., Marsh, K. L., & Baron, R. M. (2007c). Judging and actualizing intrapersonal and interpersonal affordances. *Journal of Experimental Psychology: Human Perception and Performance, 33*(4), 845.

Riley, M. A., Richardson, M. J., Shockley, K., & Ramenzoni, V. C. (2011). Interpersonal synergies. *Frontiers in Psychology, 2*, 38.

Robbins, P., & Aydede, M. (2009). A short primer on situated cognition. In *The Cambridge handbook of situated cognition* (pp. 3–10).

Roberts, M. E., & Goldstone, R. L. (2009). Adaptive group coordination. In *Proceedings of the Thirty-First Annual Conference of the Cognitive Science Society* (pp. 2698–2704).

Schippers, M. B., Roebroeck, A., Renken, R., Nanetti, L., & Keysers, C. (2010). Mapping the information flow from one brain to another during gestural communication. *Proceedings of the National Academy of Sciences, 107*(20), 9388–9393.

Searle, J. R. (1969). *Speech acts: An essay in the philosophy of language* (Vol. 626). Cambridge: Cambridge University Press.

Sebanz, N., Bekkering, H., & Knoblich, G. (2006). Joint action: bodies and minds moving together. *Trends in Cognitive Sciences, 10*(2), 70–76.

Senghas, A., & Coppola, M. (2001). Children creating language: How Nicaraguan sign language acquired a spatial grammar. *Psychological Science, 12*(4), 323–328.

Shannon, C. E. (1948). Key papers in the development of information theory. *Bell Systems Technical Journal, 27*, 623–656.

Shockley, K., Baker, A. A., Richardson, M. J., & Fowler, C. A. (2007). Articulatory constraints on interpersonal postural coordination. *Journal of Experimental Psychology: Human Perception and Performance, 33*(1), 201.

Shockley, K., Richardson, D. C., & Dale, R. (2009). Conversation and coordinative structures. *Topics in Cognitive Science, 1*(2), 305–319.

Smith, M.A. (1992). *Voices from the WELL: The logic of the virtual commons.* Master's thesis, UCLA.

Spivey, M. J., & Geng, J. J. (2001). Oculomotor mechanisms activated by imagery and memory: Eye movements to absent objects. *Psychological Research, 65*(4), 235–241.

Spivey, M. J., Tyler, M. J., Eberhard, K. M., & Tanenhaus, M. K. (2001). Linguistically mediated visual search. *Psychological Science, 12*(4), 282–286.

Spivey, M. J., Tanenhaus, M. K., Eberhard, K. M., & Sedivy, J. C. (2002). Eye movements and spoken language comprehension: Effects of visual context on syntactic ambiguity resolution. *Cognitive Psychology, 45*(4), 447–481.

Stanfield, R. A., & Zwaan, R. A. (2001). The effect of implied orientation derived from verbal context on picture recognition. *Psychological Science, 12*(2), 153–156.

Street, R. L. (1984). Speech convergence and speech evaluation in fact-finding interviews. *Human Communication Research, 11*(2), 139–169.

Tabor, W. (1995). Lexical change as nonlinear interpolation. In *Proceedings of the 17th Annual Cognitive Science Conference* (pp. 242–247).

Tanenhaus, M. K., Spivey-Knowlton, M. J., Eberhard, K. M., & Sedivy, J. C. (1995). Integration of visual and linguistic information in spoken language comprehension. *Science, 268*(5217), 1632–1634.

Theiner, G., Allen, C., & Goldstone, R. L. (2010). Recognizing group cognition. *Cognitive Systems Research, 11*(4), 378–395.

Tollefsen, D. P. (2006). From extended mind to collective mind. *Cognitive Systems Research, 7*(2), 140–150.

Turvey, M. T. (1992). Affordances and prospective control: An outline of the ontology. *Ecological Psychology, 4*(3), 173–187

Tylén, K., Weed, E., Wallentin, M., Roepstorff, A., & Frith, C. D. (2010). Language as a tool for interacting minds. *Mind and Language, 25*(1), 3–29.

Uttal, W. R. (2001). *The new phrenology: The limits of localizing cognitive processes in the brain.* Cambridge: The MIT Press.

Williams, W. M., & Sternberg, R. J. (1988). Group intelligence: why some groups are better than others. *Intelligence, 12*(4), 351–377.

Yee, E., & Sedivy, J. C. (2006). Eye movements to pictures reveal transient semantic activation during spoken word recognition. *Journal of Experimental Psychology. Learning, Memory, and Cognition, 32*(1), 1.

Zwaan, R. A., Madden, C. J., Yaxley, R. H., & Aveyard, M. E. (2004). Moving words: Dynamic representations in language comprehension. *Cognitive Science, 28*(4), 611–619.

Chapter 2
Phonological Features Mediate Object-Label Retrieval and Word Recognition in the Visual World Paradigm

Nicole Altvater-Mackensen and Nivedita Mani

2.1 Introduction: The Role of Phonological Information During Word Recognition in Toddlers

Young word learners have a considerable challenge facing them. With just a few exposures to a word, they must learn the sounds associated with this word and be able to retrieve this information when they hear a new token of this word, or see an object associated with this word. Research has long focused on the amount of detail young children store with regard to the sounds of words and a majority of studies find that children have detailed phonological representations of words (Swingley and Aslin 2000, 2002; Mani and Plunkett 2007, 2010a; White and Morgan 2008). However, it remains a matter of some discussion whether children access this phonological detail during word recognition, with a number of researchers suggesting that access to phonological detail may be restricted by the task employed by a given study, or the kinds of words being tested, or the age-group of the children (see Mani 2011, for a review of studies).

The visual world paradigm provides a particularly promising tool to investigate these questions (Tanenhaus et al. 1995). Experiments employing this paradigm typically present participants with an array of visual images on a screen followed by an auditory label, which is in most cases related to one or more of the images on the screen. Participants' eye-movements across the array of images are monitored before and after they hear the auditory stimulus and any changes in gaze-fixations subsequent to the presentation of the auditory stimulus are typically interpreted as

N. Altvater-Mackensen (✉)
Max Planck Institute for Human Cognitive and Brain Sciences, Leipzig, Germany
e-mail: altvater@cbs.mpg.de

N. Mani
University of Göttingen, Göttingen, Germany

© Springer India 2015
R.K. Mishra et al. (eds.), *Attention and Vision
in Language Processing*, DOI 10.1007/978-81-322-2443-3_2

a response to this stimulus. The paradigm has been successfully used in numerous studies to investigate mechanisms of language processing, and more specifically to tap into the phonological processes associated with word recognition in adults (see Huettig et al. 2011, for a review). For instance, Allopenna et al. (1998) presented listeners with images of a target, an onset competitor that shared the initial consonant with the target label and a rhyme competitor that rhymed with the target label. Results show that adults fixated both the target and the onset competitor upon hearing the beginning of the target label. Looks to the onset competitor decreased when the acoustic signal mismatched the phonological make-up of the onset competitor while looks to the target increased with increasing matching phonological information. Fixations of the rhyme competitor, however, only started to emerge following the offset of the target label. These findings suggest that lexical access is modulated by phonological similarity, that onset-overlapping words compete with the target label during word recognition and that rhyme overlap further constrains lexical selection. Magnuson et al. (2007) extended these findings by showing that not only phonological overlap but also word frequency and the phonological structure of the lexicon modulate word recognition. More specifically, the number of words in the lexicon that share the same onset consonant as the target label, i.e. its cohort, and the number of words that differ from the target label in only one phoneme, i.e. its neighbourhood, dynamically modulate lexical activation.

Interestingly, the co-activation of phonologically similar words does not seem to be solely influenced by phonemic overlap. Mitterer (2011) tested adults' sensitivity to subtle sub-phonemic differences between words. In this study, the target label rhymed with the competitor label but differed in either voicing or place of articulation (one-feature distance) or in both voicing and place of the initial consonant (two-feature distance). The results show that subjects looked more often at the competitor in the one- than in the two-feature condition, suggesting that adults are sensitive to the sub-phonemic overlap between words (but see Ernestus and Mak 2004; Cole et al. 1978; Connine et al. 1997, that the effect of sub-segmental overlap is not necessarily linear during lexical access). Similarly, adults have been shown to exhibit graded sensitivity to subtle phonetic differences between words, such as within-category differences in voice onset time (McMurray et al. 2002), segmental lengthening (Salverda et al. 2003) and lexical stress (Reinisch et al. 2010).

Recent work on toddler word recognition has modified the visual world paradigm to examine questions such as whether toddlers implicitly generate the labels associated with visual images (Mani and Plunkett 2010b) and whether toddlers retrieve words that sound similar or mean similar things to a heard word during word recognition (Mani and Plunkett 2011; Arias-Trejo and Plunkett 2009). Such experiments typically present children with a name-known image in silence (the prime image) followed by the presentation of a target and a distractor image, where the label for the target image is either phonologically or semantically or phono-semantically related to the label for the name-known prime image. Looks to the target image are then monitored to examine whether children's fixations to the target image vary as a result of the relationship between the target and the prime image. Indeed, phonological priming studies using the visual world paradigm suggest that—similar to adults—upon seeing an image, children retrieve and activate not only the corresponding label for this image but also other words that sound similar to the label for this image (Huang and Snedeker 2010; Mani and Plunkett 2010a, 2011; Mani et al. 2012). The results of these studies are consistent with the following conclusions: Children possess phonologically detailed representations of words and are able to access this phonological detail and, importantly for the current chapter, automatically retrieve other words that are phonologically similar to a heard or implicitly generated word during word recognition. However, the definition of phonological similarity varies in these studies leaving open the question of both what exactly is meant when we suggest that children retrieve other words that are phonologically similar to a heard word during word recognition and also the levels of representations that are involved in such co-activation. In particular, what remains undetermined is the extent to which such co-activation of other similar-sounding words is driven by sub-segmental level overlap between phonologically similar words.

Given that toddlers appear to be sensitive to small changes to the phonological features of the phonemes of a word in word recognition tasks (White and Morgan 2008), one might assume that the co-activation of phonologically similar words during word retrieval and recognition is equally influenced by sub-segmental overlap. However, sensitivity to sub-segmental detail in detecting a deviant pronunciation of a word does not necessarily imply that such detail is routinely accessed in recognising correctly pronounced words or in retrieving the label of a visually presented name-known object. In other words: Is it the case that, upon hearing a word or seeing an object, words sharing greater sub-segmental overlap with the target word are more robustly activated relative to words with lesser sub-segmental overlap? This assumption would be in line with models of lexical processing, such as TRACE (McClelland and Elman 1986), assuming that word recognition is driven by feature-mediated access to the phonemes in a word: Activation on the feature level leads to activation of the corresponding phonemes, which in turn leads to activation of lexical tokens congruent with this input (Note that next to this bottom-up activation, top-down processes such as context restrictions might also influence language processing in toddlers, see Mani and Huettig 2012). However, there is little research investigating the degree of sub-segmental detail mediating lexical-level processing in toddlers. The current chapter will review the results of a study that attempts to address this issue by examining the degree to which sub-phonemic information mediates word retrieval and recognition by toddlers. First, however, we review the literature on sub-segmental effects in toddler word recognition.

2.1.1 Phonological Feature Effects in Mispronunciation Detection Studies

There is ample evidence that toddlers are sensitive to even subtle mispronunciations of familiar and newly learned words (Bailey and Plunkett 2002; Mani and Plunkett 2007; Swingley 2009; Swingley and Aslin 2000; among others).

This has been taken as evidence that children's lexical representations contain fine phonological detail. However, a growing body of research shows that children are not equally sensitive to all types of segmental mispronunciations. Mani and Plunkett (2010b) report that 12-month-olds show less sensitivity to voicing compared to manner and place changes (for similar findings with Dutch 20-month-olds see Van der Feest 2007). Similarly, Mani et al. (2008) show that 18-month-olds are more sensitive to roundedness changes to the vowels in words relative to height or backness changes. Altvater-Mackensen et al. (2014) show that certain place and manner changes are more readily detected by 18- and 24-month-olds than others, and results by Nazzi et al. (2009) suggest that consonantal and vocalic information might play a different role during lexical access in 30-month-olds (but see Mani and Plunkett 2007, 2010b; Mani et al. 2008). Taken together, these studies indicate that infants do not treat all changes to the sounds of words equally, which might suggest that they not only encode phonemic but also more fine-grained sub-segmental information in their lexical representations of familiar words.

Given that none of the studies discussed above systematically manipulated the degree of overlap between mispronunciation and correct pronunciations in terms of phonological features or sub-segmental content, these results could be explained by assuming that toddlers detect the difference between mispronunciations and correct pronunciations based on the segmental content. Nevertheless, there is evidence that the amount of sub-segmental overlap between a mispronunciation and a correct pronunciation of a word influences toddlers' sensitivity to mispronunciations: White and Morgan (2008) tested 19-month-olds' recognition of correctly pronounced or mispronounced familiar words including mispronunciations with a one-, two- or three-phonological feature change to the initial consonant. Results show that infants' looking behaviour is modulated by the amount of feature overlap shared by the initial consonant of the mispronunciation and the correct pronunciation, i.e. infants were most sensitive to three-feature changes to the consonants, less so to two-feature changes and least sensitive to one-feature changes. Furthermore, Mani and Plunkett (2010c) find that 24-month-olds are sensitive to sub-segmental overlap in vowel mispronunciations, although the size of the mispronunciation effect was modulated by the acoustic distance between the correctly and mispronounced vowels rather than by their distance in terms of phonological features. Both studies suggest that toddlers encode sub-segmental detail in their lexical representations—be it acoustic or feature information—and that they can use this detail to estimate the match between a heard (mispronounced) and a stored label.

While mispronunciation detection studies are invaluable in broadening our knowledge about the specificity of children's early lexical representations, they do not necessarily inform us (a) how much of this detail is used during lexical processing of correctly pronounced words, and (b) whether children access this detail when retrieving the label for a visually fixated name-known image.

A mispronunciation is, typically, not a word in the toddler's lexicon. Recognition of a mispronounced word, i.e. the detection of a mispronunciation, may invoke differential access to phonological detail relative to recognition of a correctly pronounced word. For instance, because toddlers know only very few minimal pairs, such as cat and hat, mispronunciations are usually non-words. Their recognition may, thus, invoke less top-down influence from the lexical level and greater bottom-up processing relative to the recognition of correctly pronounced familiar words or the retrieval of the labels of familiar objects. Second, recognising a mispronunciation involves toddlers' detection of a subtle difference between the heard mispronunciation and the stored representation of a familiar word. The correct pronunciation and the mispronunciation presumably trigger the same lexical representation (see Altvater-Mackensen and Mani 2013). This might invoke greater involvement from the lower levels of processing, such as the segmental or sub-segmental level, relative to situations in which toddlers have to recognise a match between a correctly pronounced word and its referent or in which they retrieve the label of a seen object without matching it to a heard word. Thus, toddlers' sensitivity to sub-segmental detail in mispronunciation detection tasks do not necessarily inform us about the extent of activation of sub-segmental information in the recognition of familiar, correctly pronounced words or in the retrieval of the label of a familiar object. A more appropriate tool to tap into the processes guiding activation of a lexical item and recognition of a word might be the phonological priming paradigm, which has been used successfully with toddlers in previous studies (Mani and Plunkett 2010a, 2011).

2.1.2 Effects of Phonological Overlap in Priming Studies

There are only few studies to date that investigate the processes underlying lexical activation in toddlers. These studies indicate that, upon hearing a word or seeing an image, toddlers activate not only the corresponding word itself but also other words that are semantically (Arias-Trejo and Plunkett 2009), phonologically (Mani and Plunkett 2010a, 2011) or phono-semantically related (Mani et al. 2012) to the heard word or the label for the image. Importantly, co-activation of words in the mental lexicon of toddlers is mediated by the phonological overlap between prime and target labels. For instance, Mani and Plunkett (2011) find that 24-month-olds' recognition of a target word, such as ball, is influenced by the previous presentation of an image displaying an onset-overlapping prime, such as bed. Similarly, Mani et al. (2012) find that 24-month-olds' recognition of a target word like shoe is facilitated by previous exposure to the prime clock. These findings are interpreted as evidence that presentation of the prime clock leads to activation of the similar-sounding sub-prime sock, which in turn leads to activation of the semantically related target shoe. Since the prime was only ever presented visually in these studies, the priming effect can only have arisen from the child internally generating the label for the familiar prime image and being sensitive to the phonological overlap between the prime and sub-prime label. This effect of phonological overlap between prime and target does not appear to be bound to the lexical status of the prime. Altvater-Mackensen and Mani (2013) found that auditory presentation of not only correctly but also mispronounced primes lead to facilitated recognition of words semantically related to the prime label in 24-month-olds. Thus, not only *sock* but also its mispronunciation *fock* leads to facilitated recognition of *shoe*.

These studies, however, only coarsely manipulated the degree of phonological overlap between prime and target; they either manipulated whether prime and target shared the initial consonant (Mani and Plunkett 2010a, 2011) or the rhyme (Mani et al. 2012; Altvater-Mackensen and Mani 2013). Interestingly, this seems to lead to different priming effects. While Mani and Plunkett (2010a, 2011) find that having the very same initial consonant hinders target recognition, rhyme overlap appears to facilitate target recognition (Mani et al. 2012; Altvater-Mackensen and Mani 2013; see Sect. 2.3.1. for a discussion of the different underlying processes). This has been taken as evidence that rhyme priming effects rely on the activation of the phonemes shared between the prime and the target (see also Radeau et al. 1995; Slowiaczek and Hamburger 1992), i.e. lexical activation is mediated by phonemic information in rhyme priming. However, neither of these studies manipulated the degree of overlap between prime and target in terms of phonological features or sub-segmental content, i.e. they do not investigate whether lexical activation of familiar words is mediated by sub-phonemic or only by phonemic information. Next, we present the results of a recent study addressing this question, namely, is phonological priming systematically modulated by the amount of sub-segmental overlap between the prime and the target?

2.2 Experimental Set-up and Results: Toddlers' Use of Sub-segmental Detail in Phonological Priming

We presented 32 monolingual German 24-month-olds with a visual priming task, where participants were presented with a prime image in silence followed by the simultaneous appearance of a target and a distractor image, and the label for the target image. The labels for the prime and target images rhymed with one another but differed on the initial consonant. The difference in the initial consonant was modulated across conditions, where this initial consonant of the prime-target labels differed in two phonological features, three phonological features, or four phonological features. Following linguistic theory, phonological features are the "building blocks" of phonemes that characterise their specific properties (e.g., Chomsky and Halle 1968; Clements 1985). For instance, features can be used to describe the place of articulation of a segment, such as [labial], [coronal] or [dorsal]. The phonological features contrasted in the current study included a segment's place of articulation, manner of articulation, voicing and nasality. We expected differences in toddlers' recognition of the target across the different conditions manipulating the degree of sub-segmental feature overlap between prime and target label. In particular, we predicted that target recognition should improve,

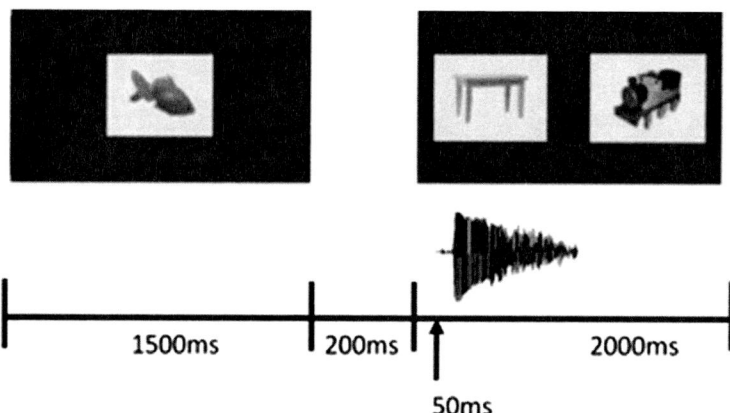

Fig. 2.1 Schematic of the trial structure. For instance, a related trial for the spoken target word Tisch 'table' displayed the image of a Fisch 'fish' (prime), followed by the side-by-side presentation of the images of a Tisch 'table' (target) and a Zug 'train' (distracter.) Original pictures were coloured

i.e. toddlers should fixate the target more, with increasing feature overlap between prime and target label. Note that using visual primes has a major advantage over using auditory primes: any priming effect that might occur necessarily involves the *lexical* activation of the prime label and cannot be attributed to pure acoustic overlap between a heard prime and target label because children have to internally generate the label for the prime image. Put differently, if we find that the priming effect is modulated by sub-segmental overlap between prime and target label, this would imply that retrieval of the prime label from the visual image entailed activation of sub-segmental detail associated with this label.

During each trial, children first saw a prime image presented in silence for 1500 ms, followed by a 200 ms inter-stimulus interval where the screen remained blank. Then target and distracter images appeared side-by-side on screen. Fifty ms following the appearance of the target and distracter images on-screen, i.e. 1750 ms into the trial, children were presented with the auditory target label. Target and distracter images stayed on-screen until the trial ended 2000 ms after the onset of the target label (see Fig. 2.1 for a trial schematic). This configuration of stimuli has proved successful in tapping into phonological effects in word recognition by 24-month-old toddlers (Mani and Plunkett 2011; Mani et al. 2012).

Each child saw four trials with a related prime and four trials with an unrelated prime. Prime, target and distracter were semantically unrelated, while we manipulated the phonological overlap between prime and target label. In related trials, prime and target rhymed and their initial consonants differed in two, three or four phonological features (see Table 2.1 for a stimulus list). The stimulus set was counterbalanced across children so that each child saw every target and distracter pair only once. We did not repeat primes or target-distracter pairs across trials to ensure that repetition effects did not distort results. The side on which the target and distracter appeared as well as the order of presentation of trials was

Table 2.1 Stimulus set

Prime		Target	Distracter
Unrelated	Related		
Haus 'house'	Buch 'book'(2: P, V)	Tuch 'scarf'	Eis 'ice'
Puppe 'doll'	Schuh 'shoe' (2: P, M)	Kuh 'cow'	Flasche 'bottle'
Hund 'dog'	Fisch 'fish' (2: P, M)	Tisch 'table'	Zug 'train'
Buch 'book'	Kamm 'comb' (3: P, M, V)	Lamm 'lamb'	Schwein 'pig'
Kamm 'comb'	Tasse 'cup' (3: P, M, V)	Wasser 'water'	Ohr 'ear'
Schuh 'shoe'	Puppe 'doll' (3: P, M, V)	Suppe 'soup'	Blume 'flower'
Tasse 'cup'	Haus 'house' (4: P, M, V, N)	Maus 'mouse'	Brille 'glasses'
Fisch 'fish'	Hund 'dog' (4: P, M, V, N)	Mund 'mouth'	Schrank 'closet'

Feature differences are listed in brackets (*P* place of articulation, *M* manner of articulation, *V* voicing, *N* nasality)

randomised. Since previous results with toddlers at 18 and 24 months of age show robust effects of phonological overlap between familiar words using similar procedures (Mani and Plunkett 2011; Mani and Plunkett 2010c), we expected that toddlers' looking behaviour will not only be influenced by the rhyme overlap between related prime and target, but also by subtler feature overlap in the initial consonant (see also White and Morgan 2008).

To estimate how children's looking behaviour was influenced by the phonological overlap between prime and target label, we calculated the amount of time that children spent looking at the prime (P), at the target (T) and at the distracter (D) throughout each trial. The proportion of target looking, $T/(T + D)$, was calculated across the time-window from 300 ms after target word offset until the end of the trial. Trials in which children did not know the prime and/or the target label (according to individual vocabulary inventory reports filled out by the parents of the children) were excluded from analysis. Furthermore, only those trials in which children looked at least once at the prime picture in the prime phase of the trial, i.e. during the first 1500 ms, and in which children looked at least once at the target post-naming were included in the final analysis. All other trials were included in the analysis, as long as the child provided data for least 50 % of trials (3 children excluded).

Figure 2.2 shows the proportion of children's fixations at the target image every 40 ms in the trial separately for related and unrelated trials. As can be seen from the graph, children fixated the target more in related trials compared to unrelated trials, i.e. when the target was primed by an image whose label rhymed with the target label (related prime) compared to an image whose label was not related to the target label (unrelated prime). A paired-samples *t*-test on the mean proportion of target looking in the critical time-window 300 ms after target word offset confirmed a significant difference between children's target looking in related and unrelated trials ($t(28) = -2.198$, $p = 0.036$) with increased target looking in related trials: Target recognition was facilitated by the rhyme overlap between the labels for the prime and target image.

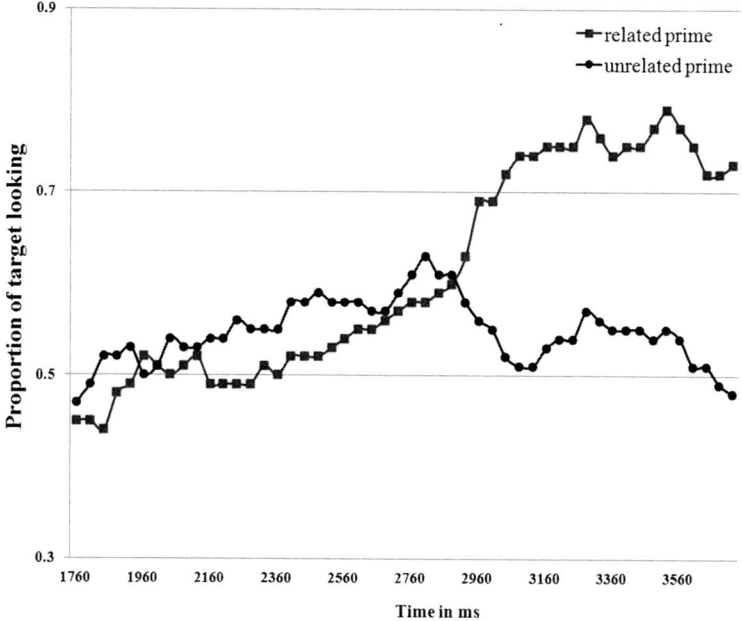

Fig. 2.2 Time course graph showing the mean proportion of target fixations in unrelated and related trials from target word onset (1750 ms) to the end of the trial

To further investigate the possible influence of feature overlap on the initial consonant of the labels for the prime and target image, we calculated the priming effect in the two-, three- and four-feature condition, i.e. the difference between target looking in related and unrelated trials, $[T/(T + D)]_{related} − [T/(T + D)]_{unrelated}$. If feature overlap modulates the priming effect, we expected to find an increase in the priming effect with increase in the amount of feature overlap in the initial consonant of the labels for the prime and target images. Figure 2.3 shows the mean difference in proportion of target looking in the two-, three- and four-feature conditions in the critical time-window after target word offset (i.e., 300 ms following target offset to the end of the trial).

As in White and Morgan (2008), we performed a trend analysis on the two-, three- and four-feature condition to examine the linearity of the effects of feature overlap. Similar to White and Morgan (2008), there was a linear trend in difference scores ($F(1, 59) = 3.495$, $p = 0.067$), but no quadratic trend ($p > 0.90$): Infants showed a larger priming effect with *increasing* feature overlap between target and prime label. This was further confirmed by a significant correlation between the size of the priming effect, i.e. the difference between target looking in related and unrelated trials, and the number of features changed ($r = −0.236$, $p_{(one-tailed)} = 0.03$). The size of the priming effect increased with increase in the degree of feature overlap between the prime and the target labels.

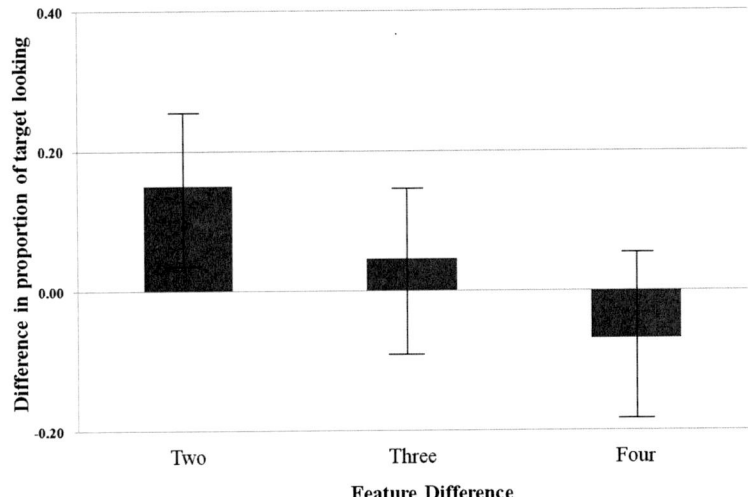

Fig. 2.3 Mean difference in proportion of target looking between unrelated and related trials after target word offset for two-, three- and four-feature distance (error bars: ±1 SE)

2.3 Discussion: Sub-segmental Detail Mediates Lexical Access in Toddlers

This chapter has provided a review of the literature on research examining toddler word recognition in the visual world paradigm as well as presented the results of a novel study examining whether toddlers' retrieval of the labels of familiar images and their recognition of correctly pronounced, familiar words involve access to the sub-segmental detail associated with the lexical representations of these words. In particular, we investigated whether the amount of feature overlap in the initial consonant between a prime and a rhyming target word modulates target word recognition. The results of this study provide evidence both for the facilitatory effects of rhyme overlap and for the activation of sub-segmental detail in toddlers' retrieval of the labels for visually presented images and recognition of familiar words.

2.3.1 Effects of Rhyme Overlap

Before we discuss the effects of sub-segmental overlap, let us first turn to the effect of rhyme overlap between words. Toddlers looked longer at the target following presentation of a visual rhyming prime relative to a prime with no obvious phonological relation to the target. This is an important finding since studies investigating phonological priming in toddlers have either focused on the effect of phonological overlap at the beginning—rather than the end—of words (Mani and Plunkett 2011), on semantically-mediated rhyme overlap (Mani et al. 2012) or on the effect of auditory non-word primes (Altvater-Mackensen and Mani 2013). Studies investigating phonological overlap at the beginnings of words show that an onset-overlapping prime interferes with target word recognition: toddlers' recognition of a target word is impaired following a prime overlapping in only the initial consonant with the target. In line with the adult priming literature, this finding is interpreted as evidence for lexical competition between words that start with the same consonant, i.e. belong to the same cohort (Mani and Plunkett 2011). In contrast to the interference effect observed in studies manipulating onset overlap, the current study finds that rhyme primes facilitate target word recognition in infants. This result is in keeping with effects of facilitated target recognition in semantically-mediated rhyme priming tasks in toddlers (Mani et al. 2012), e.g. experiments where the target (e.g., *shoe*) is semantically related to a rhyme competitor (e.g., *sock*) of the prime (e.g., *clock*); and previous studies showing that auditory non-word primes facilitate recognition of a rhyming target label (Altvater-Mackensen and Mani 2013). This result is also in keeping with results on rhyme priming in adults (see Monsell and Hirsh 1998, among others) showing that activation of a target is facilitated by previous presentation of a rhyming prime.

The different effects of onset and rhyme overlap in infants might be explained by suggesting that greater phonological overlap between prime and target aids recognition of the target: Target activation in priming tasks is sustained by the activation of the prime's phonemes because of the phonological overlap between prime and target (e.g., Radeau et al. 1995; Slowiaczek and Hamburger 1992). More specifically, when the child retrieves the prime label *Fisch* 'fish' upon seeing the picture of a fish, the corresponding phonemes /f/, /ɪ/ and /ʃ/ will be activated. The activation of the overlapping phonemes /ɪ/ and /ʃ/ in the target *Tisch* 'table' will aid subsequent activation and recognition of the target. The more overlap there is between the phonemes of the prime and the target, the more target recognition is facilitated by the prime. Note that facilitated activation of the target *Tisch* need not rely on the lexical activation of the prime *Fisch* itself in this scenario, but on the phonological-level activation that leads to the retrieval of the prime label. The interference effect observed for onset-overlapping primes, on the other hand, is typically interpreted as a consequence of the lexical-level activation of the prime that hinders activation of the target (e.g., Dufour and Peereman 2003; Segui and Grainger 1990). The different effects of rhyme- and onset-overlapping primes, thus, suggest that at least two different mechanisms modulate word retrieval and recognition in the developing lexicon: phonological-level effects that are modulated by the degree of phonological overlap between two retrieved words, and lexical-level effects that are modulated by the structure of the lexicon, i.e. the number of words in the toddler's lexicon that are phonologically similar to the retrieved words.

2.3.2 Effects of Sub-segmental Overlap

The focus of the study presented in this chapter was, however, whether retrieval and recognition of familiar words involves access to the sub-segmental detail associated with toddlers' representations of these words. Indeed, we found that the size of the priming effect did vary linearly with the amount of feature overlap; the smaller the feature overlap between the initial consonants of the prime and target, the smaller was the priming effect. Thus, the phonological priming effect was systematically modulated by the degree of sub-segmental overlap between the prime and the target label. While this resembles White and Morgan's (2008) finding of graded sensitivity to sub-segmental detail in mispronunciation detection in 19-month-olds, this result is a crucial extension of the White and Morgan findings and leads to the conclusion that both the implicit generation of the labels of visually fixated images and the recognition of correctly pronounced familiar words include access to the sub-segmental detail associated with toddlers' representations of these words.

We suggested earlier that toddlers' use of sub-segmental information in mispronunciation detection tasks does not necessarily imply the use of similar information in the recognition of a correctly pronounced, familiar word or in the implicit generation of the label of a visually fixated name-known object. In particular, we suggested that sub-segmental detail might be additionally called into play in mispronunciation detection since mispronunciations are, typically, not a word in the toddlers' lexicon and might call on more bottom-up resources relative to recognition of a word that is part of the toddlers' lexicon. The results presented in this chapter, however, show a similar influence of bottom-up sub-segmental information in toddlers' recognition of existing familiar words, i.e. words that are strongly associated with an entry in the toddlers' lexicon and for which top-down lexical-level processing may be expected to play a more dominant role. The similarity in the results of the current study and White and Morgan (2008) therefore raises questions with regard to the extent of top-down lexical-level processing in mispronunciation detection and suggests that mispronunciations trigger the lexical entries associated with the correct pronunciations (see also Altvater-Mackensen and Mani 2013, for more direct evidence that mispronunciations lead to lexical activation of the correct form of the target label).

The finding that toddlers' retrieval and recognition of familiar words involves access to the sub-segmental detail associated with the representations of these words is crucial to current models of language processing. Models of lexical processing such as TRACE (McClelland and Elman 1986) suggest that word recognition is driven by feature-mediated access to phonemes in a word. In particular, such models assume that the acoustic input leads to activation of the corresponding features at the feature level. This activation feeds through to the phoneme level so that phonemes congruent with the feature input are activated. Activation from the phoneme level then, in turn, leads to activation of lexical tokens congruent with this input. Since the prime was only ever visually presented in our task, our results further suggest that not only do toddlers rely on sub-segmental detail during auditory word recognition, but also retrieve sub-phonemic information when implicitly generating the label of an object present in the visual world around them.

Similar models of language processing have been called into force to explain the results of phonological priming studies to date (Mani and Plunkett 2011; Mani et al. 2012). However, previous phonological priming results could be explained without reference to feature-mediated lexical access given the overt phoneme overlap between the prime and the target in these studies, e.g. *Cat-Cap* versus *Cat-Book*. The results presented in this chapter, on the other hand, rely on different degrees of sub-segmental, but crucially non-phonemic overlap in the onset consonant of the prime and the target label. Therefore, the evidence reviewed in this chapter, more than other phonological priming studies to date, validate models of language processing that invoke sub-segmental or feature-mediated lexical access. Here, retrieval of the prime label leads to retrieval of the phonemes and the features corresponding to this label. Overlap between the target label and the prime label at the feature level leads to faster retrieval or processing of the target label in related trials relative to trials presenting no overlap between the prime and target label. In particular, the degree or amount of overlap in sub-phonemic features between the prime and the target label modulates the degree of the priming effect found in the current study. Note, however, that our results do not exclude an acoustic basis for toddlers' graded sensitivity to sub-segmental overlap. Mani and Plunkett's (2010c) results suggest that toddlers are sensitive to the acoustic rather than to the feature distance between words. While Mani and Plunkett's finding is based on children's responding to different degree of overlap in vowels, our finding is based on different degree of overlap in consonants. Acoustic distance in vowels can be captured in terms of formant frequencies, but identifying the relevant acoustic dimensions differentiating consonants is less straightforward. This makes them difficult to tease apart and evaluate against each other. Our findings, therefore, do not necessarily contradict an underlying acoustic basis for the current findings, inasmuch as we could not examine the influence of acoustic information on toddlers' responding in the current study. The results are therefore also compatible with models of word recognition proposing that lexical access is mediated by gradient acoustic—rather than feature and phoneme—similarity between the input and stored representations (e.g., Goldinger 1996).

2.3.3 Concluding Remarks

We have reviewed the literature on experiments using the visual world paradigm to assess infant word recognition, in particular, the amount of attention infants pay to phonological detail in word recognition. We have also presented a novel study using a modified version of the visual world paradigm to assess the extent to which toddlers access phonological detail when implicitly generating the label for a visually fixated image. The results of this study suggest that both the retrieval of an object's label and toddlers' recognition of a word involve activation of not only phonemic but also sub-segmental information associated with the lexical representation of this word. We therefore conclude that lexical access in 24-month-old toddlers is mediated by sub-phonemic information. It remains for future research to examine whether this sub-segmental content is feature-based or acoustic, perhaps by manipulating the degree of overlap at the vowel (where feature and acoustic content can be more easily separated from one another). These results have important implications for models of language processing, confirming as they do, that lexical access includes fine-grained analysis of the speech input into units of processing smaller than the phoneme.

A question that remains regards the degree to which sub-segmental information mediates lexical access at different stages of development. The adult literature is ripe with controversy with regard to the impact of sub-segmental information on word recognition in the fully developed lexicon (e.g., Cole et al. 1978; Connine et al. 1997; Ernestus and Mak 2004). Indeed, recent computational models suppose that sub-segmental information might have a larger impact on word recognition in the developing lexicon: Adapting TRACE (McClelland and Elman 1986) to model White and Morgan's (2008) data, Mayor and Plunkett (2014) show that graded sensitivity to sub-segmental detail during word recognition depends on the absence of inhibitory connections between words. Subtle effects of sub-phonemic overlap overtly impact word recognition only in small lexicons in which words do not inhibit each other during lexical access. In particular, Mayor and Plunkett predict that graded sensitivity to feature overlap will not be found in older children with sufficiently large vocabularies, since lexical inhibition effects are strengthened by increasing vocabulary size (see also Mani and Plunkett 2011; Arias-Trejo and Plunkett 2009). This does not imply that sub-segmental detail is no longer activated during lexical access. But, perhaps, once a critical mass of vocabulary knowledge is attained, lexical inhibition effects get strengthened to the extent that the perceptual similarity between words is no longer a simple linear function of overlapping features. At this stage, other factors, e.g. how *many* words overlap on certain phonological dimensions, may become more important.

References

Allopenna, P. D., Magnuson, J. S., & Tanenhaus, M. K. (1998). Tracking the time course of spoken word recognition using eye movements: Evidence for continuous mapping models. *Journal of Memory and Language, 38*, 419–439.

Altvater-Mackensen, N., & Mani, N. (2013). The impact of mispronunciations on toddler word recognition: Evidence for cascaded activation of semantically related words from mispronunciations of familiar words. *Infancy, 18*, 1030–1052.

Altvater-Mackensen, N., Van der Feest, S., & Fikkert, P. (2014). Asymmetries in children's early word recognition: The case of stops and fricatives. *Language, Learning and Development, 10*, 149–178.

Arias-Trejo, N., & Plunkett, K. (2009). Lexical-semantic priming effects in infancy. *Philosophical Transactions of the Royal Society B, 364*, 3633–3647.

Bailey, T. M., & Plunkett, K. (2002). Phonological specificity in early words. *Cognitive Development, 17*, 1267–1284.

Chomsky, N., & Halle, M. (1968). *The sound pattern of English*. New York: Harper & Row.

Clements, G. N. (1985). The geometry of phonological features. *Phonology, 2*, 225–252.

Cole, R. A., Jakimik, J., & Cooper, W. E. (1978). Perceptibility of phonetic features in fluent speech. *Journal of the Acoustical Society of America, 64*, 44–56.

Connine, C. M., Titone, D., Deelman, T., & Blasko, D. (1997). Similarity mapping in spoken word recognition. *Journal of Memory and Language, 37*, 463–480.

Dufour, S., & Peereman, R. (2003). Inhibitory priming effects in auditory word recognition: When the target's competitors conflict with the prime. *Cognition, 88*, B33–B44.

Ernestus, M., & Mak, W. M. (2004). Distinctive phonological features differ in relevance for both spoken and written word recognition. *Brain and Language, 90*, 378–392.

Goldinger, S. D. (1996). Words and voices: Episodic traces in spoken word identification and recognition memory. *Journal of Experimental Psychology. Learning, Memory, and Cognition, 22*, 166–1183.

Huettig, F., Rommers, J., & Meyer, A. S. (2011). Using the visual world paradigm to study language processing: A review and critical evaluation. *Acta Psychologica, 137*, 151–171.

Huang, Y. T., & Snedeker, J. (2010). Cascading activation across levels of representation in children's lexical processing. *Journal of Child Language, 38*, 644–661.

Magnuson, J. S., Dixon, J. A., Tanenhaus, M. K., & Aslin, R. N. (2007). The dynamics of lexical competition during spoken word recognition. *Cognitive Science, 31*, 1–24.

Mani, N. (2011). Phonological acquisition. In Kula, Botma & Nasukawa (eds.) *The Continuum Companion toPhonology*, Continuum, London UK, 278–297.

Mani, N., Coleman, J., & Plunkett, K. (2008). Phonological specificity of vocalic features at 18 months. *Language and Speech, 51*, 3–21.

Mani, N., Durrant, S., & Floccia, C. (2012). Activation of phonological and semantic codes in toddlers. *Journal of Memory and Language, 66*, 612–622.

Mani, N., & Huettig, F. (2012). Prediction during language processing is a piece of cake—but only for skilled producers. *Journal of Experimental Psychology: Human Perception and Performance, 38*, 843–847.

Mani, N., & Plunkett, K. (2007). Phonological specificity of consonants and vowels in early lexical representations. *Journal of Memory and Language, 57*, 252–272.

Mani, N., & Plunkett, K. (2010a). In the infant's mind's ear: Evidence for implicit naming. *Psychological Science, 21*, 908–913.

Mani, N., & Plunkett, K. (2010b). Twelve-month-olds know their cups from their keps and tups. *Infancy, 15*, 445–470.

Mani, N., & Plunkett, K. (2010c). Does size matter? Graded sensitivity to vowel mispronunciations of familiar words. *Journal of Child Language, 38*, 606–627.

Mani, N., & Plunkett, K. (2011). Phonological priming and cohort effects in toddlers. *Cognition, 121*, 196–206.

Mayor, J., & Plunkett, K. (2014). Infant word recognition: Insights from TRACE simulations. *Journal of Memory and Language, 71*, 89–123.

McClelland, J. L., & Elman, J. L. (1986). The TRACE model of speech perception. *Cognitive Psychology, 18*, 1–86.

McMurray, B., Tanenhaus, M., & Aslin, R. (2002). Gradient effects of within-category phonetic variation on lexical access. *Cognition, 86*, B33–B42.

Mitterer, H. (2011). The mental lexicon is fully specified: Evidence from eye-tracking. *Journal of Experimental Psychology: Human Perception and Performance, 37*, 496–513.

Monsell, S., & Hirsh, K. W. (1998). Competitor priming in spoken word recognition. *Journal of Experimental Psychology. Learning, Memory, and Cognition, 24*, 1495–1520.

Nazzi, T., Floccia, C., Moquet, B., & Butler, J. (2009). Bias for consonantal over vocalic information in french- and english-learning 30-month-olds: Crosslinguistic evidence in early word learning. *Journal of Experimental Child Psychology, 102*, 522–537.

Radeau, M., Morais, J., & Segui, J. (1995). Phonological priming between monosyllabic spoken words. *Journal of Experimental Psychology: Human Perception and Performance, 21*, 1297–1311.

Reinisch, E., Jesse, A., & McQueen, J. M. (2010). Early use of phonetic information in spoken word recognition: Lexical stress drives eye-movements immediately. *Quarterly Journal of Experimental Psychology, 63*, 772–783.

Salverda, A. P., Dahan, D., & McQueen, J. M. (2003). The role of prosodic boundaries in the resolution of lexical embedding in speech comprehension. *Cognition, 90*, 51–89.

Segui, J., & Grainger, J. (1990). Priming word recognition with orthographic neighbours: Effects of relative prime-target frequency. *Journal of Experimental Psychology: Human Perception and Performance, 16*, 65–76.

Slowiaczek, L. M., & Hamburger, M. B. (1992). Prelexical facilitation and lexical interference in auditory word recognition. *Journal of Experimental Psychology. Learning, Memory, and Cognition, 18*, 1239–1250.

Swingley, D., & Aslin, R. N. (2000). Spoken word recognition and lexical representation in very young children. *Cognition, 76*, 147–166.

Swingley, D., & Aslin, R. N. (2002). Lexical neighborhoods and the word-form representations of 14-month-olds. *Psychological Science, 13*, 480–484.

Swingley, D. (2009). Onset and codas in 1.5-year-olds' word recognition. *Journal of Memory and Language, 60*, 252–269.

Tanenhaus, M. K., Spivey-Knowlton, M. J., Eberhard, K. M., & Sedivy, J. C. (1995). Integration of visual and linguistic Information in spoken language Comprehension. *Science, 268*, 1632–1634.

Van der Feest, S.V.H. (2007). Building a phonological lexicon. The acquisition of the Dutch voicing contrast in perception and production. Doctoral Dissertation, Radboud University Nijmegen.

White, K. S., & Morgan, J. L. (2008). Sub-segmental detail in early lexical representations. *Journal of Memory and Language, 59*, 114–132.

Chapter 3
The Complexity of the Visual Environment Modulates Language-Mediated Eye Gaze

Florian Hintz and Falk Huettig

3.1 Background: The Interaction of Language, Vision, and Attention During Language-Mediated Visual Search

A remarkable characteristic about human cognition is that we are able to process visual input and spoken language at the same time and have seemingly no difficulty integrating both modalities. For instance, when walking along an unknown street and simultaneously listening to someone describe the directions on the phone, we are usually able to spot all the visual landmarks mentioned by the person on the phone quickly and with ease. Within milliseconds we can locate the "statue opposite the supermarket" and eventually navigate our way through the city. Our visual search in those situations is cued by information derived from the auditory input, which is mapped on information derived from the visual surroundings. In other words, processing spoken language activates long-term linguistic and non-linguistic mental representations just as processing visual input activates associated long-term linguistic and non-linguistic representations.

F. Hintz (✉) · F. Huettig
Max Planck Institute for Psycholinguistics, Nijmegen, The Netherlands
e-mail: florian.hintz@mpi.nl

F. Hintz
International Max Planck Research School for Language Sciences,
Nijmegen, The Netherlands

F. Huettig
Donders Institute for Brain, Cognition, and Behavior,
Radboud University, Nijmegen, The Netherlands

© Springer India 2015
R.K. Mishra et al. (eds.), *Attention and Vision
in Language Processing*, DOI 10.1007/978-81-322-2443-3_3

The general question we asked in this study is whether the nature of the visual environment has an impact on the way we process concurrent spoken language. In particular, we investigated how increased visual complexity affects the likelihood of word–object mapping at various levels of representation during language-mediated visual search. To understand how exactly language and vision interact, we must know which knowledge types are retrieved when processing both language and visual input. A useful method for the investigation of language-vision interaction is the visual world paradigm (VWP; Cooper 1974; Tanenhaus et al. 1995; see Huettig et al. 2011b, for a review). In the VWP participants hear spoken language while they look at a visual scene related to the spoken utterance. Participants' eye movements are recorded for analysis. Many recent studies have looked at the mental representations involved in word–object mapping which has led to a substantial body of literature. Allopenna et al. (1998), for example, showed that word–object mapping can occur at a phonological level of representation. The participants in that study looked at computer displays showing, for example, the pictures of a beaker (target object), a beetle (phonological onset competitor), a speaker (phonological rhyme competitor) and a carriage (unrelated distractor), while listening to the spoken instruction "Pick up the beaker". The authors observed that the participants' likelihood of fixating both the picture of the beaker and the picture of the beetle increased as they encountered the initial phonemes of the spoken target word "beaker". As the acoustic information of beaker started to mismatch with the phonological information of beetle, the likelihood of looks to the beetle decreased as the likelihood of looks to the beaker continued to rise. As the end of "beaker" acoustically unfolded, looks to the picture of a speaker started to increase. Simulations run with the TRACE model of speech perception (McClelland and Elman 1986) replicated the eye gaze pattern of the participants, consistent with the notion that the probability of fixating items within the visual display can be driven by a phonological overlap between the name of a depicted object and the target word in the auditory stimulus.

Word–object mapping can also take place at a semantic/conceptual level of representation. This has been examined in a number of studies. Huettig and Altmann (2005; see also Yee and Sedivy 2006; Yee et al. 2009; Duñabeitia et al. 2009), for instance, investigated whether semantic properties of spoken words could direct eye gaze towards objects in the visual field in the absence of any associative relationships between targets and competitors. They found that participants directed their overt visual attention towards a depicted object (e.g., trumpet) when a semantically related but not associatively related target word (e.g., "piano") acoustically unfolded, and that the likelihood of fixation was proportional to the degree of conceptual overlap (cf. Cree and McRae 2003). Similarly, Huettig et al. (2006) observed that corpus-based measures of word semantics (e.g., latent semantic analysis, Landauer and Dumais 1997) each correlated well with fixation behaviour. Based on those studies, language-mediated eye movements can be seen as a sensitive indicator of the degree of overlap between the semantic information conveyed by speech and the conceptual knowledge retrieved from the visual objects. In those experiments, phonological relationships between spoken words and visual objects were not present, hence demonstrating that semantic word–object mapping can occur in the absence of phonological mapping.

Finally, there is experimental evidence suggesting that word–object mapping occurs at a perceptual level of representation. Visual mapping, that is, increased looks to entities related for instance in visual shape, has been observed when participants were presented with the picture of a cable while listening to the spoken word "snake". The likelihood of looks to the picture of the cable increased whilst the word "snake" acoustically unfolded (Huettig and Altmann 2004, 2007; Dahan and Tanenhaus 2005). Visual mapping, likewise, was found in the absence of phonological and/or semantic mapping.

More recently, Huettig and McQueen (2007) showed that the listener's fixation behaviour during language-mediated visual search can be characterised by a *tug of war* between matches at phonological, semantic, *and* visual levels of representation. In four eye-tracking experiments, they presented participants with displays including either four visual objects (Experiments 1 and 2) or the printed word names of the same objects (Experiments 3 and 4) and concurrent spoken sentences including a critical target word which was preceded by on average seven words. The sentence preceding the critical word (e.g., "beaker") was contextually neutral (i.e., participants could not predict the target word from the sentential context). Three of the four entities in the display were related to the target word: one was related in semantics (e.g., a fork, and unrelated in phonology and visual shape), one was similar in visual shape (e.g., a bobbin, and unrelated in phonology and semantics) and the name of the third object overlapped phonologically in the first syllable with the target (e.g., beaver, and was unrelated in semantics and visual shape). In Experiments 1 and 4, participants were presented with the visual display from the beginning of the sentence but in Experiments 2 and 3, they only had a 200 ms preview of the display before the critical word acoustically unfolded. In Experiment 1, the phonological overlap between the critical spoken word and the visually presented phonological competitor object resulted in shifts in eye gaze to that object for the duration of the overlap. As the spoken target word unfolded beyond the overlapping first syllable and indicated that the competitor object was not part of the sentence, participants shifted their eye gaze to the shape and semantic competitors. When there was only 200 ms to look at the same display prior to the onset of the critical spoken word (Experiment 2), participants did not look preferentially at the phonological competitors. Instead, they made more fixations to the shape competitors and then to the semantic competitors. Huettig and McQueen (2007) interpreted the absence of an attentional bias to the phonological competitors in Experiment 2 as revealing that participants had not yet retrieved the names of the pictures before the onset of the spoken word. Hence, picture processing had not advanced to a phonological level of representation and by the time a picture name would have been retrieved, the evidence in the speech signal had already indicated that the phonological competitor was not part of the sentence. When the pictures in Huettig and McQueen (2007) were replaced with their printed word names (Experiments 3 and 4), the authors observed attentional shifts to the phonological competitors only, both with short and long previews of the display. This suggested that the likelihood of mapping between representations derived from the language input and representations derived from the visual input was contingent upon the nature of the visual stimuli (i.e. printed words vs. pictures).

Huettig and McQueen (2011) investigated this issue further and examined whether semantic and visual-shape representations are routinely retrieved from printed-word displays and used during language-mediated visual search. They used the same sentences as in the earlier study and printed word displays with no phonological competitors present. The study found evidence for semantic mapping with printed word displays (when phonological matches between the speech signal and the visual objects were not present) but not for shape mapping even though participants looked at these competitors when they were presented as pictures (Huettig and McQueen 2007, Experiments 1, 2). Huettig and McQueen argued that shape information about the objects appears not to be used in online search of printed-word displays whereas it is used with picture displays suggesting that the nature of the visual environment modulates word–object mapping.

In summary, when we are faced with spoken language and visual input at the same time, matches between representations derived from either modality can happen at phonological, semantic and visual levels of representation. The listener's fixation behaviour during language-mediated visual search seems to be determined by a tug of war between all these types of word knowledge. However, the exact level of representation at which word–object mapping takes place appears to be determined by the timing of processing in both the language and the visual processing system, the temporal unfolding of the speech signal, and by the nature of the visual environment. In the present study, we further investigated how the nature of the visual environment impacts on on-line word–object mapping.

The studies described above suggested that there are important differences in online word–object mapping between displays of visual objects and displays of printed words. Moreover, most of the research using the VWP has either used simple object displays (usually four objects, one in each corner of the screen) or its written-word equivalent. With such 'simple displays' the interpretation of fixation behaviour could only be based on the properties of the individual objects. Using complex visual scenes in those studies would have made the evaluation of the findings very difficult because the effects of scene-specific influences on fixation behaviour (e.g., scene schema knowledge) could not have been easily separated from influences of lexical effects of, e.g. semantic similarity (see for instance, the semantic influences on object identification reported by Boyce and Pollatsek 1992; De Graef 1998).

A recent study investigated word–object mapping using photographs of real world scenes (Andersson et al. 2011). Participants viewed cluttered scenes containing a large number of objects (e.g., a scene depicting a garage sale) while listening to three-sentence-passages that varied in speech rate. The authors showed that effects of language-mediated eye gaze appear to be very robust as the participants directed their visual attention to objects mentioned in the speech even under demanding conditions (e.g., a fast speech rate). What we cannot tell from those findings is at which levels of representation word–object mapping takes place in complex visual scenes because this was not part of Andersson et al.'s manipulation. As the objects mentioned in the speech signal were present in the visual scene, it is possible that matches happened at all three levels of representation (e.g., phonological, semantic, visual). However, it is also possible that word–object mapping in realistic scenes and word–object mapping in simple four-object displays are fundamentally different.

In the present series of experiments, we examined how semi-realistic visual scenes affect the likelihood of matches at phonological, semantic and visual shape levels of representation. This question has considerable real life relevance as we typically do not view objects in visually impoverished simple displays but rather in more complex surroundings. In other words, the way we experience the visual environment in our daily life is much more complex than is simulated in most experiments conducted using the VWP. In order to approximate natural language-vision interaction, we must know how exactly word–object mapping, i.e. the tug of war between phonological, semantic and visual shape information is influenced by more complex visual environments.

3.2 Word–Object Mapping in Complex Visual Scenes

Printed word displays have been shown to induce implicit biases during language-mediated visual search, as with such displays mappings occur mainly at phonological levels of representation. Huettig and McQueen (2011) argued that with printed-word displays, there is particularly easy access to the phonological form of words (van Orden et al. 1988; Frost 1998). Here, we tested how the increased complexity of semi-realistic scenes impacts on phonological, semantic and shape word–object mapping.

3.2.1 Experiment 1

Thirty participants with normal or corrected to normal vision participated. The same visual objects were used as in Huettig and McQueen (2007).[1] We embedded those objects in semi-realistic line drawings including human-like cartoon characters with either a narrow path running through the scene or three implied walls indicating the contours of a room. Four different characters (two male and two

---

[1]See Huettig and McQueen (2007) for a detailed description of the materials and the results of seven norming studies. Five of the original item sets were removed from both Experiment 1 and all subsequent experiments, because they contained pictures of body parts present in the human-like characters.

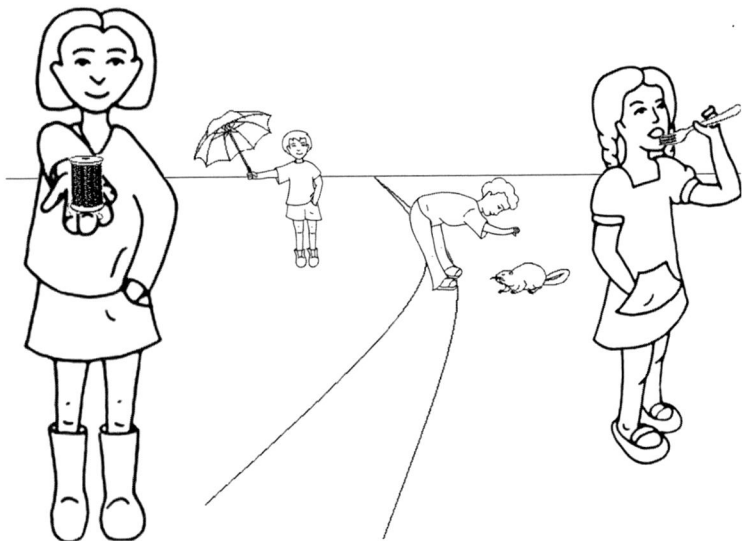

Fig. 3.1 Example display used in Experiment 1. For the spoken word "beker", *beaker*, the display consisted of pictures of a beaver (the phonological competitor), a bobbin (the visual-shape competitor), a fork (the semantic competitor) and an umbrella (the unrelated distractor)

female) in different postures were drawn. A random combination of four of those was present in each scene and shown to interact with the visual objects (hold, lean down to, pet, etc.). Huettig and McQueen's (2007) stimulus materials were created to avoid any semantic relationship between the four objects. The scenes (Fig. 3.1, for an example) were hence composed such that scene schema information (i.e., contextual knowledge of objects that might be expected within a specific scene; for example, shower gel, sponge, and soap are items that one might expect to see in a bathroom scene and in particular locations, Strik and Underwood 2007) was minimised. This was done to separate effects of scene schema information from effects of the visual complexity and from effects of character–object interactions.

After a three-second preview, our participants heard single spoken target words while looking at semi-realistic scenes and were asked to indicate the presence or absence of the target object. That is, they were asked to produce "Ja" (Yes) when the target was present and "Nee" (No) when the target was absent. During filler trials, the target objects (and three unrelated distractor objects) were present, but during experimental trials they were absent and the display contained an unrelated distractor object (an umbrella, *paraplu*) and various competitor objects. For example, given the spoken target "beaker" (*beker*), the display contained a phonological (a beaver, *bever*), a shape (a bobbin, *klos*), and a semantic (a fork, *vork*) competitor.

Given the robust nature of language-mediated orienting (cf. Andersson et al. 2011), we expected that our manipulation would not result in a breakdown of word–object mapping. Compared to Huettig and McQueen (2007, Experiment 1,

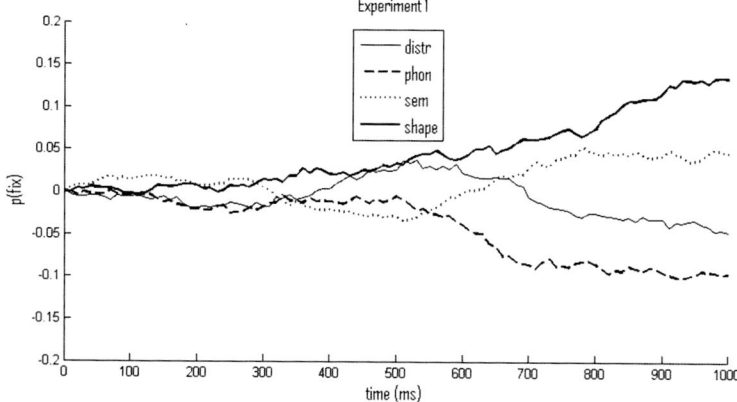

Fig. 3.2 Time course graph showing change in fixation probabilities to phonological competitors, visual-shape competitors, semantic competitors and unrelated distractors for Experiment 1 (semi-realistic scene)

four objects in four corners of the screen), the displays in the current experiment contained more visual entities. Also, the cartoon characters were shown to interact with the visual objects possibly supplying additional semantic information, which was not present in the earlier experiment. We hypothesised that enhanced visual and semantic complexity would lead to mapping biases at semantic and visual levels at the expense of mapping at the phonological level.

Figure 3.2 shows a time course graph illustrating the change in fixation probabilities for Experiment 1,[2] for each of the four objects, for 1 s after the acoustic onset of the spoken target word. The proportion of trials with a fixation at the acoustic onset of the target word served as a baseline. Each subsequent data point reflects the proportion of trials with a fixation at that moment minus the baseline (cf. Huettig and Altmann 2005). Negative values thus reflect moves away from objects that were already fixated at the onset.

Trials on which participants had responded incorrectly were removed from the analysis.[3] For the statistical analysis, we calculated ratios between the proportion of fixations made to a particular competitor (phonological, semantic, or shape) and the sum of proportion of fixations made to the distractor object and that competitor. A ratio greater than 0.5 suggests that of all the fixations directed to a particular

[2]Prior to Experiment 1 (and Experiment 2) participants carried out an object naming task during which their eye movements were recorded. The task was independent of the subsequent main experiment and required participants to look at one object at a time presented at the centre of the computer screen and name it as fast as possible. Sixty objects which were not used in the main experiment had to be named. The task lasted around 5 min and we observed no obvious impact on participants' performance in either Experiment 1 or 2 nor did they report anecdotal effects.

[3]There was one item on which more than 50 % of the participant sample had responded incorrectly. This item was removed from further analyses, and was removed from the subsequent experiments.

competitor and the distractor, the competitor attracted more than 50 % of those fixations. Conversely, a ratio smaller than 0.5 reflects that of all the fixations directed to the competitor and the distractor, the distractor attracted more than 50 % of those fixations. Mean ratios were computed by participants and items for 100 ms time bins starting at the acoustic onset of the target word. Given the time necessary for programming and initiating an eye movement (Saslow 1967), we can assume that fixations during the 0–99 ms time window were not influenced by information from the spoken target word. Pairwise t-tests were carried out comparing the 0–99 ms bin (baseline, hereafter) to nine subsequent time bins (until 1 s after the spoken word onset). We tested, for the data in each window, whether the competitor–distractor ratio was significantly different from fixations made during the baseline. These analyses provide estimates of when competitor and distractor fixation proportions diverge (and perhaps later converge) over the time window of interest. The average duration of the spoken target words was 500 ms. The time bin analysis hence spanned the acoustic lifetime of the spoken word and additional 500 ms after the spoken word offset.

Figure 3.2 suggests a replication of the visual shape and semantic biases reported by Huettig and McQueen (2007, Experiment 1).[4] Importantly, however, there was no sign of a bias in looks to the phonological competitor as in Huettig and McQueen (2007, Experiment 1). The statistical analysis revealed that fixations to the shape competitor became significant during the time bin starting 800 ms after the spoken word onset (800–900 ms: $t1(29) = -2.49$, $p = 0.019$; $t2(33) = -2.29$, $p = 0.029$; 900–1000 ms: $t1(29) = -3.89$, $p = 0.001$; $t2(33) = -3.77$, $p = 0.001$). Fixations to the semantic competitor were significant by participants and approached statistical significance by items ($t1(29) = -2.81$, $p = 0.009$; $t2(33) = -1.44$, $p = 0.159$). There were no increased looks to the phonological competitors during the earlier time windows (200–300 ms: $t1(29) = 1.07$, $p = 0.296$; $t2(33) = 1.13$, $p = 0.267$; 300–400 ms: $t1(29) = 0.88$, $p = 0.387$; $t2(33) = 0.81$, $p = 0.425$). We observed, however, some evidence for inhibition of shifts in eye gaze to the phonological competitors (i.e., more looks to the unrelated distractor than to the phonological competitor) during late time bins (600–999 ms; 600–699 ms bin: $t1(29) = 2.47$, $p = 0.02$; $t2(34) = 1.81$, $p = 0.079$) suggesting that the phonological forms (i.e. the word names) had been retrieved.

In sum, in Experiment 1, we examined the impact of semi-realistic visual environments on the tug of war between phonological, semantic and visual shape information. We used the same materials as Huettig and McQueen (2007) but instead of presenting the visual objects in simple 2 × 2 arrays, we embedded them in semi-realistic scenes including four human-like characters, which were shown to interact with the objects. Participants showed increased fixations to visual-shape competitors. However, there was no hint of an initial bias in shifts to phonological competitors, and the bias in shifts to the semantic competitor was reduced and not statistically robust in the item analysis.

---

[4]Note that our main aim interest was not in the exact timing of the shifts to semantic and shape competitors. What is clear from the data (see Fig. 3.2) is that participants started to shift their eye gaze to both competitors after the target word had been heard.

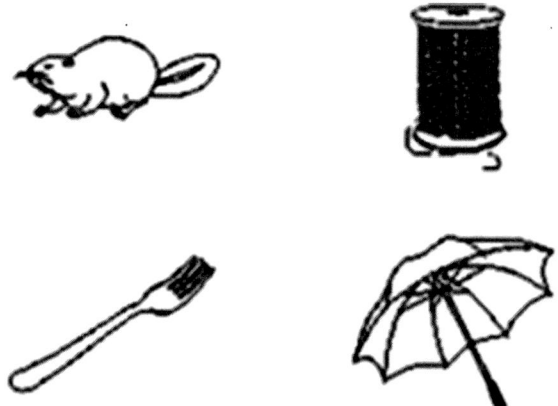

Fig. 3.3 Example display used in Experiment 2 (cf. Huettig and McQueen 2007, Experiment 1). For the spoken word "beker", *beaker*, the display consisted of pictures of a beaver (the phonological competitor), a bobbin (the visual-shape competitor), a fork (the semantic competitor), and an umbrella (the unrelated distractor)

Experiment 2 was conducted to rule out an alternative explanation namely that the differences between the present results and those of Huettig and McQueen (2007, Experiment 1) were due to differences in the tasks used. Huettig and McQueen (2007) asked participants to simply look at the displays while listening to the spoken language. In the present study, we asked participants to pursue an active search task, i.e. to indicate (by saying yes or no) whether the visual object referred to by the spoken target word was present in the display or not. Hence, we cannot rule out that the observed differences in the results between the two studies were due to task differences. In Experiment 2, we presented participants with the same simple object arrays as used in Huettig and McQueen (2007, Experiment 1, cf. Fig. 3.3, for an example) but instructed them to carry out the same task as in the present Experiment 1. If the differences in results are due to task differences, then the data of Experiment 2 should be similar to the results of the present Experiment 1. If on the other hand the difference in the nature of the visual environment is crucial, Experiment 2 should replicate the data pattern of Huettig and McQueen (2007, Experiment 1).

3.2.2 Experiment 2

Thirty subjects who had normal or corrected to normal vision and had not participated in Experiment 1 were tested in Experiment 2. The results revealed that task differences are unlikely to account for the differences between the present Experiment 1 and Experiment 1 of Huettig and McQueen (2007). Figure 3.4 and the statistical analyses show that with simple four object displays, using an active task, participants' fixations to the phonological competitor objects (300–400 ms: $t1(29) = -2.3$,

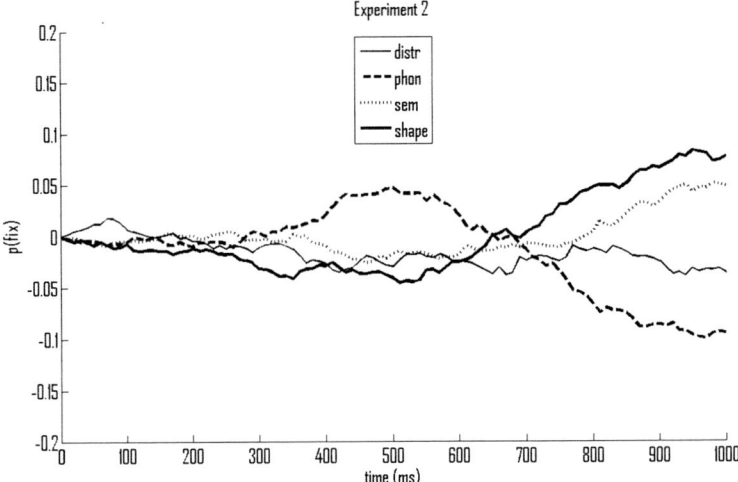

Fig. 3.4 Time course graph showing change in fixation probabilities to phonological competitors, visual-shape competitors, semantic competitors and unrelated distractors for Experiment 2 (simple object displays)

$p = 0.029$; t2(33) $= -2.96$, $p = 0.006$) preceded those to shape (e.g., 900–999 ms: t1(29) $= -2.91$, $p = 0.007$; t2(33) $= -2.15$, $p = 0.039$) and semantic competitors (e.g., 900–999 ms: t1(29) $= -2.81$, $p = 0.009$; t2(33) $= -1.44$, $p = 0.159$). The results of Experiment 2 were therefore a close replication of Huettig and McQueen (2007, Experiment 1). Hence, we can rule out that the observed differences between the present Experiment 1 and Experiment 2 were due to an active task being used instead of a passive look-and-listen task. More likely, these differences can be attributed to the varying nature of the visual environment in those experiments.

The findings are intriguing, indicating substantial differences in word–object mapping between semi-realistic scenes and 2 × 2 object arrays. The data pattern in Experiment 1 suggests that participants show an increased preference for visual mapping with the increased visual complexity of the semi-realistic scenes. Why might participants show a preference of visual mapping during language-vision interactions involving complex visual scenes?

One possibility is that in the more complex display, the objects were less salient (i.e., took more time to find) than in the simpler displays. This could have had two implications: First, this could delay the retrieval of the objects' phonological representations such that by the time the onset of the spoken words occurred, picture processing had not cascaded to levels at which phonological forms are retrieved (cf. Huettig and McQueen, Experiment 2). We believe that to be unlikely. Participants had sufficient preview of the visual scenes (3 s) before the spoken words were heard. Perhaps more importantly, our data show some evidence for phonological inhibition during the 600–999 ms time window. This suggests that the participants had retrieved the phonological forms of the objects.

Second, one might argue that the lack of visual salience of the objects in the semi-realistic scene affected the time-course of the mapping process of language-derived and vision-derived representations. That is, when the target word (e.g., "beaker") acoustically unfolded, participants were not able to locate the phonological competitors quickly. Note that such an account predicts that all types of competitors should be equally affected. However, this was not the case. We found a strong and robust bias for mapping at the visual level of representation and a clear (albeit reduced) tendency for semantic mapping.

What then are the mechanisms modulating word–object mapping in semi-realistic scenes? One could argue that our semi-realistic scenes did not substantially increase the 'semantic content' in the displays as the character–object couplings were rather arbitrary and all four character–object pairs did not belong to a semantically coherent scene, thus limiting the extent of semantic mapping. However, as indicated above, the employment of visual displays, where scene schema information is present, is generally difficult as lexical effects cannot be differentiated from effects of scene schema knowledge. In the semi-realistic scenes, visual complexity however was substantially increased as compared to the 2 × 2 displays. If visual complexity resulted in the visual bias then we should expect a replication of the pattern of Experiment 1, even if the characters are replaced with meaningless shapes.

3.2.3 Experiment 3

In Experiment 3, we therefore, removed the character–object interactions by replacing the human-like drawings with unnamable, meaningless black shapes. Those shapes have been used in earlier studies on statistical learning of higher order temporal structures (cf. Fiser and Aslin 2002, see Fig. 3.5, for an example display used in the current study). That way, the additional four visual entities cannot be interpreted as interacting with the objects, yet we kept the scene visually complex. In all other respects, the set-up was identical to Experiment 1. Thirty subjects who had not participated in either Experiment 1 or 2 were tested.

The fixation graph in Fig. 3.6 and the statistical analysis[5] revealed that while there were robust biases to shape (700–799 ms: $t1(29) = -3.43, p = 0.002$; $t2(32) = -2.13, p = 0.041$) and semantic (800–899 ms: $t1(29) = -2.92, p = 0.007$; $t2(32) = -2.01, p = 0.053$) competitors, there was not a tendency for looks to the phonological competitors. As in Experiment 1, we found some evidence for phonological inhibition ($t1(29) = 2.74, p = 0.01$; $t2(32) = 1.39, p = 0.175$). These results are consistent with our predictions that increased visual complexity induces a bias of word–object mapping at the visual level of representation.

---

[5]Due to an error, one experimental item had to be removed from the analysis.

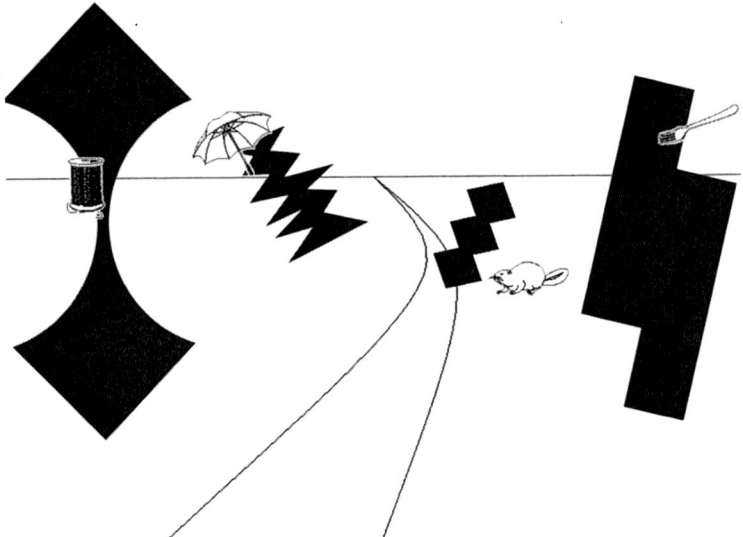

Fig. 3.5 Example display used in Experiment 3. For the spoken word "beker", *beaker*, the display consisted of pictures of a beaver (the phonological competitor), a bobbin (the visual-shape competitor), a fork (the semantic competitor) and an umbrella (the unrelated distractor). The cartoon characters were replaced with meaningless *black shapes*

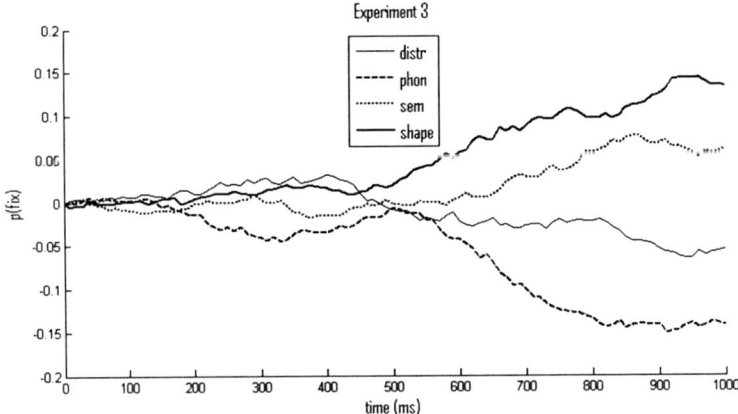

Fig. 3.6 Time-course graph showing change in fixation probabilities to phonological competitors, visual-shape competitors, semantic competitors and unrelated distractors in Experiment 3 (cartoon characters replaced with meaningless shapes)

3.3 General Discussion

The present findings provide further evidence that during language-mediated visual search with picture displays, there is a tug of war between multiple types of mental representations (e.g., phonological, semantic, visual shape, cf. Huettig and McQueen 2007). Our main aim in the present study was to assess the influence of more complex visual environments on this tug of war. To this end, we showed identical visual objects either in more complex visual environments including four human-like cartoon characters or four meaningless black shapes, or as simple four object arrays. Participants heard single spoken target words while looking at the different displays and were asked to indicate the presence or absence of the target objects. We hypothesised that the more complex visual information and the semantic information intrinsic to the semi-realistic scenes would induce a mode of processing yielding matches at the visual and semantic level. We assumed that this mode of processing would lead to a modulation of mapping behaviour at the phonological level, in other words, to a reduced likelihood of phonological mapping.

In Experiment 1, we observed an attentional bias in looks to the visual-shape competitors and a tendency for a bias for the semantic competitors, but there were no shifts in eye gaze towards phonological competitors when the objects were embedded in semi-realistic scenes. When the objects were presented in simple four object displays (Experiments 2), however, we replicated the clear early attentional bias to phonological competitors found in earlier research (Huettig and McQueen 2007, Experiment 1). This showed that task differences (active vs. look-and-listen task) could not account for the absence of shifts in attention to phonological competitors with semi-realistic scenes. Crucially, we observed fixation behaviour very similar (biases for visual-shape and semantic mapping) to that in the present Experiment 1, when the human-like cartoon characters in the earlier experiment were replaced with meaningless black shapes (Experiment 3).

This suggests that the pattern of results was not driven by the objects being presented in interaction with the human-like cartoon characters but can most likely be attributed to the increased visual complexity in the scene.

3.3.1 Why Do More Complex Visual Environments Reduce the Likelihood of Word–Object Mapping at the Phonological Level of Representation?

While increasing the complexity of the visual scene, we re-arranged the objects' regular distribution over the display. Usually, those are arranged in a square and the distances between all objects are the same. In the semi-realistic scenes we used, this was not the case (compare Figs. 3.1 and 3.3). One could argue that this might have affected the mapping process as saccades might have been longer or shorter as compared to 'regular-arranged' object displays. But if a regular arrangement of objects in a symmetrical square was crucial for the observed eye gaze behaviour, all types of competitors should be affected. However, for the visual-shape and semantic competitors, we observed similar biases as in the experiments with simple object displays.

We conjecture that the mode of processing towards mapping of visual-shape and semantic features of objects in the present experiments with more complex visual scenes was induced by the increased amount of visual information present in the visual scene. That is, increased visual processing led participants to a mode where matches at visual (and semantic) levels are preferred over matches at the phonological level. The character–object formations (Fig. 3.1) and the black shape–object formations (Fig. 3.5) are visually more complex than the same objects being presented in isolation. That is, with more visual information present in the displays, visual processing was enhanced, shifting word–object mapping preferences.

Importantly, Experiment 3 showed that the mere presence of additional visual entities is sufficient to induce this mode of processing and was more important in modulating word–object mapping than the semantic information inherent to the character–object couplings. In fact, those might have even hindered the extent of semantic mapping as they were not contributing to a semantically coherent scene. Võ and Wolfe (2013) recently showed that viewing semantically altered scenes elicits electrophysiological responses similar to when semantically implausible sentences are comprehended (e.g., N400 deflections). We suggest that semantically fully coherent visual scenes (e.g., a kitchen scene) may induce an enhanced bias towards word–object mapping at a semantic level of representation. Future work could usefully explore this hypothesis.

3.3.2 Inhibition of Phonological Word–Object Mapping

In Experiment 1 and Experiment 3 we found some evidence for inhibition in looks to the phonological competitors, i.e. fewer looks to the competitor than to the distractor during late time windows. This pattern might reveal general insights into eye gaze behaviour during language-mediated visual search in more complex visual environments. This is interesting because to our knowledge effects of inhibition during language-mediated search have previously not been demonstrated (but see McQueen and Huettig 2014, for evidence from three cross-modal priming experiments for interference of spoken word recognition through phonological priming from visual objects).

The current results strongly suggest that language-mediated eye movements are (at least partially) under substantial control processes and that a complete account of language-mediated eye gaze will have to include inhibitory mechanisms. We suggest that processing in the current experiments was contingent upon attentional control over how processing is distributed across different levels of representation (cf. Stolz and Besner 1998). Indeed substantial amounts of cognitive control during language-mediated visual search have recently been predicted by a working memory model of language-vision interactions (Huettig et al. 2011a). The authors proposed that working memory plays a central role during language-mediated eye movements, because it grounds linguistic, cognitive, and perceptual processing in space and time by providing short-term connections between objects (cf. Knoeferle and Crocker 2007; Spivey et al. 2004). If language-attention interactions are mediated by working memory, such interactions are likely to be subject to a substantial amount of cognitive control. Han and Kim (2009) showed recently in a (non-language) visual search task that although working memory appears to bias visual selection towards matching stimuli, participants exerted some control over which items are ignored in the search display especially when search was slow. As language-mediated visual search tends to be slower than a standard visual search task, it is likely to be under increased cognitive control. Future research could usefully examine the nature of the inhibition effects observed in the present study and explore underlying mechanisms and conditions in which they occur.

3.3.3 Conclusion

Given our results, one may ask to what extent word–object mapping at the phonological level of representation occurs during real world language–vision interactions. A strong conclusion from our data would be that in complex visual surroundings word–object mapping at a phonological level of representation is the exception rather than the rule and limited to situations with very simple visual environments. However, such a conclusion may be premature. Our results indicate that the dynamics of the representational level at which online word–object mapping occurs is determined by, among other things, the complexity of the visual environment. There are many other factors (e.g., cascaded processing in the spoken word and picture recognition systems; the temporal unfolding of the spoken language, the particular task goals, etc.) also co-determining this mapping behaviour. The present findings do not rule out that there are situations in which mapping at a phonological representational level is particularly potent even in complex visual environments. Another mediating factor for instance appears to be literacy skills. Huettig et al. (2011c) found robust evidence for word–object mapping at the phonological level in high literates. In low literates (who had no reading or other cognitive impairments), however, they observed that word–object mapping (with four object displays) takes place primarily at the semantic level.

In sum, word–object mapping is contingent upon the nature of the visual environment. More complex visual environments induce visual modes of processing during language-mediated visual search. The data suggest further that word–object mapping is under substantial cognitive control.

Acknowledgments We thank Anna Gastel for drawing the semi-realistic scenes, Neil Bardhan for providing the artificial shapes and Johanne Tromp for assistance in running the experiments.

References

Allopenna, P. D., Magnuson, J. S., & Tanenhaus, M. K. (1998). Tracking the time course of spoken word recognition using eye movements: Evidence for continuous mapping models. *Journal of Memory and Language, 38*(4), 419–439.

Andersson, R., Ferreira, F., & Henderson, J. M. (2011). I see what you're saying: The integration of complex speech and scenes during language comprehension. *Acta Psychologica, 137*(2), 208–216.

Boyce, S. J., & Pollatsek, A. (1992). Identification of objects in scenes: The role of scene background in object naming. *Journal of Experimental Psychology. Learning, Memory, and Cognition, 18*(3), 531–543.

Cooper, R. M. (1974). Control of eye fixation by meaning of spoken language: New methodology for real-time investigation of speech perception, memory, and language processing. *Cognitive Psychology, 6*(1), 84–107.

Cree, G. S., & McRae, K. (2003). Analyzing the factors underlying the structure and computation of the meaning of chipmunk, cherry, chisel, cheese, and cello (and many other such concrete nouns). *Journal of Experimental Psychology: General, 132*(2), 163–201.

Dahan, D., & Tanenhaus, M. K. (2005). Looking at the rope when looking for the snake: Conceptually mediated eye movements during spoken-word recognition. *Psychonomic Bulletin and Review, 12*(3), 453–459.

De Graef, P. (1998). Prefixational object perception in scenes: Objects popping out of schemas. In G. Underwood (Ed.), *Eye guidance in reading and scene perception* (pp. 313–336). Oxford, UK: Elsevier.

Duñabeitia, J. A., Avilés, A., Afonso, O., Scheepers, C., & Carreiras, M. (2009). Qualitative differences in the representation of abstract versus concrete words: Evidence from the visual-world paradigm. *Cognition, 110*(2), 284–292.

Fiser, J., & Aslin, R. N. (2002). Statistical learning of higher-order temporal structure from visual shape sequences. *Journal of Experimental Psychology: Learning, Memory, and Cognition, 28*(3), 458–467.

Frost, R. (1998). Toward a strong phonological theory of visual word recognition: True issues and false trails. *Psychological Bulletin, 123*(1), 71–99.

Han, S. W., & Kim, M. S. (2009). Do the contents of working memory capture attention? Yes, but cognitive control matters. *Journal of Experimental Psychology: Human Perception and Performance, 35*(5), 1292–1302.

Huettig, F., & Altmann, G. T. M. (2004). The online processing of ambiguous and unambiguous words in context: Evidence from head-mounted eye-tracking. In M. Carreiras, & C. Clifton (Eds.), *The on-line study of sentence comprehension: Eyetracking, ERP and beyond* (pp. 187–207). New York: Psychology Press.

Huettig, F., & Altmann, G. T. M. (2005). Word meaning and the control of eye fixation: Semantic competitor effects and the visual world paradigm. *Cognition, 96*(1), 23–32.

Huettig, F., & Altmann, G. T. M. (2007). Visual-shape competition during language-mediated attention is based on lexical input and not modulated by contextual appropriateness. *Visual Cognition, 15*(8), 985–1018.

Huettig, F., & McQueen, J. M. (2007). The tug of war between phonological, semantic and shape information in language-mediated visual search. *Journal of Memory and Language, 57*(4), 460–482.

Huettig, F., & McQueen, J. M. (2011). The nature of the visual environment induces implicit biases during language-mediated visual search. *Memory and Cognition, 39*(6), 1068–1084.

Huettig, F., Olivers, C. N. L., & Hartsuiker, R. J. (2011a). Looking, language, and memory: Bridging research from the visual world and visual search paradigms. *Acta Psychologica, 137*(2), 138–150.

Huettig, F., Quinlan, P. T., McDonald, S. A., & Altmann, G. T. M. (2006). Models of high-dimensional semantic space predict language-mediated eye movements in the visual world. *Acta Psychologica, 121*(1), 65–80.

Huettig, F., Rommers, J., & Meyer, A. S. (2011b). Using the visual world paradigm to study language processing: A review and critical evaluation. *Acta Psychologica, 137*(2), 151–171.

Huettig, F., Singh, N., & Mishra, R. (2011c). Language-mediated visual orienting behavior in low and high literates. *Frontiers in Psychology, 2*, 285.

Knoeferle, P., & Crocker, M. W. (2007). The influence of recent scene events on spoken comprehension: Evidence from eye movements. *Journal of Memory and Language, 57*(4), 519–543.

Landauer, T. K., & Dumais, S. T. (1997). A solution to plato's problem: The latent semantic analysis theory of acquisition, induction, and representation of knowledge. *Psychological Review, 104*(2), 211–240.

McClelland, J. L., & Elman, J. L. (1986). The trace model of speech perception. *Cognitive Psychology, 18*(1), 1–86.

McQueen, J. M., & Huettig, F. (2014). Interference of spoken word recognition through phonological priming from visual objects and printed words. *Attention, Perception, and Psychophysics, 76*, 190–200.

Saslow, M. G. (1967). Latency for saccadic eye movement. *Journal of the Optical Society of America, 57*(8), 1030.

Spivey, M. J., Richardson, D. C., & Fitneva, S. A. (2004). Thinking outside the brain: Spatial indices to visual and linguistic information. In J. Henderson & F. Ferreira (Eds.), *The interface of language, vision, and action: Eye movements and the visual world* (pp. 161–190). San Diego: CA: Academic Press.

Stolz, J. A., & Besner, D. (1998). Levels of representation in visual word recognition: A dissociation between morphological and semantic processing. *Journal of Experimental Psychology: Human Perception and Performance, 24*(6), 1642.

Strik, J. A., & Underwood, G. (2007). Low-level visual saliency does not predict change detection in natural scenes. *Journal of Vision, 7*(10), 1–10.

Tanenhaus, M. K., Spivey-Knowlton, M. J., Eberhard, K. M., & Sedivy, J. C. (1995). Integration of visual and linguistic information in spoken language comprehension. *Science, 268*(5217), 1632–1634.

Van Orden, G. C., Johnston, J. C., & Hale, B. L. (1988). Word identification in reading proceeds from spelling to sound to meaning. *Journal of Experimental Psychology: Learning, Memory, and Cognition, 14*(3), 371.

Võ, M. L.-H., & Wolfe, J. M. (2013). Differential electrophysiological signatures of semantic and syntactic scene processing. *Psychological Science, 24*(9), 1816–1823.

Yee, E., Overton, E., & Thompson-Schill, S. L. (2009). Looking for meaning: Eye movements are sensitive to overlapping semantic features, not association. *Psychonomic Bulletin and Review, 16*(5), 869–874.

Yee, E., & Sedivy, J. C. (2006). Eye movements to pictures reveal transient semantic activation during spoken word recognition. *Journal of Experimental Psychology. Learning, Memory, and Cognition, 32*(1), 1–14.

Chapter 4
Visually Situated Language Comprehension in Children and in Adults

Pia Knoeferle

4.1 Introduction

Prompted by the desire to test claims about procedural modularity of the language and vision systems (Fodor 1983), psycholinguistic research has examined the interplay of language comprehension with visual perception. This interplay is rapid, incremental, and closely temporally coordinated. It further appears to be bidirectional such that language guides visual attention and attended non-linguistic visual information in turn affects comprehension (henceforth 'visually situated' language comprehension). Information from a visual context can crucially inform syntactic disambiguation within a few hundred milliseconds, a finding that suggests core comprehension processes are not procedurally modular (Spivey et al. 2002; Tanenhaus et al. 1995). These and other findings have shaped accounts of visually situated language processing in which language guides (visual) attention and attended non-linguistic information can rapidly influence comprehension processes (e.g., Altmann and Kamide 2007; Knoeferle and Crocker 2006, 2007).

However, most eye-tracking evidence on this temporally coordinated interplay comes from studies with healthy university students (approximately 18–31 years of age), thus focusing on a short interval of adult life and on a small population segment. To ensure the generality of language comprehension accounts, we could test them more broadly. This includes tests across the lifespan (e.g., in infancy, childhood, young adulthood, and older age, e.g., Carminati and Knoeferle 2013; Trueswell et al. 1999; Zhang and Knoeferle 2012), on diverse social population segments (e.g., working class people, academics, illiterates, or dialect speakers, e.g.

P. Knoeferle (✉)
Research Group "Language and Cognition", CITEC, Cognitive Interaction Technology Excellence Center, Bielefeld University, Room 2.036, 33615 Bielefeld, Germany
e-mail: knoeferle@cit-ec.uni-bielefeld.de

© Springer India 2015
R.K. Mishra et al. (eds.), *Attention and Vision in Language Processing*, DOI 10.1007/978-81-322-2443-3_4

Huettig et al. 2011, 2012), and for different levels of cognitive function (e.g., good vs. poor comprehenders or people with high vs. low working memory, e.g. Nation et al. 2003; Knoeferle et al. 2011b). This would bring us closer towards including a model of the comprehender (and ultimately also, of the speaker) into visually situated language comprehension accounts and permit us to refine their predictions.

With regard to insights across the lifespan, a number of studies examining young infants and children could inform us about this interplay. However, relatively few studies have undertaken a "direct" (i.e., within-item) comparison of visually situated child and adult language comprehension. Strictly speaking, this is necessary to exclude the possibility that between-group differences in the time course or manner of processing result from stimulus variation. The results from one influential within-item comparison in 5-year olds and adults suggested marked differences between these two groups (Trueswell et al. 1999; see also Snedeker and Trueswell 2004). Overall, the children relied more on their linguistic knowledge for syntactic structuring than the adults. By contrast, children failed to exhibit an adult-like reliance on the visual referential context for syntactic structuring and disambiguation.

These results suggest that the non-linguistic referential context is of limited importance for at least some processes in child language comprehension (e.g., real-time syntactic disambiguation of local structural ambiguity). The rapid, temporally coordinated interplay of language comprehension and visual attention in adults also seems to emerge gradually in infants. While 24-month-olds did not rapidly relate visual referential contrast to an unfolding utterance, 36-month-olds resembled adults in that they shifted their visual attention more quickly to a target picture upon hearing "blue…" ("blue car") when the context contained only one blue object (a blue car) than when it contained two blue objects (Fernald et al. 2010).

The insights into the limited role of the visual context for real-time language comprehension seem to contrast with its role in language learning. Reference from nouns to objects across different learning instances, for instance, plays an influential role for language learning (e.g., Smith and Yu 2008; Yu and Smith 2010). Other cues such as object sequences also seem to be important for guiding infants' visual attention to, and their learning about, objects (e.g., Wu et al. 2011). Infants are further sensitive to actions and to goal-related information before they complete the first year of their life (e.g., Woodward and Sommerville 2000). In addition, non-linguistic behaviours such as joint attention episodes seem positively related to young infants' vocabulary size (e.g., Tomasello and Farrar 1986; Tomasello and Todd 1983). Thus, subtle cues in the non-linguistic visual context appear to play an important role for learning about language and objects.

It is possible that these differences in comprehension compared with learning result from different grain sizes in the time course of these two processes. For language comprehension, children must orient towards a visual stimulus within a few hundred milliseconds. Comprehension studies often do not repeat individual stimuli, and the child has a window of no more than a few hundred milliseconds to relate the visual context to language. Language learning success, by contrast, is often measured offline. And in those studies that measured eye gaze, stimuli were repeated and rapid orienting to a mentioned object could thus have emerged over time.

Another possibility is that non-linguistic visual context plays a role only for some cognitive processes (e.g., for establishing reference but not for syntactic disambiguation). The picture may further be complicated by variation as to when in the child's development visual cues affect specific comprehension processes (see Trueswell et al. 1999, pp. 122ff. for discussion of children's reliance on linguistic knowledge and their insensitivity to the visual referential context).

4.2 Summary

In sum, the role of the non-linguistic context for incremental language comprehension across the lifespan remains unclear. And yet, this is an important point for refining predictions of visually situated language comprehension accounts with a model of the comprehender. This chapter accordingly argues in favour of examining and modelling the realtime interplay of language comprehension and visual attention more broadly. I will illustrate this argument by comparing visually situated language comprehension in children and in adults. Visual context could serve merely as a backdrop to children's language-mediated visual attention. Alternatively, it could play a more active role, not just in language learning but also in comprehension. A first section motivates the active role of the visual context for comprehension by appealing to insights from learning about language, objects, and events (sect. 4.3). A sub-sequent section reviews insights into the interplay of language comprehension with visual attention, as well as into visual context effects on language comprehension (sect. 4.4). Based on this review, I will argue that (attention to objects and events in) the non-linguistic visual context plays a fundamental role not only for learning about language and objects but also for child language comprehension.

4.3 Learning About Objects and About Language in Visual Context

For a temporally coordinated interplay between language comprehension, visual attention, and visual context effects, children must be able to rapidly map nouns onto objects, and actions onto verbs. One pre-requisite for this is that children can identify words and objects from the stream of auditory and visual events. Indeed, infants can segment words from the speech stream through, for instance, statistical regularities. 8-month-olds listened to a stream of artificial speech containing "words" (e.g., "tilado") which could be detected based on transitional probabilities[1] of syllable pairs (Saffran et al. 1996). Within words, the transitional probability of

---

[1]The transitional probability (X|Y) of a syllable pair XY is given by the frequency of the pair XY divided by the frequency of X.

syllable pairs was set to 1.0 (e.g., for "tilado", "la" always followed "ti"), and across word boundaries, it was set to 0.3. Infants' listening times to words compared with non-words were inferred from how long they fixated a blinking light on a side-wall of the test booth. Crucially, they fixated the blinking light longer when listening to word than non-word stimuli, suggesting word recognition.

Infants' sound processing is further finely attuned to the rhythmic structure of their language, and it has been suggested that this sensitivity plays a role for word segmentation. Höhle et al. (2009) played CVCV sequences (e.g., "gaba") with either trochaic or iambic stress to German 6-month-olds. Both stress patterns had a lengthened second syllable and a higher-pitched first syllable. They differed, however, in the degree to which they exhibited these two patterns. For iambic (compared with trochaic) metre, the increased duration of the second over the first syllable was more pronounced; and for trochaic (compared with iambic) metre, the pitch of the first syllable was higher. The German 6-month-olds preferred to fixate a blinking light on the side-wall of the test booth longer for the trochaic than iambic stimuli, a preferential looking behaviour that generalised neither to German 4-month-old infants (but see Friederici et al. 2007) nor to French 6 month-olds. It seems then that the specific rhythmic pattern of German modulated the German infants' use of stress cues, a factor that can influence word segmentation (see also Jusczyk et al. 1993, 1999).

Infants can also learn verbs from a very early age, a process that benefits from the sentential syntactic structure (e.g., Fisher et al. 1994; Gleitman 1990; Naigles 1990). Children inspected scenes (e.g., a rabbit feeding an elephant with a spoon) and responded to questions about the meaning of novel verbs (e.g., "zorking") in one of three syntactic contexts (transitive, intransitive, and uninformative verb contexts, Fisher et al. 1994). The 2-year-olds interpreted the novel verb more often as reflecting feeding when the syntax supported feeding (i.e., "The bunny is …ing the elephant.") than when it supported an intransitive event ("The elephant is …ing."). Thus, children can assign meaning to a novel verb based on its syntactic context.

There has been discussion as to when abstract syntactic knowledge emerges. While some scientists advocate a late emergence and an early reliance on lexical learning (e.g., Tomasello 2000; Tomasello and Brooks 1998), others argue that abstract syntactic knowledge (e.g., of verb transitivity) is key for early verb learning (e.g., Gleitman 1990; Fisher 1996, 2002; Pinker 1994). Either way, children begin to learn verbs such as "dance" and "open" by around 10 months of age (e.g., Fenson et al. 1994), and verb-related syntactic knowledge from approximately 2 years of age, if not before (Fisher 2002; Golinkoff and Hirsh-Pasek 2008).

Learning of statistical regularities appears to be domain-general and extends to object sequences (Kirkham et al. 2002). After infants (2-month-olds, 5-month-olds, and 8-month-olds) had inspected object sequences with different transitional probabilities (within-pair: 1.0; between-pair: 0.3), they looked longer at novel than highly familiar object sequences (i.e., with 1.0 transitional probability). Infants' age had no reliable effect on their novelty preference. However, another study observed longer inspection of novel than known circle sequences in 11-month but not in 8-month-olds (Kirkham et al. 2007, Experiment 1).

Results on the learning of object regularities generalised even to within-object feature-changes (Wu et al. 2011). In a first experiment, Wu et al. familiarised 9-months-olds with how objects split into parts by showing them two instances of an object's splitting behaviour. During testing, the infants saw either a consistent or an inconsistent split of a familiar object. They gazed significantly longer at objects splitting in an inconsistent than in a familiar way. Beyond information from the objects themselves, the infants used a speaker's eye-gaze for learning object features. Learning improved and children preferred the object with the inconsistent (vs. consistent) split, when the speaker had inspected it (but not when no speaker was visible, Wu et al. 2011). This generalised both when only one object was present and when two objects (a target and a distractor) competed for attention.

Just as infants can learn object-based regularities, they can also learn about actions and events (Sharon and Wynn 1998; Wynn 1996). In a habituation paradigm, 6-months-olds inspected a puppet jumping either two or three times. At test, they were able to discriminate these two events from a sequence of two- and three-jump events. By 14–17-months of age, they were also able to discriminate motion from path events (Pulverman et al. 2008) and 18-month-olds anticipated the goal of incomplete actions (Meltzoff 1995). Six-to-nine-month-olds habituated to actions in which a human agent (vs. an inanimate rod) reached for one of two presented toys. During testing, an experimenter switched the location of the two toy objects and the actor either executed the action with a different arm trajectory or grasped the other toy. Infants inspected a changed toy longer than a changed arm trajectory and this gaze pattern emerged for animate agents only (Woodward 1998).

Interestingly, infants can also use familiar actions to interpret novel and potentially ambiguous actions. Twelve-month-olds inspected a hand touching the lid of a clear box containing a toy animal. That action could be interpreted as directed at either the box or the toy animal (Woodward and Sommerville 2000). In one condition, the actor touched the lid but did not open the box. In another condition, the actor touched the box, opened it, and grabbed the toy. During testing, the actor touched either the old box (containing a new toy), or a new box. Infants inspected the new box for the same time as the old box if the actor had merely touched the old box during habituation. However, if he had instead taken the toy, they inspected the old box longer than the new box. Grabbing a toy appeared to influence infants' visual attention when observing a novel ambiguous action. This result failed to replicate when the toy was outside of the box (i.e., when touching the lid of the box was no longer related to taking the toy). Simply seeing the actor touch the lid of the box with the toy nearby did not affect the interpretation of the ambiguous action.

Overall, children are thus exquisitely sensitive to regularities and structure in the linguistic and non-linguistic input. If they were unable to identify both words and objects, they could not relate these two information sources in real-time. With this ingredient, however, infants could learn to rapidly relate words to objects, and to exploit this link during real-time language comprehension.

Just as children can recruit regularities in the linguistic and non-linguistic visual context from individual learning instances, they can also learn word-object correspondences from cross-situational occurrences. In one recent study, 12-month and

14-month old infants inspected two objects per trial and heard two names. Within a trial, the mapping from names to objects was ambiguous (Smith and Yu 2008) but across trials reference was unambiguous. An infant would see two novel objects during training and hear "bosa" and "gasser". On a later trial, the infant would see the referent of "bosa" together with a new object and hear "bosa" and "colat". Based on cross-trial co-occurrences of an object and a name (one object always occurred together with the word "bosa"), the infant could deduce the reference for "bosa". During testing, the authors monitored infants' attention to two pictures in response to object names. The infants inspected the named object longer than the other object. Despite referential ambiguity for individual trials, the infants related the name of an object to its appropriate referent based on cross-trial statistics.

It appears then that infants are not only finely tuned to regularities in their linguistic and non-linguistic environment but that they can also relate at least a small number of novel nouns to novel objects through cross-situational statistics. These findings alone, however, would not necessarily support the view that visual context can play an important role for child language *comprehension*. During language comprehension, words are processed in a rapid sequence. Relating them in real-time to objects in the visual context requires an attentional system that responds rapidly to spoken words. Adults inspect relevant visual context information within a few hundred milliseconds during language comprehension, and this relationship holds even when scenes are cluttered and objects are mentioned in rapid succession (Andersson et al. 2011). In addition, attended information in the visual context rapidly affects their comprehension and visual attention (e.g., Chambers et al. 2004; Knoeferle et al. 2005, 2008; Tanenhaus et al. 1995). To predict that visual context plays an important role for child language comprehension, we would want to see some evidence that a similarly close temporal coordination between seeing an object, hearing its name, and inspecting it, also contributes to successful language learning.

Recent evidence for this view comes from a study on cross-situational word-referent mapping. Yu and Smith (2010) recorded the eye movements of 14-month-olds in a statistical learning task and analysed the relationship between individual differences in eye-gaze pattern and learning success. During learning, thirty slides showed pictures of two novel objects that were named (e.g., "gasser", "bosa"). Word-object reference was ambiguous for a given slide, and correct word-object pairs occurred ten times during learning. Results from a preferential-looking task showed that despite within-trial ambiguity, most infants learned more than half of the words through cross-trial statistics.

However, some infants learned hardly any word-referent mappings (weak learners) while others seemed to master five out of the six words (strong learners). Strong learners switched less often between the two objects than weak learners and made longer fixations to the attended object during training. These differences were most pronounced in the middle of the learning phase. Weak compared with strong learners had higher entropy of eye movements per trial (i.e., more attention switches between the objects within a trial and more evenly-distributed fixation times across the two objects). They crucially also had a higher entropy time-locked to word presentation. Thus, success in cross-situational learning of word-object mappings seems to be related to how the infants inspect an object during learning.

In summary, children are sensitive to subtle statistical regularities in their visual environment. They can exploit information from both referenced objects and speakers for language learning. Importantly, strong learners seemed to exhibit a temporal coordination between hearing an object name and inspecting the named object (Yu and Smith 2010). Temporal synchrony was also important for word learning in 7- and 8-month-olds (Gogate 2010, Experiment 1). An actor pronounced syllables such as "gah" and "tah" either together with moving an object (downward, laterally, or forward) or asynchronously with object motion (e.g., in the pauses between moving the objects). 8- but not 7-month-olds learned sound-object mappings in the synchronous but not in the asynchronous presentation condition (see also Gogate et al. 2006).

Much of the reviewed evidence comes from learning about nouns and objects. As discussed above, research on how infants acquire the meaning of novel verbs highlights how sentential syntactic structure contributes to verb learning (e.g., Fisher et al. 1994; Gleitman 1990; Naigles 1990). Learners also appear to be most successful in learning nouns when both the referential visual context and language contain corresponding systematic pattern (e.g., Moeser and Olson 1974 and references therein). Indeed, two key pre-requisites for enabling non-linguistic visual context effects during child language comprehension are likely children's sensitivity to fine-grained regularities in the linguistic and non-linguistic input, as well as the role that (the timing of) attention (to object naming) plays for successful noun learning.

4.4 Visually Situated Language Comprehension in Young Infants and Adults

Based on these insights from language learning, sect. 4.4 argues that the non-linguistic visual context and its interaction with linguistic cues can play an important role for child language comprehension.

4.4.1 How Language Comprehension Guides Visual Attention in Children and Adults

To examine the real-time interplay between language comprehension and visual attention in infants, several studies have monitored infants' eye movements in picture contexts during spoken language comprehension. Six-to-nine-month-olds rapidly shifted attention to a named object (e.g., "Look at the banana!") in a display showing a picture of a banana and of a head (Bergelson and Swingley 2012). And when watching videos of their parents, 6-month-olds looked more often at the correct parent upon hearing "mommy" or "daddy", a behaviour that did not emerge with videos of unfamiliar adults (Tincoff and Jusczyk 1999). Six-month-olds were even able to visually orient towards adult body parts upon hearing them named (hands compared with feet, Tincoff and Jusczyk 2012). Interestingly, 15-month-olds rapidly oriented their eye-gaze to a familiar referent (e.g., a dog) but they did so only after they had heard the entire name (e.g., "doggie", Fernald et al. 1998). By contrast, 24-month-olds—similar to adults—began to shift their eye-gaze to a referent *before* they had heard its entire name. By the age of two, children thus resembled adults in that even incomplete words guided their visual attention to objects. When adults listened to a word such as "beetle", they inspected the picture of a beetle more often than unrelated targets from around 200 ms after word onset (e.g., Allopenna et al. 1998; see also Dahan 2010; Tanenhaus et al. 1995).

The rapid interplay of spoken comprehension and information from visual context is also evident in event-related brain potentials (ERPs): Friedrich and Friederici (2004) compared semantic processing in 19-month-olds and adults. A picture of an object accompanied by an incongruous word (vs. the object name) elicited more negative mean amplitude ERPs at right hemisphere and midline sites (from approximately 300 ms), as well as locally over temporal sites (from 100 to 250 ms) in the adults. The continued greater negativity for incongruous relative to congruous stimuli resembled the N400 effect observed for semantically incongruous relative to congruous words in sentence contexts (Kutas and Hillyard 1980, 1984). For the 19-month-olds, incongruous words triggered a broadly distributed negativity compared with congruous words which overall resembled the N400-like effect observed in the adults. The emergence of the same component in both of these groups highlights similarity in their semantic interpretation mechanisms. However, the infant N400 effect occurred 400 ms later, lasted somewhat longer, and had a different topography than the adult N400. Children are thus subtly slower in noun-object mapping, and the topography of the N400 suggests some differences in their interpretation mechanisms relative to the adults.

Children's visual attention seems to be guided rapidly also by their grammatical knowledge. Spanish-learning children (aged 34–42 months) listened to sentences such as (*Encuentra la pelota*, 'Find the ball'), while inspecting related objects in the visual context. Upon hearing 'the ball', they inspected the target (a ball) earlier when the object names differed in grammatical gender ("la pelota", 'ball [feminine]'; "el zapato", 'shoe [masculine]'), than when they had the same gender ("la pelota", 'ball [feminine]'; "la galleta", 'cookie [feminine]', Lew-Williams and Fernald 2010; see also Van Heugthen and Shi 2009 for similar evidence in 2-year-olds). Children's rapid use of gender marking in finding an object resembles that of adults. When adult participants had to click on one out of four objects, and two of these had similar-sounding name onsets ('bouteille' and 'bouton'), they inspected the objects with similar names more often than the phonologically-unrelated objects for a brief time interval after word onset. This effect disappeared when a gender-marked article differentiated between the referents with similar name onsets ('le bouton' vs. 'la bouteille', Dahan et al. 2000).

Just as children can rapidly relate nouns to objects, they can also predict an object in the visual context based on verb information. When 10–11-year-olds inspected clipart scenes in which a verb (e.g., "eat") restricted the domain of reference to just one object (a cake), they began to anticipate that object before its mention, and more often than when the verb was non-restrictive (e.g., "choose",

Nation et al. 2003). This was true independent of whether the children were skilled or less skilled comprehenders. However, compared with highly skilled comprehenders, the less skilled ones made more fixations and spent less time inspecting the target. Adults' time course of anticipating an edible object for "eat" relative to "move" resembles that of 10–11-year-olds (Altmann and Kamide 1999). Crucially, this predictive capacity is present from an early age. When 2-year-olds listened to sentences such as "The boy eats a big cake", they began to inspect a depicted cake soon after they had heard a semantically restrictive verb (and before "cake" was mentioned, Mani and Huettig 2012).

Even linguistic cues to abstract temporal aspects of a context rapidly influenced 3–5-year-olds' visual attention (Zhou et al. 2014). The children and adults listened to sentences in Mandarin Chinese about an old lady planting a flower. The verb 'plant' appeared either together with the particle "le", indicating the perfective aspect of the event (e.g., "zhong-le", 'has planted'), or with the particle "zhe", indicating that the event was ongoing (e.g., "zhong-zhe", 'is planting'). During comprehension, the participants inspected a computer screen showing two pictures. One of them depicted the completed version of the event (the flower was in the soil and the old lady was walking away) while the other depicted the old lady as she was planting the flower. Both, the children (3-, 4-, and 5-year-olds) and the adults began to inspect the completed event picture more often approximately 200–400 ms after the onset of "le" than "zhe", and they began to inspect the ongoing event more often 200–400 ms after the onset of "zhe" compared with "le". This gaze pattern did not vary with age, suggesting that aspectual markers can guide both young children and adults' visual attention to the temporal structure of depicted events.

Children moreover resemble adults in how lexical cues guide their attention during syntactic disambiguation but they can experience delay in exploiting prosodic cues. In Snedeker and Yuan (2008), 4–6-year-olds inspected four objects (e.g., a candle, a feather, a frog with a feather, and a leopard with a candle), and were instructed that they "can feel the frog with the feather". Sentences in Experiment (1) had either instrument prosody (with an intonational phrase break after the object noun) or modifier prosody (with an intonational phrase break after the verb). Looks to, and actions with, the instrument were taken to reflect interpretation of the ambiguous prepositional phrase "with the feather" as an instrument. The children inspected the target instrument (the feather) more often from around 700 ms after the onset of the prepositional phrase ("with the feather"), and used the feather more often for action execution when they heard the utterance in instrument rather than modifier prosody.

In a second related study, the authors manipulated verb bias in addition to prosody.[2] The verb either biased towards a modifier interpretation (e.g., "choose the cow with the stick"), was neutral ("feel") or biased towards the instrument

---

[2]The prosodic manipulation was similar to Experiment 1; prosodic analyses ascertained accent differences between the instrument (mostly H* on the verb and noun and a pitch accent on "with") and the modifier intonation (mostly an L + H* accent on the verb, a clear H* on the noun, and no pitch accent on "with").

interpretation ("tickle the pig with the feather"). Children, much like the adults, used the verb bias within 200 ms after the onset of "feather" for structural disambiguation, but were delayed in their visual response to prosodic cues by approximately 500 ms relative to the adults (see also Weber et al. 2006 for relevant prosodic effects in adults).

Prosodic cues such as contrastive pitch accent is used rapidly by adults and young children alike, although children benefit from additional time in their prosodic processing. Ito et al. (2012) presented Japanese 6-year-olds with 2-utterance sequences in which the first singled out one among many depicted objects (e.g., a pink cat). The second utterance mentioned another object which was either of the same category (e.g., a green cat) or of another category (e.g., an orange monkey), and the noun phrase referring to that object either carried a pitch accent on the pre-nominal colour adjective or not. When adults and children processed these kinds of stimuli, the contrastive pitch accent prompted faster looks to the green cat when "green" was accentuated. Adults (but not children) showed garden-pathing when the utterance sequences were not contrastive (i.e., the second utterance mentioned the orange monkey). In this case the adults temporarily fixated the target signalled by the contrastive pitch (the orange cat) while children showed no such effect. When they were given more time between the two utterances, however, the older among the 6-year-olds began to show garden-pathing similar to that evident in the adults. Thus, the children seem to process these prosodic cues rapidly when they are felicitous, and when they are infelicitous, they can use them incrementally if they are awarded extra time.

When prosody served a different purpose (signalling the illocutionary status of an utterance as a statement or a question), children relied on it as rapidly as adults. Zhou et al. (2012) presented Mandarin Chinese utterances to 4–5-year-olds and to adults. The utterances were identical but intonation disambiguated them as either a statement (level intonation on the "wh"-phrase, e.g., literally 'Xiaoming not pick what fruit', sense: 'Xiaoming did not pick any fruit') or a question (rising intonation on the same phrase 'what fruit', sense: 'What fruit did Xiaoming not pick?'). The visual context showed a boy with bananas, two distractor animals, and two further pieces of fruit (e.g., a pear and an orange). When the utterance was disambiguated as a question (vs. statement), participants more often inspected the fruit that the boy had not picked (the pear and the orange) and responded to the question. For statement compared with question intonation, they inspected the boy with the bananas more often and decided whether the sentence matched the depiction. Importantly, the children did not differ from the adults in how rapidly prosody affected their visual attention, suggesting similarities in children and adults' real-time use of prosodic cues for the disambiguation of illocutionary force during comprehension.

By contrast, pronounced differences in the time course of child and adult language processing seem to emerge for pragmatic inferences. Huang and Snedeker (2009b) showed their adult participants pictures of two boys and one girl, and an experimenter distributed nine socks evenly among them (Experiment 3). Upon hearing "Point to the girl that has some of the socks", the adults rapidly inspected the girl that had three socks. By contrast, when "some of the" was referentially ambiguous (the boy and one girl were each given two socks and another girl received three balls), adults inspected the girl with two socks substantially later for "some" (around 1000 ms after quantifier onset) compared with "all" and compared with "two" or "three" as scalars (target inspection was above chance 200 ms after quantifier onset, Experiments 1 and 2). The authors attributed this delay to the computation of scalar implicature since gaze pattern suggested that "some" was interpreted without delay when its meaning was sufficient to disambiguate refer-ence. Compared with the adults, 5–9-year-olds interpreted the quantifier "some" much later, after phonological disambiguation of the target noun ("socks"), sug-gesting that they, unlike the adults failed to compute pragmatic implicature in real-time (Huang and Snedeker 2009a).

Thus, children can relate words to objects from as early as 6 months of age. They employ their grammatical knowledge as well as semantic information related to adjectives and nouns similar to the adults from approximately 24 to 36 months of age. For verbs, adult-like visual inspection of objects associated with the verb emerges also around 24 months of age. Lexical (verb bias) information affects 4–6-year-olds' structural disambiguation as rapidly as adults' structural dis-ambiguation. Children's use of prosodic cues during comprehension, however, appears to be somewhat more variable. When intonational phrase breaks and dif-ferences in accentuation served as cues to structural disambiguation, visual atten-tion shifts to the target objects were subtly delayed in 4–6-year-olds relative to adults. Similarities between children and adults emerged, however, in Japanese 6-year-olds' use of contrastive pitch accent when that accent was contextually felicitous, and also in Mandarin Chinese 4–5-year-olds when prosody cued the illocutionary force of an utterance. Clear age differences emerged for complex pragmatic processes. Even much older children (5–9 years of age) failed to com-pute scalar implicature in realtime, a finding hinting at differences in child and adult language comprehension at the pragmatic level.

4.4.2 Non-linguistic Visual Context Effects on Comprehension and Visual Attention

In the preceding section, we reviewed how language guides visual attention. This section focuses on how visual context influences language comprehension once it has been identified as relevant by language. One key question for accounts of visu-ally situated language comprehension is to which extent the non-linguistic visual context modulates children's language comprehension in *real-time*. For adults, different visual cues are integrated within a few hundred milliseconds. Among these is information about an object's size, colour (Sedivy et al. 1999; Huettig and Altmann 2011) and shape (Dahan and Tanenhaus 2005) but also depicted clipart events (Knoeferle et al. 2005), real-world action events (Knoeferle et al. 2011a) and action affordances (Chambers et al. 2004). For noun-object relationships, the language learning literature supports the prediction of rapid visual context effects also in child language comprehension. For verbs and actions, the case is less clear. If the children do resemble adults in language comprehension, however, rapid visual context effects should emerge both when a noun and when a verb identifies relevant aspects of the visual context. For adults, it has even been argued that they ground their language comprehension in the immediate or recent events in preference over relying on their linguistic and world knowledge (Knoeferle and Crocker 2006, 2007). Below we discuss to which extent these characteristics of adult comprehension extend to children.

Sekerina and Trueswell (2012), for instance, failed to observe rapid visual context effects in Russian 6-year-olds. They presented the Russian children with spoken utterances (e.g., 'Put the red butterfly in the bag') while the children inspected a visual context depicting nine objects. The visual context either contained only one contrastive pair (a red and a purple butterfly) and a distractor (a red fox); or it contained a second contrastive pair (a red fox and a grey fox). The utterances further varied in focus, which was realised either through a cleft construction (literally: 'red put butterfly' vs. 'red butterfly put') and/or through pitch accent placement (early: on 'red' or late: on 'butterfly'). Russian adults rapidly used the contrastive pitch on the adjective for anticipating the referent of the ensuing noun 'butterfly', and they were even faster when the visual context contained only one contrastive object pair (the red butterfly and the purple butterfly). The children, by contrast, waited for the noun 'butterfly' before inspecting the target, even when both the early pitch accent on the sentence-initial adjective and the visual context (one contrastive pair of objects) should have sped up their visual attention to the butterfly.

Another example of limited visual context effects in young children comes from an experiment in which Trueswell et al. (1999) examined whether young children (5-year-olds) rely on the so-called 'referential principle'[3] for disambiguating a local structural ambiguity. In the sentence "Put the apple on the towel…" the prepositional phrase "on the towel" can either modify "the apple", indicating its location, or the verb phrase, specifying the destination of the action. Adults prefer the destination interpretation (and inspect an empty napkin to which the apple can be moved) but rapidly switch to the location interpretation (inspecting the apple located on the towel) when the referential context supports this (e.g., when one of two apples is on a towel, Spivey et al. 2002; Tanenhaus et al. 1995).

Five-year-olds (4.8–5.1 years) by comparison did not apply this referential principle online. When listening to "Put the frog on the napkin in the box", they frequently inspected a potential destination of the action (an empty napkin) instead of the frog on the napkin even when the context supported the location interpretation (one of two frogs was on a napkin). They did not even revise their initial analysis when executing the instruction, and put the frog onto the napkin (instead of into the box) on 60 % of the trials. The authors concluded that children were not able to revise their initial syntactic analysis and suggested their more limited processing capacities relative to those of the adults may lead them to discard

---

[3]When more than one syntactic analysis is possible, the referentially supported analysis is preferred.

infrequent alternative structures and interpretations early on in favour of the dominant (destination) interpretation (Trueswell et al. 1999). A capacity account seems plausible since children can employ the referential principle provided they are given more time. Three-to-five-year-olds exhibited adult-like performance in a post-sentence act-out task (i.e., they moved the frog that was on the red napkin into the box) when they had listened to a similar sentence with their eyes closed (Meroni and Crain 2003).

Alternatively, children must engage in pragmatic processing to apply the referential principle. They must know which objects are present, notice the initial referential ambiguity (there are 2 frogs), and infer that "on the napkin" could disambiguate reference. At age 5, however, they may not yet be able to compute pragmatic inferences during realtime language comprehension. This would be in line with the observed delay in 5–9-year-olds computation of pragmatic implicature (Huang and Snedeker 2009a).

Yet another possibility is that the experimental stimuli discourage children's reliance on the visual context (Zhang and Knoeferle 2012). When children heard "… on the napkin…" they could either inspect the empty napkin (a potential referent) or the frog located on the napkin. It is not implausible to assume that children pursue primarily a referential strategy (mapping "napkin" onto its referent), leading them to inspect the empty napkin (vs. another object on a napkin). If so, then children would be garden-pathed even more since a referential strategy would guide their attention to the incorrect destination (the empty napkin). If this were the reason for children's failure to rapidly rely on the visual context, the results would no longer reflect an inability to rapidly rely on the visual context but rather garden-pathing precisely *because* children rely on the visual context (relating nouns to objects).

Indeed, when Zhang and Knoeferle (2012) examined visual context effects in a situation when a sentential verb referred to a depicted action event, the events rapidly affected 5-year-olds' thematic role assignment and syntactic structuring. The events depicted, for instance, a bear pushing a bull and a worm painting the bear (Fig. 4.1). As they inspected this scene, adults and 5-year-olds listened to either an unambiguous subject-verb-object (SVO, "Der Bär schubst sogleich den Stier", 'The bear (subj) pushes soon the bull (obj)') or an object-verb-subject (OVS) sentence ("Den Bär malt sogleich der Wurm", 'The bear (obj) paints soon the worm (subj)').[4] Adults anticipated the event agent (the bull) upon hearing 'pushes' (Zhang and Knoeferle 2012). Five-year olds exhibited a strikingly similar eye-movement pattern. They also anticipated the agent of the painting event more when the verb was 'paints' than 'pushes', and they inspected the patient of the pushing event more when the verb was 'pushes' rather than 'paints'.

In children, this gaze pattern emerged later (during the post-verbal adverb) than for the adults, but still before the second noun phrase disambiguated the correct role filler. The similarities in the eye-movement pattern for the children and the adults suggest that 5-year-olds *can* rely on the non-linguistic visual context

---

[4]Object-initial word order is grammatical in German but non-canonical, and elicits processing difficulty (e.g., the case-marking on the determiner of the noun phrases elicits longer reading times).

Fig. 4.1 Example for an
event scene from Zhang and
Knoeferle (2012, p. 2595)

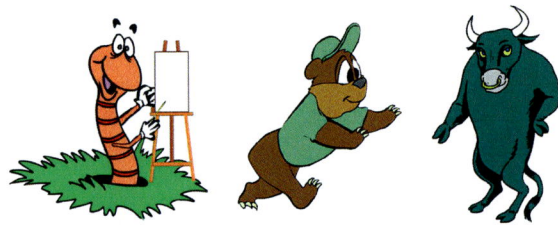

(depicted events) for thematic role assignment and syntactic structuring. Note,
however, that the sentences were structurally unambiguous. It remains to be seen
whether depicted events also help children to rapidly disambiguate local structural
ambiguity (Zhang and Knoeferle in progress).

Five-year-olds resembled adults also in their preference to rely on recently
inspected events. Adults preferentially ground their spoken language comprehension
in recent compared with future events. They inspected a clipart scene depicting a
waiter polishing candelabra and moving away from them (Knoeferle and Crocker
2007, Experiment 3). Other objects (crystal glasses) also afforded polishing. An
ensuing spoken German sentence referred either to the recent event (literal translation: 'The waiter polished recently the candelabra') or to a potential future event
(literal translation: 'The waiter polishes soon the crystal glasses'). The initial noun
and the verb (up to the last two letters) did not reveal the tense of the event (past vs.
future). Adults made more inspections to the target of the recently depicted than the
future event (e.g., polishing the crystal glasses), a preference which generalised to
real-world stimuli (Knoeferle et al. 2011a), and to experiments in which the future
events were much more frequent than the recent events (Abashidze et al. 2013).

When two further participant groups (5-year-olds and adults) were each shown
similar stimuli, analyses replicated the results from Knoeferle and Crocker (2007,
Experiment 3). Participants saw a red barn, and a horse depicted as galloping to a
blue barn. They listened to German sentences such as 'The horse galloped to the
blue barn' (Zhang et al. 2012). The adults invariably inspected the blue rather than
the red barn during the verb. The children exhibited a qualitatively similar but subtly delayed pattern, and inspected the blue barn post-verbally.

4.5 Summary

Not surprisingly infants and adults differ in how rapidly they relate language to
the "world". Infants often lag somewhat behind adults in their language-mediated
eye-movement behaviour. This lag may reflect younger children's limited processing capacity under the assumption that processing capacity affects the speed
of language processing (e.g., Just and Carpenter 1992). Clear differences emerged
regarding pragmatic and inferential processes, whereby adults but not children
computed pragmatic inferences online (but see Papafragou and Musolino 2003).

With regard to language-world mapping, however, even young infants' language-mediated visual attention behaviour resembled that of adults, and the literature on language processing documents their emerging ability to rapidly relate an unfolding utterance to objects in the visual context. While 5-year-olds may not always rely on the visual referential context, visual cues rapidly affected their thematic role assignment and syntactic structuring when mediated directly by language (e.g., a verb referring to an action). Five-year-olds also resembled adults in their preferred inspection of a recently depicted (over another future) action target but their eye-movement response was subtly slower than for adults.

4.6 Conclusions

This chapter has argued for an approach that strives to include a model of the comprehender into situated language processing accounts. To illustrate this approach I have discussed age-related variation in visually situated language processing. I have argued that visually situated language comprehension in young children resembles this process in adults. To corroborate this point, I have reviewed empirical research on (a) learning about language, objects and actions and on (b) language processing.

Insights from language learning can inform predictions for language comprehension. The literature on visually situated language comprehension suggests that contrast between objects can not enable rapid syntactic disambiguation in young children. This could be seen at odds with the important role of noun-object correspondences for language learning. One possibility is that certain processes such as syntactic disambiguation are exempt from visual context effects in child comprehenders. However, if we assume a similar role of visual context for language learning and comprehension, then object-based information should rapidly affect language comprehension. Assume, for instance, that children see a visual context in which one dog sits on a cushion while another dog sits on a rock. The children listen to "Den Hund auf dem Felsen füttert gleich der Mann." (literal translation: 'The dog on the rock (obj) feeds soon the man (subj)'). Object-first sentences are difficult to understand, but can be felicitous when they establish reference through contrast ('on the rock/cushion'). If children can rapidly use that contrast for syntactic structuring, then they should anticipate the upcoming agent (the man) earlier in a context with two dogs than with one dog (and another animal). To the extent that these and related predictions are borne out, they would corroborate that a comparison of language learning and comprehension can help us to gain insight into age-related variation of visually situated comprehension, with the goal of establishing a model of the comprehender.

Acknowledgments This research was funded by the Cognitive Interaction Technology Excellence Center 277 (CITEC, German Research Council).

References

Abashidze, D., Knoeferle, P., & Carminati, M. N. (2013). Do comprehenders prefer to rely on recent events even when future events are more likely to be mentioned? In *Proceedings of the Conference on Architectures and Mechanisms for Language Processing*. Marseille, France.

Allopenna, P., Magnuson, J. S., & Tanenhaus, M. K. (1998). Tracking the time course of spoken word recognition using eye movements: Evidence for continuous mapping models. *Journal of Memory and Language, 38*, 419–439.

Altmann, G. T. M., & Kamide, Y. (1999). Incremental interpretation at verbs: restricting the domain of subsequent reference. *Cognition, 73*, 247–264.

Altmann, G. T. M., & Kamide, Y. (2007). The real-time mediation of visual attention by language and world knowledge: linking anticipatory (and other) eye movements to linguistic processing. *Journal of Memory and Language, 57*, 502–518.

Andersson, R., Ferreira, F., & Henderson, J. (2011). I see what you're saying: The integration of complex speech and scenes during language comprehension. *Acta Psychologica, 137*, 208–216.

Bergelson, E., & Swingley, D. (2012). At 6–9 months, human infants know the meanings of many common nouns. In *Proceedings of the National Academy of Sciences of the USA, 109*, 3253–3258.

Carminati, M. N., & Knoeferle, P. (2013). Effects of speaker emotional facial expression and listener age on incremental sentence processing. *PLoS ONE, 8*(9), e72559. doi:10.1371/journal.pone.0072559.

Chambers, C. G., Tanenhaus, M. K., & Magnuson, J. S. (2004). Actions and affordances in syntactic ambiguity resolution. *Journal of Experimental Psychology. Learning, Memory, and Cognition, 30*, 687–696.

Dahan, D., Swingley, D., Tanenhaus, M. K., Magnuson, J. (2000). Linguistic gender and spoken-word recognition in French. *Journal of Memory and Language, 42*, 465–480.

Dahan, D., & Tanenhaus, M. K. (2005). Looking at the rope when looking for the snake: Conceptually mediated eye movements during spoken-word recognition. *Psychonomic Bulletin & Review, 12*, 453–459.

Dahan, D. (2010). The time course of interpretation in speech comprehension. *Current Directions in Psychological Science, 19*, 121–126.

Fenson, L., Dale, P., Reznick, J., Bates, E., Thal, D., & Pethick, S. (1994). Variability in early communicative development. *Monographs of the Society for Research on Child Development, 59*, 1–189.

Fernald, A., Thorpe, K., & Marchman, V. A. (2010). Blue car, red car: Developing efficiency in online interpretation of adjective-noun phrases. *Cognitive Psychology, 60*, 190–217.

Fernald, A., Pinto, J. P., Swingley, D., Weinberg, A., & McRoberts, G. W. (1998). Rapid gains in speed of verbal processing by infants in the second year. *Psychological Science, 9*, 72–75.

Fisher, C. (1996). Structural limits on verb mapping: The role of analogy in children's interpretation of sentences. *Cognitive Psychology, 31*, 41–81.

Fisher, C. (2002). Structural limits on verb mapping: the role of abstract structure in 2.5-year-olds' interpretations of novel verbs. *Developmental Science, 5*, 55–64.

Fisher, C., Hall., D. G., Rakowitz, S., & Gleitman, L. (1994). When it is better to receive than to give: Syntactic and conceptual constraints on vocabulary growth. *Lingua, 92*, 333–375.

Fodor, J. (1983). *The modularity of mind*. Cambridge, MA: MIT Press.

Friederici, A. F., Friedrich, M., & Christophe, A. (2007). Brain responses in 4-month-old infants are already language specific. *Current Biology, 17*, 1208–1211.

Friedrich, M., & Friederici, A. D. (2004). N400-like semantic incongruity effect in 19-month-olds: Processing known words in picture contexts. *Journal of Cognitive Neuroscience, 16*, 1465–1477.

Gleitman, L. (1990). The structural sources of verb meanings. *Language Acquisition, 1*, 3–55.

Gogate, L. J., Bolzani, L., & Betancourt, E. (2006). Attention to maternal multimodal naming by 6- to 8-month-old infants and learning of word–object relations. *Infancy, 9*, 259–288.

Gogate, L. J. (2010). Learning of syllable–object relations by preverbal infants: the role of temporal synchrony and syllable distinctiveness. *Journal of Experimental Child Psychology, 105*, 178–197.

Golinkoff, R., & Hirsh-Pasek, K. (2008). How toddlers learn verbs. *Trends in Cognitive Science, 12*, 397–403.

Höhle, B., Bijeljac-Babic, R., Herold, B., Weissenborn, J., & Nazzi, T. (2009). Language specific prosodic preferences during the first half year of life: Evidence from German and French infants. *Infant Behavior and Development, 32*, 262–274.

Huang, Y. T., & Snedeker, J. (2009a). Semantic meaning and pragmatic interpretation in 5-year-olds: Evidence from real-time spoken language comprehension. *Developmental Psychology, 45*, 1723–1739.

Huang, Y. T., & Snedeker, J. (2009b). Online interpretation of scalar quantifiers: Insight into the semantics–pragmatics interface. *Cognitive Psychology, 58*, 376–415.

Huettig, F., & Altmann, G. T. M. (2011). Looking at anything that is green when hearing "frog": How object surface colour and stored object colour knowledge influence language-mediated overt attention. *The Quarterly Journal of Experimental Psychology, 64*, 122–145.

Huettig, F., Mishra, R. K., & Olivers, C. N. (2012). Mechanisms and representations of language-mediated visual attention. *Frontiers in Psychology, 2*, 394. doi:10.3389/fpsyg.2011.00394.

Huettig, F., Singh, N., & Mishra, R. K. (2011). Language-mediated visual orienting behavior in low and high literates. *Frontiers in Psychology, 2*, 285. doi:10.3389/fpsyg.2011.00285.

Ito, K., Jincho, N., Minai, U., Yamane, N., & Mazuka, R. (2012). Intonation facilitates contrast resolution: Evidence from Japanese adults and 6-year olds. *Journal of Memory and Language, 66*, 265–284.

Jusczyk, P. W., Houston, D. M., & Newsome, M. (1999). The beginnings of word segmentation in English-learning infants. *Cognitive Psychology, 39*, 159–207.

Jusczyk, P. W., Cutler, A., & Redanz, N. (1993). Preference for the predominant stress patterns of English words. *Child Development, 64*, 675–687.

Just, M. A. & Carptenter, P. (1992). A capacity theory of comprehension: Individual differences in working memory. *Psychological Review, 99*, 122–149.

Kirkham, N. Z., Slemmer, J. A., & Johnson, S. P. (2002). Visual statistical learning in infancy: Evidence of a domain general learning mechanism. *Cognition, 83*, B35–B42.

Kirkham, N. Z., Slemmer, J. A., Richardson, D. C., & Johnson, S. P. (2007). Location, location, location: Development of spatiotemporal sequence learning in infancy. *Child Development, 78*, 1559–1571.

Knoeferle, P., Crocker, M. W., Scheepers, C., & Pickering, M. J. (2005). The influence of the immediate visual context on incremental thematic role-assignment: evidence from eye-movements in depicted events. *Cognition, 95*, 95–127.

Knoeferle, P., & Crocker, M. W. (2006). The coordinated interplay of scene, utterance, and world knowledge: Evidence from eye tracking. *Cognitive Science, 30*, 481–529.

Knoeferle, P., & Crocker, M. W. (2007). The influence of recent scene events on spoken comprehension: Evidence from eye-movements. *Journal of Memory and Language, 75*, 519–543.

Knoeferle, P., Habets, B., Crocker, M. W., & Muente, T. F. (2008). Visual scenes trigger immediate syntactic reanalysis: Evidence from ERPs during situated spoken comprehension. *Cerebral Cortex, 18*, 789–795.

Knoeferle, P., Carminati, M. N., Abashidze, D., & Essig, K. (2011a). Preferential inspection of recent real-world events over future events: Evidence from eye tracking during spoken sentence comprehension. *Frontiers in Psychology, 2*, 376. doi:10.3389/fpsyg.2011.00376.

Knoeferle, P., Urbach, T., & Kutas, M. (2011b). Comprehending how visual context influences incremental sentence processing: Insights from ERPs and picture-sentence verification. *Psychophysiology, 48*, 495–506.

Kutas, M., & Hillyard, S. A. (1980). Reading senseless sentences: Brain potentials reflect semantic incongruity. *Science, 207*, 203–205.

Kutas, M., & Hillyard, S. A. (1984). Brain potentials during reading reflect word expectancy and semantic association. *Nature, 307*, 161–163.

Lew-Williams, C., & Fernald, A. (2010). Real-time processing of gender-marked articles by native and non-native Spanish speakers. *Journal of Memory and Language, 63*, 447–464.

Mani, N., & Huettig, F. (2012). Prediction during language processing is a piece of cake—but only for skilled producers. *Journal of Experimental Psychology: Human Perception and Performance, 38*(4), 843–847.

Meltzoff, A. N. (1995). Understanding the intentions of others: Re-enactment of intended acts by 18-month-old children. *Developmental Psychology, 31*, 838–850.

Meroni, L. & Crain, S. (2003). On not being led down the kindergarten path. In *Proceedings of the 27th Boston University Conference on language development* (pp. 531–544), Somerville, MA: Cascadilla Press.

Moeser, S. D., & Olson, J. A. (1974). The role of reference in children's acquisition of a miniature artificial language. *Journal of Experimental Child Psychology, 17*, 204–218.

Naigles, L. (1990). Children use syntax to learn verb meaning. *Journal of Child Language, 17*, 357–374.

Nation, K., Marshall, C., & Altmann, G. T. M. (2003). Investigating individual differences in children's real-time sentence comprehension using language-mediated eye movements. *Journal of Experimental Child Psychology, 86*, 314–329.

Newport, E. L., & Aslin, R. (2004). Learning at a distance I: Statistical learning of non-adjacent dependencies. *Cognitive Psychology, 48*, 270, 127–162.

Papafragou, A. & Musonlino, J. (2003). Scalar implicatures: experiments at the semantics–pragmatics interface. *Cognition, 86*, 253–282.

Pinker, S. (1994). How could a child use verb syntax to learn verb semantics. *Lingua, 92*, 377–410.

Pulverman, R., Sootsman, J., Golinkoff, R., & Hirsh-Pasek, K. (2008). Manners matter: Infants' attention to manner and path in non-linguistic dynamic events. *Cognition, 108*, 825–830.

Saffran, J., Aslin, R., & Newport, R. (1996). Statistical learning by 8-month-old infants. *Science, 274*, 1926–1928.

Sharon, T., & Wynn, K. (1998). Infants' individuation of actions from continuous motion. *Psychological Science, 9*, 357–362.

Sedivy, J. C., Tanenhaus, M. K., Chambers, C. G., & Carlson, G. N. (1999). Achieving incremental semantic interpretation through contextual representation. *Cognition, 71*, 109–148.

Sekerina, I. A., & Trueswell, J. C. (2012). Interactive processing of contrastive expressions by Russian children. *First Language, 32*, 63–87.

Smith, L., & Yu, C. (2008). Infants rapidly learn word-referent mappings via cross-situational statistics. *Cognition, 106*, 1558–1568.

Snedeker, J., & Trueswell, J. C. (2004). The developing constraints on parsing decisions: The role of lexical-biases and referential scenes in child and adult sentence processing. *Cognitive Psychology, 49*, 238–299.

Snedeker, J., & Yuan, S. (2008). Effects of prosodic and lexical constraints on parsing in young children (and adults). *Journal of Memory and Language, 58*, 574–608.

Spivey, M. J., Tanenhaus, M. K., Eberhard, K. M., & Sedivy, J. C. (2002). Eye-movements and spoken language comprehension: Effects of visual context on syntactic ambiguity resolution. *Cognitive Psychology, 45*, 447–481.

Tanenhaus, M. K., Spivey-Knowlton, M. J., Eberhard, K. M., & Sedivy, J. C. (1995). Integration of visual and linguistic information in spoken language comprehension. *Science, 268*, 1632–1634.

Tincoff, R., & Jusczyk, P. (1999). Some beginnings of word comprehension in 6-month-olds. *Psychological Science, 10*, 172–175.

Tincoff, R., & Jusczyk, P. (2012). Six-month-olds comprehend words that refer to parts of the body. *Infancy, 17*, 432–444.

Tomasello, M., & Farrar, J. (1986). Joint attention and early language. *Child Development, 57*, 1454–1463.

Tomasello, M., & Todd, J. (1983). Joint attention and lexical acquisition style. *First Language, 4*, 197–211. doi:10.1177/014272378300401202.

Tomasello, M., & Brooks, P. (1998). Young children's earliest transitive and intransitive constructions. *Cognitive Linguistics, 9*, 379–395.

Tomasello, M. (2000). Do young children have adult syntactic competence? *Cognition, 74*, 209–253.

Trueswell, J. C., Sekerina, I., Hill, N., & Logrip, M. (1999). The kindergarten-path effect: Studying online sentence processing in young children. *Cognition, 73*, 89–134.

Van Heugthen, M., & Shi, R. (2009). French-learning toddlers use gender information on determiners during word recognition. *Developmental Science, 12*, 419–425.

Weber, A., Grice, M., & Crocker, M. W. (2006). The role of prosody in the interpretation of structural ambiguities: A study of anticipatory eye movements. *Cognition, 99*, B63–B72.

Woodward, A. L. (1998). Infants selectively encode the goal object of an actor's reach. *Cognition, 69*, 1–34.

Woodward, A., & Sommerville, J. (2000). Twelve-month-old infants interpret actions in context. *Psychological Science, 11*, 73–77.

Wu, R., Gopnik, A., Richardson, D. C., & Kirkham, N. Z. (2011). Infants learn about objects from statistics and people. *Developmental Psychology, 47*, 1220–1229.

Wynn, K. (1996). Infants' individuation and enumeration of actions. *Psychological Science, 7*, 164–169.

Yu, C., & Smith, L. (2010). What you learn is what you see: Using eye movements to study infant cross-situational word learning. *Developmental Science, 14*, 165–180.

Zhang, L., & Knoeferle, P. (2012). Visual context effects on thematic role assignment in children versus adults: Evidence from eye tracking in German. In Naomi Miyake, David Peebles, & Richard P. Cooper (Eds.), In *Proceedings of the annual meeting of the cognitive science society* (pp. 2593–2598). Boston, USA: The Cognitive Science Society.

Zhang, L., & Knoeferle, P. (in progress). Can depicted events disambiguate local structural ambiguity in German SVO / OVS sentences?

Zhang, L., Kornbluth, L., & Knoeferle, P. (2012). The role of recent versus future events in children's comprehension of referentially ambiguous sentences: Evidence from eye tracking. In N. Miyake, D. Peebles, & R. P. Cooper, In *Proceedings of the Annual Meeting of the Cognitive Science Society* (pp. 1227–1232), Boston, USA: The Cognitive Science Society.

Zhou, P., Crain, S., & Zhan, L. (2014). Grammatical aspect and event recognition in children's online sentence comprehension. *Cognition, 133*, 262–276.

Zhou, P., Crain, S., & Zhan, L. (2012). Sometimes children are as good as adults: The pragmatic use of prosody in children's online sentence processing. *Journal of Memory and Language, 67*, 149–164.

Chapter 5
Vision and Language in Cross-Linguistic Research on Sentence Production

Elisabeth Norcliffe and Agnieszka E. Konopka

5.1 Introduction

A classic assumption in the cognitive sciences has been the existence of an invariant cognitive architecture underlying language processing. Perhaps for this reason, the early days of modern psycholinguistics saw little engagement with cross-language data. Indeed, despite the vitality of the discipline in the 1960s and 1970s, it is striking that the language in which experiments were conducted were seldom explicitly considered as an important potential variable of interest. As Cutler (1985) observes, during this period, experiments undertaken in one language could be supported or refuted by experiments in another language, without consideration of whether the particular language could have affected the processes under study. Similarly, the major psycholinguistic textbooks of the day did not make reference to cross-linguistic data or comparative argumentation (see, e.g., Fodor et al. 1974; Glucksberg and Danks 1975).[1]

Beginning in the 1980s, this picture began to change, as researchers in the field of speech perception began to consider cross-linguistic differences more closely. In the process, the blanket universalist assumption was challenged as it was revealed that certain critical cross-linguistic differences can, in fact, affect language processing (Cutler et al. 1983, 1986, 1989; Mehler et al. 1993, 1996). Mehler et al. (1981) found, for example, that French speakers responded faster in

---

[1]It is interesting to observe that this contrasts starkly with the flurry of cross-linguistic research that was undertaken in the sister field of language acquisition during the same period, in large part due to the pioneering work of Dan Slobin.

E. Norcliffe (✉) · A.E. Konopka
Max Planck Institute for Psycholinguistics, Nijmegen, The Netherlands
e-mail: elisabeth.norcliffe@mpi.ni

© Springer India 2015
R.K. Mishra et al. (eds.), *Attention and Vision in Language Processing*, DOI 10.1007/978-81-322-2443-3_5

a syllable detection task when the target corresponded to the first syllable of the stimulus word, compared to targets that consisted of a segment longer or shorter than the first syllable. This was evidence that speakers segment the speech into syllabic units prior to lexical access. Strikingly, however, the results did not generalise to English: Cutler et al. (1983) failed to find a syllable advantage effect for English speakers when they performed an equivalent task. On the basis of these different response patterns, Cutler et al. (1986) proposed that speakers of languages with different rhythmic properties parsed speech differently: for languages such as French, with clear syllabic boundaries, listeners use a syllabic representation to segment speech. For stress languages, such as English, such a representation is not used. Thus, listeners from different language backgrounds appear to rely on different processing routines. This and other seminal work launched a new focus on reconciling the language specific and the universal in speech processing.

In contrast with speech processing, most current models of language production have tended to continue to emphasise the universal aspects of the process (Levelt 1989). Here too, however, there has been scattered evidence of language-mediated processes. To date, most of these findings come from studies of noun phrase production. For example, Costa et al. (1999), Miozzo and Caramazza (1999), and Caramazza et al. (2001) demonstrate cross-linguistic differences in the time-course of determiner production. In German and Dutch, determiners agree in gender with the noun they combine with. For example, in Dutch, *de* is used for common gender nouns (e.g. *de tafel*, 'the table'), and *het* is used for neuter gender nouns (e.g. *het boek*, 'the book'). In Romance languages, such as Catalan, Spanish, Italian and French, determiners are selected not only on the basis of the gender of the noun, but also on the phonological form of the onset of the word that immediately follows it. For example, in Catalan, the masculine determiner *el* is used when the following word begins with a consonant (*el got*, 'the glass', *el meu ull*, literally "the my eye"), and with *l'* when the following word begins with a vowel (*l'ull* 'the eye'). In picture-word interference tasks, Dutch and German speakers are slower to name pictures of objects when a printed distractor phrase mismatches in gender with that of the depicted object (Schriefers 1993; Schiller and Caramazza 2003). While this so-called 'gender congruency' effect is robustly attested for German and Dutch, it has not been found for speakers of Romance languages. Miozzo and Caramazza (1999; see also Caramazza et al. 2001) suggest that this may reflect differences in the timing of determiner selection during noun phrase production in the two sets of languages. The authors propose that the gender congruency effect reflects competition between determiners; the selection of the target determiner is slowed when a different determiner is simultaneously activated by the distractor word. In Romance languages, the lack of gender congruency effect reflects the fact that determiner selection takes place later in the production process because it requires access not just to lemma-level information of the noun (gender information), but also the phonological form of the following word. As a result of this time lag, potentially conflicting information from the distractor determiner has already dissipated. In sum, this body of research suggests that languages differ in the extent to which information at different levels of processing (conceptual, grammatical and phonological) interacts during the selection of closed class words.

Similarly, cross-linguistic differences in the *order* of words within noun phrases also influence the timing of word retrieval. Janssen et al. (2008) reported that linear word order can be responsible for differences in the timing of phonological activation in noun-adjective combinations; in French, where nouns typically precede adjectives, noun phonology was activated earlier than in English, where adjectives appear before nouns. This indicates that noun phrase production can proceed in a highly incremental fashion (word for word), allowing for language-specific variation in the time-course of formulation.

Interestingly, cross-linguistic differences in word order appear to influence not just the timing of grammatical-level processes, but even conceptual formulation. Brown-Schmidt and Konopka (2008) tested whether speakers of English and Spanish incorporate size information into modified expressions like *the small butterfly* and *la mariposa pequeña* at different points in time, consistent with the surface linear order of nouns and modifiers in the two languages. Eye-tracked speakers described highlighted object pictures (e.g., *butterfly*) presented in large displays. Speakers were expected to mention object size if they noticed a second referent in the display that differed from the target referent only in size (i.e., a size contrast: a large butterfly). The results showed that, when speakers produced modified noun phrases, fixations to the size contrast occurred on average later in Spanish (where modifiers follow nouns) than in English (where modifiers precede nouns). This suggests that linear word order afforded more flexibility in the timing of generation of the preverbal message in Spanish than in English.

Studies such as these suggest that, at least at the phrasal level, cross-linguistic differences in the nature of the syntactic dependencies between elements in phrases, or differences in the relative ordering of those elements, can influence processing routines. Such cross-linguistic differences can systematically affect the time-course of the computations involved in conceptual and linguistic planning.

In this chapter we consider the question of whether and how the planning processes involved in producing whole sentences—i.e., utterances with multiple referents and a more complex hierarchical structure—might be fine-tuned to language-specific properties. Specifically, we ask to what extent language structure can affect the breadth and order of the conceptual and linguistic encoding operations that take place during sentence formulation. We survey the small body of cross-linguistic research that bears on this question, focusing in particular on recent evidence from eye-tracking studies. The relatively recent application of visual world eye-tracking techniques to language production research (Griffin and Bock 2000; Griffin 2004; Meyer et al. 1998) has yielded important insights into the time-course of sentence formulation. Because eye-tracking methods provide a very fine-grained temporal measure of how conceptual processing and utterance planning unfold in real time, they serve as an important complement to standard approaches based on coarser temporal measures such as speech onset latencies, or offline measures such as structure choice. Significantly, the development of portable eye-trackers in recent years has, for the first time, allowed eye-tracking techniques to be used with language populations that are located far away from university laboratories. This has created the exciting opportunity to extend the typological base of vision-based psycholinguistic research. Illustrating these advances, we describe results from studies carried out in the field with two verb-initial languages: Tzeltal (Mexico) and Tagalog (Philippines).

5.2 Incremental Sentence Formulation

Producing spoken language requires transforming an abstract idea or a communicative intention into a linear string of words. According to most models of language production (e.g., Levelt 1989), the first stage involves formulating a *message*, i.e. an abstract, preverbal representation of the information that the speaker wants to express. The message must then undergo *linguistic encoding* in preparation for articulation. Linguistic encoding itself involves several component processes, including selecting and retrieving the words appropriate for conveying the message, and integrating them into a sentence structure. It is generally assumed that this entire process unfolds *incrementally* (Kempen and Hoenkamp 1987; Levelt 1989): we do not plan everything we say in advance of opening our mouths. Rather, in an incremental system, speech can begin once some minimal chunk of the utterance is prepared, with the planning of subsequent material taking place as speaking unfolds over time.

Given the assumption of incrementality, the central debates in sentence production research revolve largely around the question of how much information speakers *can* and *do* plan at the conceptual level (i.e., the preverbal message) and at the sentence level before initiating overt production. This question has a venerable tradition in psycholinguistic research, dating back to the very genesis of the discipline. One view, first articulated by Paul (1886/1970), and reflected in modern 'word-driven' or 'linearly incremental' approaches to formulation, holds that speaking is a highly opportunistic process, in which the relative availability of individual concepts in a message determines the order in which words are retrieved. On this view, increments at the message level and at the sentence level can be very small (perhaps as small as a single concept or word): speakers may encode as little as one content word before speech onset, and the structure of the rest of the sentence is automatically constrained by whichever content word happens to be retrieved first. An alternative view, first espoused by Wundt (1900), and recapitulated in modern 'structure-driven' theories of formulation, holds that formulation begins with the generation of a larger conceptual representation of the message and, from there, a structural representation of the sentence. This structural plan in turn guides the order of subsequent word retrieval operations. Empirically, differences between these views have been addressed by considering implications of different planning strategies for the selection of *starting points* (MacWhinney 1977): when preparing an utterance, what (and how much) do speakers plan first?

Linearly incremental ('word-driven') formulation is supported by the robust cross-linguistic finding that speakers make structural choices that allow them to place *accessible* (roughly, more easily retrievable) information earlier in sentences (Arnold et al. 2000; Bock and Warren 1985; Branigan and Feleki 1999; Ferreira and Yoshita 2003; MacWhinney and Bates 1978; see Jaeger and Norcliffe 2009, for a review). Accessibility may depend, for example, on a referent's *perceptual* salience and can be enhanced by exogenous attention-capturing cues (Gleitman et al. 2007; Ibbotson et al. 2013; Myachykov and Tomlin 2008; Tomlin 1995, 1997). Referents may also differ in their *conceptual accessibility*, which includes such features as animacy, imageability or givenness. For example, speakers of English are more likely to produce passive structures (where the patient is expressed as the sentence-initial subject), when the patient is animate (Bock et al. 1992) or imageable (Bock and Warren 1985). For example, they are more likely to say "the man was hit by the ball", than "the ball hit the man", as this allows the human argument to be expressed as the sentence-initial subject. Effects like these are compatible with the view that speakers begin formulation by retrieving the first readily available word, and that this initial choice constrains the structure of the rest of the sentence.

This interpretation is supported by evidence from visual-world eye-tracking studies. In these paradigms, speakers describe pictures of simple events while their eyes are tracked. As noted by Bock et al. (2004), eye-tracking is particularly well suited to examining theories about incrementality in sentence formulation because speakers typically look at the things they want to talk about. Thus, the distribution of attention and the timing of gaze shifts to the various characters in an event provide fine-grained temporal information about when various elements of the message and sentence are planned (see discussions in Henderson and Ferreira 2004). Gleitman et al. (2007) used this method in combination with an implicit visual cueing procedure. Participants' attention was directed to one or another character in the event by means of a fleeting, subliminal visual cue (a black square). Gleitman et al. found that English speakers preferentially fixated the visually cued character within 200 ms of picture onset and that they tended to select that character to be the first-mentioned referent in their sentence. This result suggests that sentence formulation can indeed begin with the conceptual and linguistic encoding of as little as a single referent. Such results are also generally consistent with theories assuming that the order in which various encoding operations are performed depends on relative states of *activation* at different levels of representation in the production system.

An important constraint on interpreting such findings and generalising them across languages, however, is the fact that languages vary considerably on a number of grammatical dimensions that can be relevant for incremental formulation. One of these dimensions is linear word order: a significant complication in interpreting accessibility effects like the ones described by Gleitman et al. (2007) for English is that the first-mentioned element in the sentence also happens to be the subject of the sentence. Thus in subject-initial languages like English, it is difficult to tease apart whether accessibility influences *linear word order* directly or whether it influences *subject assignment* (Bock and Warren 1985; McDonald et al. 1993), and only indirectly word order. A strong or 'radical' version of linear incrementality (Gleitman et al. 2007) would hold that accessibility directly drives lexical encoding and that early formulation involves little grammatical encoding (assignment of grammatical functions); on this view, subject assignment *follows* from whichever element is lexically retrieved first. The alternative view would be that planning the first character and retrieving the first content word involves not only the lexical encoding of one message element, but also the assignment of that element to the subject function: subject assignment implies some advance planning of the relational structure of the event (who is doing what to whom) as well as some grammatical-level processing.

Studies of languages that allow word order scrambling and thus do not confound subject position and sentence-initial position provide support for both possibilities. Some work has found that accessible concepts are more likely to become subjects, rather than simply sentential starting points (Christianson and Ferreira 2005, for Odawa). Other work (both experimental and corpus-based) has shown that conceptual accessibility can directly affect word order, even when grammatical function (subjecthood) is controlled for (Branigan and Feleki 1999, for Greek; Ferreira and Yoshita 2003, for Japanese; Kempen and Harbusch 2004, for German; MacWhinney and Bates 1978, for Italian and Hungarian). There is also recent evidence to suggest that within a language, both word order *and* grammatical function assignment may be influenced by conceptual accessibility (Tanaka et al. 2011, for Japanese).

In contrast, other eye-tracking evidence from English is more compatible with the structure-driven view of formulation. Using an eye-tracked picture description task, Griffin and Bock (2000) found that English speakers did not preferentially fixate either character in the depicted events within the first 400 ms of picture onset. Only after 400 ms did they direct their gaze preferentially to the character they would mention first. The authors interpret this as evidence of an early pre-linguistic 'gist apprehension' phase, in which speakers encode the relationship between event characters before beginning linguistic encoding of the first-mentioned character. On this account, early gist apprehension allows for the generation of a larger message representation and, on this basis, selection of a suitable structural frame; this information, in turn, controls the order in which speakers encode individual event characters linguistically. More generally, unlike word-driven formulation, the 'structure-driven' view predicts that visual or conceptual salience of individual characters plays a subordinate role to 'wholistic' message-planning processes: speakers look to the character they will mention first not because their attention was initially drawn to it (contrary to Gleitman et al. 2007), but because their eyes were guided there by the structural framework generated shortly after picture onset (Bock et al. 2004).

Further support for structure-driven formulation comes from a study by Lee et al. (2013), who examined the structure of advanced planning in English using a picture description task. Analysis of speech onset times and word durations showed that when producing relative clause constructions (*the student of the teacher who is raising her hand*), structurally dependent lexical items were planned together, suggesting that formulation involved advance hierarchical planning of a sentence structure.

5.2.1 Flexibility

In sum, there is a range of evidence to support both the word-driven and the structure-driven view of sentence formulation. Recently, evidence has accumulated to suggest that mixed findings like these can also reflect the fact that the time-course of formulation is flexible: while speakers are *able* to prepare increments consisting of multiple referents before initiating overt production, they may plan either more or less information before initiating speech under different conditions. Under certain circumstances, speakers might begin formulation by encoding isolated bits of information; while under other circumstances, they may begin by encoding the entire relational structure of a message, with linguistic formulation accordingly affected by the nature of the initial conceptual planning.

Factors that contribute to reductions in the scope of advance planning include extra-linguistic variables like time pressure (Ferreira and Swets 2002), cognitive load (Wagner et al. 2010) and differences in working memory capacity (Swets et al. 2008)—all of which can constrain the amount of information that speakers can encode in parallel in a given time window. Another set of factors concerns production processes proper, for example, resource constraints affecting the coordination of lexical and structural processes (Konopka 2012), or the relative ease of formulating a message plan. Kuchinsky and Bock (2010) found, for example, that attentional cueing had an effect on first mention (replicating Gleitman et al. 2007) for events for which the relation between the characters was difficult to conceptualise or interpret. In other words, for hard-to-interpret events, directing attention to one character in the event resulted in early mention of this character in the sentence, consistent with word-driven formulation. For easily encodable events, by contrast, attentional cueing had no effect on first mention. This suggests that fast encoding of a rudimentary message structure, and not character accessibility, mediated subject selection. Thus, different formulation strategies may be induced by differences in how 'hard' or 'easy' it is to apprehend the relational content of a message.

More generally, evidence of flexibility in the incremental preparation of messages and sentences motivates one key conclusion and makes one important prediction for research on sentence formulation across languages. The conclusion is that differences across studies may be a natural outcome of differences in the way that speakers coordinate encoding or prioritise encoding of different types of information (individual elements of a message versus the message "as a whole") when preparing their utterances. The prediction then is that details of this coordination should be sensitive to the order in which words must be ultimately produced in an utterance. Incrementality naturally assumes that some parts of a message or sentence are encoded before other parts of a message or sentence undergo encoding; thus, to produce language efficiently, formulation can benefit from speakers' ability to prioritise encoding those parts of a message and sentence that must be expressed first. This implies that the time-course of formulation should vary across languages with different basic word orders, because language-specific constraints on word order should license allocation of resources to encoding different parts of a message or sentence at different points in time. In the next section, we review evidence suggesting that the order of encoding operations during sentence formulation may indeed depend on the grammatical properties of the target language—and that this may naturally result in planning patterns that resemble either word-driven or structure-driven planning.

5.3 Cross-Linguistic Differences

To what extent can reliance on different planning strategies be driven by *grammar*? To a certain degree, it may seem fairly unquestionable that the formulation process would be influenced by language-specific constraints, given that the target structures of linguistic encoding are language-specific. A key question for theories of incrementality, however, is where and how far up in the production system language-specific properties might be expected to exert an influence on formulation. We address this question by considering how grammar influences encoding of complex relationships between elements of a message. We first review a set of studies that suggest that the grammars of languages may differ in the extent to which they are compatible with word-driven formulation. Then we turn to the special case of verb-initial languages, and ask whether the sentential position of the verb, as well as its morphological properties, can exert an influence not just on the timing of linguistic-level formulation processes, but also on message-level formulation itself.

5.3.1 Different Grammars, Different Formulation Preferences

To date, research on the time-course of sentence formulation comes largely from work on English. Arguably, the grammar of English affords a high degree of flexibility in planning. Sentences typically begin with subjects, which are not morphologically dependent on any other element in the sentence. As such, speakers may begin by selecting and retrieving a single noun lemma, without engaging in any advance planning of the rest of the message or planning of a sentence frame (consistent with radical, word-driven incrementality). Alternatively, nothing in the grammar prevents a structure-driven formulation process either: speakers may, in principle, begin formulating their sentences by encoding some of the hierarchical relationships between message elements early in the formulation process.

However, while linear incrementality is compatible with the syntax of English, it is apparently more problematic for other types of grammars. Evidence for this conclusion comes from a set of cross-linguistic studies that have employed the attentional cueing paradigm to study the effects of perceptual accessibility on structure choice. Myachykov et al. (2010) compared the performance of English and Finnish speakers in a task modelled on Gleitman et al. (2007). While the data from English participants replicated earlier results (speakers were more likely to begin their sentence by mentioning the cued referent first), the authors failed to find any effect of perceptual salience in Finnish: Finnish speakers consistently produced transitive SVO sentences, regardless of the position of the cued referent. Notably, Finnish is a *case-marking* language: the authors suggest that early commitment to a case-marker requires a larger degree of pre-planning compared to a language like English that lacks case marking on nouns. In Finnish, then, reliance on word-driven formulation may be attenuated by its case-marking properties.

Further empirical support for this possibility comes from Korean, which, like Finnish, is a case-marking language. Hwang and Kaiser (2009) found for Korean that priming patient characters with semantic prime words (to increase their conceptual accessibility) or employing visual cues (to increase their perceptual accessibility) did not influence structure choice. Thus, just as in the case of Finnish, attentional salience did not affect speakers' choice of sentential starting points.

In sum, it seems, logically, that in order to produce an initial case-marked noun phrase, speakers need to have already engaged in more than simple word retrieval to begin production: the selection of the appropriate case-marker on a sentence-initial noun should necessitate the early selection of a grammatical function for this noun. This would require some advance planning of the relational structure of the target message and some grammatical-level processing. As a result, not all languages allowing early mention of sentence subjects may equally support a radically incremental, word-driven formulation process. While English speakers can and do engage in word-driven formulation, this tendency does not generalise across languages in similar experimental paradigms.

There is also evidence that languages may differ in the *extent* to which they rely on a given formulation strategy. Myachykov and Tomlin (2008) employed an explicit cueing procedure to study the effects of attentional salience on Russian structure choice. The cueing procedure they employed was modelled on an earlier study on English by Tomlin (1995), which made use of an animated programme referred to as the "Fish Film". In this task, participants viewed and described a series of animations of two differently coloured fish swimming towards each other, culminating with one (the agent) eating the other (the patient). In each trial, an arrow appeared above one of the fish, and participants were explicitly instructed to look at the cued fish, and then describe the scene however they liked. Tomlin found that English speakers very consistently began their sentences with the cued fish (producing nearly 100 % actives when the agent was cued, and passives when the patient was cued). Myachykov and Tomlin (2008) repeated the study with Russian speakers to test which structural preferences would be revealed in a language that allowed more structural choices: Russian has a passive alternation like

English, but it also allows scrambling (object-subject as well as subject-object word order). The authors found that speakers tended to produce active subject-first constructions when the agent was cued (i.e., allowing the cued character to be the sentence-initial element), and active object-first constructions when the patient was cued (again, allowing the cued character to be the sentence-initial element). Notably, this effect was much smaller (around 20 %) compared to the almost 100 % effect size observed for English speakers. Interestingly, the passive was produced very rarely (only around 2 % of the time).

Several conclusions can be drawn from these findings. First, the fact that speakers typically started their sentence with the cued character is evidence that, as in English, speakers of Russian can adopt a word-driven formulation strategy. Second, the fact that the effect size was much smaller in Russian suggests that different languages accommodate attentional effects differently. One possible explanation for the cross-linguistic difference in effect size may be that Russian, like Korean and Finnish, is a case-marking language. Alternatively (or additionally), it could stem from differences in the relative frequencies of the different structural options in the two languages. In Russian there was a greater overall tendency to rely on canonical active SVO sentence structures, regardless of the position of the cue: this may reflect the overall high frequency of active SVO structures in Russian, compared to other structural alternatives (especially compared to the passive, which is reportedly very rare; Myachykov et al. 2011).

In this vein, MacDonald (2013) suggests that some cross-linguistic differences in production strategies may emerge from differences in how strongly specific structures are favoured in a given language. It is robustly attested that speakers have a tendency to reuse recently produced structures. This tendency, referred to as structural persistence, or syntactic priming, is often assumed to be the result of long-term implicit learning of structure-building procedures (Bock and Griffin 2000; Bock et al. 2007; Chang et al. 2006; Jaeger and Snider 2013). On this view, speakers constantly learn from their own productions and the productions of others: the more often a structure is used or heard, the more likely it is to be used again. Such structural biases may, therefore, induce a structure-driven formulation strategy over a word-driven strategy, by facilitating the mapping between a message and an abstract structural representation. Evidence of this relationship already exists for English and Dutch (Konopka 2012; Konopka and Meyer 2014; Van de Velde et al. 2014). On the assumption that languages differ in terms of the strength (and direction) of their overall structural biases, it is possible that these differences may also give rise to cross-linguistic differences in the extent to which speakers' structural choices are driven by lexical availability (see also Gennari et al. 2012).[2]

In sum, evidence from attentional cueing studies suggests that structural choices are not affected by perceptual salience equally across languages. In some languages, such as English, entities that are made accessible via visual cueing exert an influence on structural choices, consistent with word-driven incremental

---

[2]This of course leaves open the interesting question of what gives rise to such cross-linguistic differences in frequency distributions to begin with.

formulation. Other languages appear to show little sensitivity to perceptual sali-ence, suggesting that linearization in these languages is not affected by the acces-sibility of individual message entities in the same manner. Such cross-linguistic differences in reliance on word-driven formulation may be due to grammatical dif-ferences: as reviewed above, one set of languages that has, to date, been found to exhibit little or no effects of perceptual accessibility are case-marking languages. Plausibly, case-marking is not readily compatible with a strongly word-driven for-mulation process as it necessitates the early assignment of grammatical functions to arguments. Of course, the strong version of word-driven formulation is not ten-able for longer utterances in languages like English either: English speakers may certainly *begin* utterances with accessible words, but word order in the rest of the utterance must obey certain grammatical constraints. However, the simple fact that there *are* reported differences across languages with respect to effects of percep-tual salience on subject selection suggests that this aspect of sentence formulation may be modulated by language-specific properties.

5.3.2 A View from Verb-Initial Languages

The cross-linguistic studies discussed so far have all shared a common property: they all concern subject-initial languages. Subject-initial languages in fact make up the vast majority of languages of the world. According to the World Atlas of Language Structures, SOV and SVO languages together constitute around 76 % of the world's languages (41 and 35 % respectively). It is therefore unsurprising that, to date, most psycholinguistic studies have centred on this language type. Far rarer, and far more under-studied, are languages whose basic sentences do not start with subjects, or indeed, with nouns of any grammatical function: i.e., verb-initial languages. VSO and VOS languages together make up around 8 % of the world's languages (6 and 2 % respectively). They offer a particularly interesting test case for studying the effects of grammar on sentence formulation: in order to produce a verb-initial sentence, relational information presumably *must* be planned early in order to retrieve an appropriate sentence-initial verb. Comparing the time-course of sentence formulation for verb-initial and subject-initial languages provides a unique means of assessing the extent to which message and sentence formulation may be influenced by a language's basic word order (also see Hwang and Kaiser 2014, for evidence from a verb-final language).

As outlined above, it is of course self-evident that to a certain extent, formula-tion will be affected by linear word order. Eye-tracking studies have already estab-lished empirically, moreover, that *within* English, the order of words in sentences affects the order in which they are encoded linguistically. For example, when pre-paring to produce an active sentence, speakers first fixate the agent (the sentence-initial subject) and then the patient (Griffin and Bock 2000). This suggests that, at least in the context of simple picture description tasks, speakers lexically encode the noun phrases in their sentences in order of mention. Similar left-to-right order effects are observed within noun phrases as well (Janssen et al. 2008). It seems reasonable to assume, then, that *across* languages, word order differences would also affect the order of encoding operations involved in linguistic formulation.

Could word order influence the time-course of *message* formulation? According to top-down models of sentence production, this possibility is in fact ruled out on theoretical grounds: given the principles of information encapsulation and unidirectionality, message preparation should unfold without recourse to information encapsulated at linguistic levels of formulation (Bock and Levelt 1994; Garrett 1980; Levelt 1989). This predicts that message-level ordering decisions should not vary as a consequence of language-specific word order constraints.

As we discussed above, there is already evidence at the level of noun phrase production to suggest, contrary to the predictions of top-down models, that even message-level encoding operations may be affected by word order (Brown-Schmidt and Konopka 2008). It remains an empirical question whether or not we should expect to find such effects in longer utterances. In fact, neither of the two theories of incrementality we have considered so far would predict an effect of word order on message-level processes. According to radical, word-driven incrementality, linearization is controlled by the relative availability of individual elements of a message: the resulting word order of an utterance is thus assumed to be constrained by the properties of the message, and not the other way around. According to structure-driven formulation, speakers begin formulation by generating a 'wholistic' message plan that triggers building of a structural sentence plan and then word retrieval. In Griffin and Bock's (2000) version of this theory, the initial phase of message formulation ('gist apprehension') is assumed to be isolated from subsequent linguistic processes. Thus, the time-course of message formulation itself would not be predicted to vary as a consequence of the linear word order of the target utterance.

5.3.3 Tzeltal

To address this question, Norcliffe et al. (in press) conducted an eye-tracked picture description task in Tzeltal, a Mayan language spoken in Mexico by over 400,000 speakers (Polian 2013). Tzeltal's basic word order is VOS. The language also optionally permits SVO word order, thus allowing a within-language contrast of how sentence formulation might vary as a consequence of the linear position of subjects and verbs. For a direct comparison with an SVO language, the same experiment was also carried out with speakers of Dutch. The methodology was modelled on previous picture description studies (Griffin and Bock 2000; Konopka and Meyer 2014): speakers described pictures of simple transitive events involving familiar actions and characters while their speech and gaze were tracked.

Speakers described simple pictured events (e.g., a woman chasing a chicken) eliciting transitive descriptions, of the type exemplified below. [1] shows an example sentence with VOS word order, and [2] shows the alternative SVO word order (the inflected verb stem, together with the preceding aspect marker, is underlined in both examples):

[1] ya̲ ̲ ̲s-nuts-ø me'mut te ants=e
INC[3] 3S.ERG-chase-3S.ABS chicken the woman=CL
"The woman is chasing a chicken"
(VERB-OBJECT-SUBJECT)

[2] te ants=e ya̲ ̲ ̲s-nuts-ø me'mut
the woman=CL INC 3S.ERG-chase-3S.ABS chicken
"The woman is chasing a chicken"
(SUBJECT–VERB–OBJECT)

We hypothesised that if word order mediated the relationship between the uptake of visual information in an event and the formulation of a description of that event, then early verb placement would require earlier encoding of relational information. The degree to which speakers engage in encoding of relational information can be assessed in terms of patterns of *divergence* or *convergence* of fixations to event characters (agents and patients) before speech onset: while encoding of individual characters at the outset of formulation is reflected in preferential and sustained fixations on a single character (see Gleitman et al. 2007), relational encoding should be indexed by distributed fixations *between* the two characters (as relational information is presumably 'distributed' between characters in an event; see Griffin and Bock 2000).

Importantly, the aim was to test how early an effect of word order would arise. If formulation is modulated by linguistic structure from the outset of formulation, then gaze patterns in verb-initial and subject-initial sentences should reflect word order differences immediately after picture onset (0–400 ms). If, by contrast, word order does not influence early formulation, then word order should only shape the distribution of fixations after 400 ms, that is, in time windows associated primarily with linguistic encoding.

The results supported the first possibility, both within Tzeltal and in comparisons between Tzeltal and Dutch: time-course analyses revealed effects of verb placement on the time-course of formulation from the earliest time-windows until articulation. In both Tzeltal and in Dutch, subject-initial sentences were formulated in a similar way to English sentences with the same word order (Gleitman et al. 2007; Griffin and Bock 2000; Kuchinsky and Bock 2010): formulation began with a rapid divergence of fixations to the two characters immediately after picture onset, and speakers continued fixating the first-mentioned character until speech onset. This cross-linguistic similarity in the formulation of subject-initial

---

[3]The following abbreviations are used: INC = incompletive aspect, 3S = third person singular, ERG = ergative, ABS = absolutive, CL = clitic.

sentences demonstrates that when the linear order of words in event descriptions is the same across languages, so is the time-course of formulation. The formulation of Tzeltal verb-initial sentences was markedly different: speakers distributed their gaze between agents and patients across a very broad window before speech onset. Formulation of active sentences began with a short-lived spike of fixations to the agent within 300 ms of picture onset and was followed by a convergence of fixations between agents and patients until speech onset. Formulation of passive sentences showed a similar pattern (although speakers generally preferred fixating the agent over the patient, consistent with the robust finding that speakers generally attend to agents more than patients; see Cohn and Paczynski 2013, for a review).

Taken together, these results demonstrate that from a very early stage of formulation, the word order that was under production strongly influenced how speakers constructed their sentences online. This suggests that, very rapidly after picture onset, speakers are able to generate a rudimentary structural plan and this plan can then guide subsequent conceptual and linguistic encoding operations. Supporting the conclusion of fast message-level encoding, a number of recent studies have demonstrated that very brief presentations (40–300 ms) of event pictures are in fact sufficient for speakers to identify event categories, as well as the role and identity of characters in the event (Dobel et al. 2007; Hafri et al. 2013). Identification of such information is presumably sufficient to allow for the generation of a conceptual and linguistic structural frame, which can direct the eye to efficiently sample information from the scene as the structure calls for it. Such tight parallels between fixation patterns and linguistic structure from the earliest stages of conceptual formulation, suggest, ultimately, that there may be no strict separation between processes related to conceptualization and those related to linguistic formulation.

5.3.4 Tagalog

An interesting question is whether the nature of early relational encoding for verb-initial structures also differs across languages as a function of the properties of verbs themselves. In Tzeltal, the extensive prioritising of early relational encoding may be driven not only by the verb's placement, but also by its complex morphology, which specifies information about both participants in the event. Further evidence supporting the possibility that verbal morphology can affect the early stages of formulation in verb-initial languages comes from Tagalog, an Austronesian language spoken in the Philippines by 23 million speakers.

The preferred word order for transitive sentences in Tagalog is also verb-initial. Interestingly, Tagalog requires marking the semantic role of one of the arguments (the privileged syntactic argument, or PSA) on the verb. This is illustrated in the examples below (two sentences describing an event where a child is kicking a ball). In [3], the PSA (marked with the prefix *ang*) is the actor (the agent in the event), so the verb takes 'actor voice' (AV) marking. In [4], where the PSA is the undergoer (the patient), the verb takes 'undergoer voice' (UV) marking. The order of postverbal arguments is not fixed, thus either the PSA or the non-PSA argument may occur directly after the verb (here we only show examples with the PSA in final position):

[3] s<um>isipa   ng=bola   ang=bata
    <AV>kick[4]   NPSA=ball   PSA=child
    predicate   undergoer   actor
    "The child kicks the ball."

[4] s<in>ispa   ng=bata   ang=bola
    <UV>kick   NPSA=child   PSA=ball
    predicate   actor   undergoer
    "The child kicks the ball."

From the perspective of formulation, this system of verbal marking implies that speakers must engage in fairly extensive encoding of relational information early in the formulation process. Besides having to select a suitable verb to begin producing a sentence (as in Tzeltal), Tagolog speakers must make a commitment to treat one of the arguments of the verb as the PSA. Crucially, they must do this at the outset of formulation, even though they do not need to encode the PSA character itself linguistically and produce it until after they have produced the verb (i.e., typically after speech onset).

Sauppe et al. (2013) tested whether this grammatical requirement results in different gaze patterns during formulation of sentences that mark either the agent or the patient in the event as the PSA. Tagalog speakers performed an eye-tracked picture description task similar to the tasks described above in English, Dutch, and Tzeltal. Comparisons of fixation patterns to agents and patients across different sentence types showed that speakers briefly fixated the PSA character within an early time window (0–600 ms) and then fixated the two characters in the order of mention. As in other languages, fixations in the early time window can be seen as reflecting processes involved in the apprehension of the gist of the to-be-described event and generation of a structural framework, and fixations in later time windows index the order of lexical retrieval operations. Thus an effect of PSA marking on early eye movements suggests an early effect of linguistic structure on formulation (specifically, on processes at the interface of message formulation and linguistic encoding).

5.4 Conclusion

Production research carried out in the last several decades has shown that message and sentence formulation proceed incrementally. Importantly, however, it has recently become obvious that the timecourse of incremental message and sentence

---

[4]The following abbreviations are used: AV = actor voice, NPSA = non-privileged syntactic argument, PSA = privileged syntactic argument, UV = undergoer voice.

formulation is relatively flexible. While flexibility can be observed *within* languages under different conditions, the most striking demonstrations of flexibility are arguably provided by cross-linguistic comparisons. In this respect, the studies reviewed in this chapter have shown, first, that incrementality is a general principle of production that applies cross-linguistically and, second, that incremental encoding can be controlled by those aspects of the language that are responsible for linearization—i.e., grammar. In short, differences in language-specific grammatical constraints on word order result in differences in the order of encoding operations performed to produce grammatically correct utterances. These effects are observed in utterances ranging from simple noun phrases, which express relatively short messages, to full sentences, which can convey a wider range of complex concepts and relations.

As noted, most of the support for these conclusions comes from eye-tracking studies. The value of this methodology is that eye movements 'illustrate' incrementality in ways that other dependent measures cannot: speakers look at the referents they will describe, so eye movements can 'track' the incremental assembly of messages and sentences in real time. Crucially, the relationship between *looking* and *speaking* appears to be constant (or stable) across languages: speakers of different languages look at referents in a display in the order in which they will mention them (there is, quite strikingly, not yet any documented exception to this pattern). The stability of this relationship allows interpretations of differences in fixation patterns during sentence production in different languages in terms of underlying cross-linguistic differences in the time-course of encoding proper.

As such, eye-tracking as a methodology has provided important insight into a number of questions relevant for formulation. First, eye movements can reveal aspects of language that matter for formulation. The results show that cross-linguistic differences at both syntactic and morphosyntactic levels influence the time-course of formulation. Examples include syntactic features such as verb placement (as shown in Tzeltal) as well as morphosyntactic features such as language-specific agreement-marking on verbs (as shown in Tagalog). Second, eye movements can reveal *when* a particular linguistic feature influences formulation. Again, the results show that the timing of encoding depends on linear order: speakers prioritise encoding of the information that must be expressed next in the sentence shortly before it must be articulated.

The significance of cross-linguistic differences for theories of formulation depends on what *type* of information the target language requires speakers to express early on in a sentence. As described, an important contribution of eye-tracking to studies of formulation concerns the theoretical distinction between word-driven and structure-driven formulation. Since eye movements can be influenced both by lower-level factors like salience and accessibility (people look at objects or referents that attract their attention) and by higher-level factors like communicative goals (people look at objects or referents that they want to say something about), eye-tracking provides some of the most detailed data needed to distinguish between accounts assuming lexical guidance and accounts assuming structural guidance in formulation. Eye movements thus reveal whether speakers talk about referents that they happen to fixate first in a display or whether speakers look at referents in a display in a goal-directed fashion—or, for present purposes, in a manner reflecting guidance from a linguistic framework. The results from numerous studies converge on a similar conclusion: language, or more specifically linguistic structure, can exert a strong influence on what speakers encode with priority at various points during formulation. If the information that receives priority is character-specific information (e.g., the subject of a sentence), the time-course of encoding resembles word-driven formulation; if languages require expressing relational information early on (e.g., the sentence verb or agreement marking on the verb), the time-course of encoding shows evidence of early relational encoding. Thus languages may inherently differ in the extent to which they 'allow' word-driven or structure-driven formulation.

At the same time, we note that these conclusions are based on a relatively small set of cross-linguistic comparisons. In principle, there are also other theoretical possibilities to consider, e.g. encoding patterns that lie somewhere between word-driven and structure-driven formulation. There may be as many different ways of assembling sentences incrementally as there are language-specific instantiations of linear ordering and dependency relations. Language-specific grammatical constraints may apply to encoding at different levels in the production system: some may have to do with higher-level conceptual groupings, while other may apply to smaller, local dependencies. As in the case of most experimental methods, eye-tracking has some limitations (see Irwin 2004) which may or may not make it suitable to study some of these fine-grained distinctions (the first of these limitations is that, of course, we have to use visual stimuli to elicit speech spontaneously). Nevertheless, there are still numerous targeted comparisons of individual language contrasts that can plausibly be addressed with this methodology.

With the advent of portable eye-trackers, eye-tracking research is no longer restricted to laboratories on university campuses. We now have the means to conduct eye-tracking studies in the field, with different groups of speakers and languages. The value of visual-world eye-tracking as a 'field-friendly' method has been demonstrated already through its successful application in a small, but diverse sample of languages and cultures (e.g. Huettig et al. 2011; Mishra et al. 2012; Norcliffe et al. in press; Sauppe et al. 2013). For language production research, this is an important advancement. It allows us to extend the typological base of vision-based research, in order to assess the extent to which our current models of formulation can adequately allow for language-specific instantiations of general principles. Current research has, of course, only scraped the surface of the astonishing range of linguistic diversity exhibited by the world's languages (Evans and Levinson 2009), so this remains an exciting empirical question.

References

Arnold, J. E., Wasow, T., Losongco, T., & Ginstrom, R. (2000). Heaviness vs. Newness: The effects of structural complexity and discourse status on constituent ordering. *Language, 76*, 28–55.

Bock, J. K., & Warren, R. K. (1985). Conceptual accessibility and syntactic structure in sentence formulation. *Cognition, 21*, 47–67.

Bock, J. K., Irwin, D. E., & Davidson, D. J. J. (2004). Putting first things first. In F. Ferreira & M. Henderson (Eds.), *The integration of language, vision, and action: Eye movements and the visual world* (pp. 249–278). New York: Psychology Press.

Bock, J. K., Dell, G. S., Chang, F., & Onishi, K. H. (2007). Persistent structural priming from language comprehension to language production. *Cognition, 104*, 437–458.

Bock, K., & Griffin, Z. M. (2000). The persistence of structural priming: Transient activation or implicit learning? *Journal of Experimental Psychology: General, 129*, 177–192.

Bock, K., & Levelt, W. J. M. (1994). Language production: Grammatical encoding. In M. A. Gernsbacher (Ed.),*Handbook of Psycholinguistics* (pp. 945–984). London: Academic Press.

Bock, K., Loebell, H., & Morey, R. (1992). From conceptual roles to structural relations: Bridging the syntactic cleft. *Psychological Review, 99*, 150–171.

Branigan, H. P., & Feleki, E. (1999). Conceptual accessibility and serial order in Greek speech production. *Proceedings of the 21st Cognitive Science Society Conference*. Vancouver.

Brown-Schmidt, S., & Konopka, A. E. (2008). Little houses and casas pequeñas: Message formulation and syntactic form in unscripted speech with speakers of English and Spanish. *Cognition, 109*, 274–280.

Caramazza, A., Miozzo, M., Costa, A., Schiller, N., & Alario, F.-X. (2001a). The gender congruity effect: Evidence from Spanish and Catalan. *Language and Cognitive Processes, 14*, 381–391.

Caramazza, A., Miozzo, M., Costa, A., Schiller, N., & Alario, F.-X. (2001b). A cross-linguistic investigation of determiner production. In E. Dupoux (Ed.), *Language, brain and cognitive development: Essays in Honor of Jacques Mehler* (pp. 209–226). Cambridge, MA: MIT Press.

Chang, F., Dell, G. S., & Bock, J. K. (2006). Becoming syntactic. *Psychological Review, 113*, 234–272.

Christianson, K., & Ferreira, F. (2005). Conceptual accessibility and sentence production in a free word order language (Odawa). *Cognition, 98*, 105–135.

Cohn, N., & Paczynski, M. (2013). Prediction, events, and the advantage of Agents: The processing of semantic roles in visual narrative. *Cognitive Psychology, 67*, 73–97.

Costa, A., Sebastian-Galles, N., Miozzo, M., & Caramazza, A. (1999). The gender congruity effect: Evidence from Spanish and Catalan. *Language and Cognitive Processes, 14*, 381–391.

Cutler, A. (1985). Cross-language psycholinguistics. *Linguistics, 23*, 659–667.

Cutler, A., Mehler, H., Norris, D. G., & Segui, J. (1983). A language-specific comprehension strategy. *Nature, 204*, 159–160.

Cutler, A., Mehler, J., Norris, D., & Segui, J. (1986). The syllable's differing role in the segmentation of French and English. *Journal of Memory and Language, 25*, 385–400.

Cutler, A., Mehler, J., Norris, D., & Segui, J. (1989). Limits on bilingualism. *Nature, 340*, 229–230.

Dobel, C., Gumnior, H., Bölte, J., & Zwitserlood, P. (2007). Describing scenes hardly scene. *Acta Psychologica, 125*, 129–143.

Evans, N., & Levinson, S. C. (2009). The myth of language universals: Language diversity and its importance for cognitive science. *Behavioral and Brain Sciences, 32*(5), 429–492.

Ferreira, F., & Swets, B. (2002). How incremental is language production? Evidence from the production of utterances requiring the computation of arithmetic sums. *Journal of Memory and Language, 46*, 57–84.

Ferreira, V. S., & Yoshita, H. (2003). Given-new ordering effects on the production of scrambled sentences in Japanese. *Journal of Psycholinguistic Research, 32*, 669–692.

Fodor, J. A., Bever, T. G., & Garrett, M. F. (1974). *The psychology of language*. New York: McGraw-Hill.

Garrett, M. F. (1980). Levels of processing in sentence production. In B. Butterworth (Ed.), *Language production* (Vol. 1). London: Academic Press.

Gennari, S. P., Mirković, J., & MacDonald, M. C. (2012). Animacy and competition in relative clause production: A cross-linguistic investigation. *Cognitive Psychology, 65*, 141–176.

Gleitman, L. R., January, D., Nappa, R., & Trueswell, J. C. (2007). On the give and take between event apprehension and utterance formulation. *Journal of Memory and Language, 57*, 544–569.

Glucksberg, S., & Danks, J. H. (1975). *Experimental psycholinguistics: An introduction*. Hillsdale, N. J.: Erlbaum.

Griffin, Z. M. (2004). Why look? Reasons for eye movements related to language production. In J. Henderson & F. Ferreira, (Eds.), *The integration of language, vision, and action: Eye movements and the visual world* (pp. 213–247). New York: Taylor and Francis.

Griffin, Z. M., & Bock, K. (2000). What the eyes say about speaking. *Psychological Science, 11*, 274–279.

Hafri, A., Papafragou, A., & Trueswell, J. C. (2013). Getting the gist of events: Recognition of two-participant actions from brief displays. *Journal of Experiment Psychology: General, 142*, 880–905.

Henderson, J. M., & Ferreira, F. (Eds.). (2004). *The interface of language, vision, and action: Eye movements and the visual world.* New York: Psychology Press.

Huettig, F., Singh, N., & Mishra, R. K. (2011). Language-mediated visual orienting behavior in low and high literates. *Frontiers in Psychology, 2*, 285.

Hwang, H., & Kaiser, E. (2009). *The effects of lexical vs. perceptual primes on sentence production in Korean: An on-line investigation of event apprehension and sentence formulation.* Paper presented at the 22nd CUNY Conference on Human Sentence Processing, Davis, CA.

Hwang, H., & Kaiser, E. (2014). The role of the verb in grammatical function assignment in English and Korean. *Journal of Experimental Psychology: Learning, Memory and Cognition.* June 2 (Epub ahead of print).

Ibbotson, P., Lieven, E., & Tomasello, M. (2013). The attention-grammar interface: Eye-gaze cues structural choice in children and adults. *Cognitive Linguistics, 24*.

Irwin, D. E. (2004). Fixation location and fixation duration as indices of cognitive processing. In J. M. Henderson & F. Ferreira (Eds.), *The interface of language, vision, and action: Eye movements and the visual world* (pp. 105–133). New York, NY: Psychology Press.

Jaeger, T. F., & Norcliffe, E. (2009). The cross-linguistic study of sentence production. *Language and Linguistic Compass, 3*(4), 866–887.

Jaeger, T. F. & Snider, N. (2013) Alignment as a consequence of expectation adaptation: Syntactic priming is affected by the prime's prediction error given both prior and recent experience. *Cognition, 127*, 57–83.

Janssen, N., Alario, F.-X., & Caramazza, A. (2008). A word-order constraint on phonological activation. *Psychological Science, 19*, 216–220.

Kempen, G., & Harbusch, K. (2004). A Corpus study into word order variation in German subordinate clauses: Animacy affects linearization independently of grammatical function assignment. In T. Pechmann (Ed.), *Language Production* (pp. 173–181). Berlin: Mouton.

Kempen, G., & Hoenkamp, E. (1987). An incremental procedural grammar for sentence formulation. *Cognitive Science, 11*, 201–258.

Konopka, A. E. (2012). Planning ahead: How recent experience with structures and words changes the scope of linguistic planning. *Journal of Memory and Language, 66*, 143–162.

Konopka, A. E., & Meyer, A. S. (2014). Priming sentence planning. *Cognitive Psychology, 73*, 1–40.

Kuchinsky, S. E., & Bock, K. (2010). *From seeing to saying: Perceiving, planning, producing.* Paper presented at the 23rd meeting of the CUNY Human Sentence Processing Conference, New York, NY.

Lee, E. K., Brown-Schmidt, S., & Watson, D. W. (2013). Ways of looking ahead: Incrementality in language production. *Cognition, 129*, 544–562.

Levelt, W. J. M. (1989). *Speaking: From intention to articulation.* Cambridge, MA: MIT Press.

MacDonald, M. C. (2013). How language production shapes language form and comprehension. *Frontiers in Psychology, 4*, 1–16.

MacWhinney, B. (1977). Starting points. *Language, 53*, 152–168.

MacWhinney, B., & Bates, E. A. (1978). Sentential devices for conveying givenness and newness: A cross-cultural developmental study. *Journal of Verbal Learning and Verbal Behavior, 17*, 539–558.

McDonald, J. L., Bock, K., & Kelly, M. H. (1993). Word and world order: Semantic, phonological, and metrical determinants of serial position. *Cognitive Psychology, 25*, 188–230.

Mehler, J., Dommergues, J. Y., Frauenfelder, U., & Segui, J. (1981). The syllable's role in speech segmentation. *Journal of Verbal Learning and Verbal Behavior, 20*, 298–305.

Mehler, J., Dupoux, E., Nazzi, T., & Dehaene-Lambertz, G. (1996). Coping with linguistic diversity: The infant's viewpoint. In J. L. Morgan & K. Demuth, et al. (Eds.), *Signal to syntax: Bootstrapping from speech to grammar in early acquisition* (pp. 101–116). Mahwah, NJ: Lawrence Erlbaum Associates, Inc.

Mehler, J., Sebastian, N., Altmann, G., Dupoux, E., Christophe, A., & Pallier, C. (1993). Understanding compressed sentences: The role of rhythm and meaning. In P. Tallal, A. M. Galaburda et al. (Eds.), *Temporal information processing in the nervous system: Special reference to dyslexia and dysphasia. Annals of the New York Academy of Sciences* (Vol. 682, pp. 272–282). New York, NY: New York Academy of Sciences.

Meyer, A. S., Sleiderink, A. M., & Levelt, W. J. M. (1998). Viewing and naming objects: Eye movements during noun phrase production. *Cognition, 66*, B25–B33.

Miozzo, M., & Caramazza, A. (1999). The selection of lexical-syntactic features in noun phrase production: Evidence from the picture-word interference paradigm. *Journal of Experimental Psychology: Learning, Memory, and Cognition, 25*, 907–922.

Mishra, R. K., Singh, N., Pandey, A., & Huettig, F. (2012). Spoken language-mediated anticipatory eye movements are modulated by reading ability: Evidence from Indian low and high literates. *Journal of Eye Movement Research, 5*(1), 3, 1–10.

Myachykov, A., & Tomlin, R. S. (2008). Perceptual priming and structural choice in Russian sentence production. *Journal of Cognitive Science, 6*, 31–48.

Myachykov, A., Garrod, S., & Scheepers, C. (2010). Perceptual priming of structural choice during english and finnish sentence production. In R. K. Mishra & N. Srinivasan (Eds.), *Language & cognition: State of the art* (pp. 54–72). Munich: Lincom Europa.

Myachykov, A., Thompson, D., Scheepers, C., & Garrod, S. (2011). Visual attention and structural choice in sentence production across languages. *Language and Linguistic Compass, 5*, 95–107.

Norcliffe, E., Konopka, A. E., Brown, P., & Levinson S. C. (in press). Word order affects the time-course of sentence formulation in Tzeltal. *Language, Cognition, and Neuroscience.*

Paul, H. (1886/1970). The sentence as the expression of the combination of several ideas. In A. L. Blumenthal (Ed. & Trans.), Language and psychology: Historical aspects of psycholinguistics (pp. 34–37). New York: Wiley.

Polian, G. (2013). *Gramática del tseltal de Oxchuc*. Mexico, D.F.: Centro de Investigaciones y Estudios Superiores en Antropología Social.

Sauppe, S., Norcliffe, E., Konopka, A. E., Van Valin, R. D. Jr., & Levinson, S. C. (2013). Dependencies first: Eye-tracking evidence from sentence production in Tagalog. In: M. Knauff, M. Pauen, N. Sebanz, & E. Wachsmuth (Eds.), *Proceedings of the 35th annual meeting of the Cognitive Science Society* (pp. 1265–1270). Austin, Texas: Cognitive Science Society.

Schiller, N., & Caramazza, A. (2003). Grammatical feature selection in noun phrase production: Evidence from German and Dutch. *Journal of Memory and Language, 48*, 169–194.

Schriefers, H. (1993). Syntactic processes in the production of noun phrases. *Journal of Experimental Psychology: Learning, Memory, and Cognition, 19*, 841–850.

Swets, B., Jacovina, M. E., & Gerrig, R. J. (2008). *Individual differences in the planning scope of language production.* Paper presented at the 49th meeting of the Psychonomic Society, Chicago, IL (November).

Tanaka, M. N., Branigan, H. P., McLean, J. F., & Pickering, M. J. (2011). Conceptual influences on word order and voice in sentence production: Evidence from Japanese. *Journal of Memory and Language, 65*, 318–330.

Tomlin, R. (1995). Focal attention, voice, and word order: An experimental, cross-linguistic study. In M. Noonan & P. Downing (Eds.), *Word order in discourse* (pp. 521–558). Amsterdam: John Benjamins.

Tomlin, R. (1997). Mapping conceptual representations into linguistic representations: the role of attention in grammar. In J. Nuyts & E. Pederson (Eds.), *Language and conceptualization* (pp. 162–189). Cambridge: Cambridge University Press.

Van de Velde, M., Meyer, A. S., & Konopka, A. E. (2014). Message formulation and structural assembly: Describing "easy" and "hard" events with preferred and dispreferred structures. *Journal of Memory and Language, 71*, 124–144.

Wagner, V., Jescheniak, J. D., & Schriefers, H. (2010). On the flexibility of grammatical advance planning during sentence production: Effects of cognitive load on multiple lexical access. *Journal of Experiment Psychology: Learning, Memory, and Cognition, 36*, 423–440.

Wundt, W. (1900). *Völkerpsychologie: Eine Untersuchung der Entwicklungsgesetze von Sprache, Mythus und Sitte* (Vol. 1). *Die Sprache* [Language]. Leipzig: Kroner-Engelmann.

Part II
Attention and Vision in Reading

Chapter 6
Capturing Reading Processes in Connected Texts with Eye Movements and a Letter Detection Task

Jean Saint-Aubin and Raymond M. Klein

It is widely acknowledged that investigating reading processes is quite a challenge. Part of the challenge comes from the necessity of using experimental paradigms that must involve a trade-off between avoiding disturbing normal reading processes and collecting information about specific decisions made by the reader (Smith and Pattison 1982). As suggested by Smith and Pattison, at one end of the continuum, eye movement monitoring is a relatively unintrusive technique, but by itself it may not provide all the information required for testing theories. At the other end of the continuum, the lexical decision task provides elegant evidence about the specific information processes by a reader, but the application of the findings to normal reading of continuous texts has been called into question (see, e.g., Balota and Chumbley 1984; Hyönä et al. 2002; Kambe 2004; Pollatsek and Hyönä 2005; Rayner 1999).

The letter detection task as a means of investigating reading processes originates from the pioneer work of Corcoran (1966). In the founding article, Corcoran simply asked participants to read a magazine article and to circle all occurrences of the letter *e*. He found that readers missed more *e*s in *the* than in any other words. While Corcoran must be credited for discovering that, in connected texts, letter detection accuracy varies as a function of word status, Read (1983) must get credit for popularising the effect by giving it almost the status of a visual illusion with this, now famous, sentence in which readers must find all instances of the letter *f*: "FINISHED FILES ARE THE RESULT OF YEARS OF SCIENTIFIC STUDY COMBINED WITH THE EXPERIENCE OF MANY YEARS". Even though there

J. Saint-Aubin (✉)
Université de Moncton, Moncton, Canada
e-mail: jean.saint-aubin@umoncton.ca

R.M. Klein
Dalhousie University, Halifax, Canada

© Springer India 2015
R.K. Mishra et al. (eds.), *Attention and Vision in Language Processing*, DOI 10.1007/978-81-322-2443-3_6

are six occurrences of the letter *f*, between 85 and 90 % of adult readers detect only three *f*s at their first attempt to read the sentence. In this example, *of* differs from *finished*, *files*, and *scientific* with regards to word frequency, function and length, as well as target letter location and pronunciation. Studies conducted over the last four decades have well established that when controlling for all those possible confounds, readers are more likely to omit the target letter when it is embedded in high- than in low-frequency words (Assink et al. 2003; Greenberg et al. 1998; Healy 1976; Minkoff and Raney 2000), and in function than in content words (Koriat and Greenberg 1991; Koriat et al. 1991; Saint-Aubin and Poirier 1997). This dual effect of word function and word frequency on omission rate has been coined the *missing-letter effect*. The missing-letter effect nicely shows that the inclusion of a letter detection task while reading allows the investigator to collect information about processing of individual words similar to the lexical decision task, but in contrast the information is collected during reading of connected text.

The relationship between the missing-letter effect and eye movements was raised very early in the literature. In fact, Corcoran (1966) suggested that omissions might be a by-product of eye movements by proposing that the higher omission rate for the target letter embedded in *the* arises "because 'the' is a highly redundant word, which may be 'taken for granted' and thus not scanned" (p. 658). This hypothesis is well grounded in the eye movement literature revealing that function words are more likely to be skipped in reading than content words of similar length (Carpenter and Just 1983; Chamberland et al. 2013; Gautier et al. 2000; O'Regan 1979).

The hypothesis that the missing-letter effect is caused by this differential rate of skipping is based on the assumption that the inclusion of a letter detection requirement does not prevent readers from skipping function words more frequently than content words. This assumption has been challenged in the field of reading (see, e.g., Rayner and Pollatsek 1989). We will return, in the next section, to the question of whether skipping causes the missing-letter effect, but first it is important to address this challenge.

The critical evidence cited against independence of eye movements from the letter detection task is that different patterns of eye movements are observed in visual search and reading tasks. In two studies that are often cited in this context (Rayner and Raney 1996; Spragins et al. 1976), participants are either required to read the text for comprehension or to search for a predesignated target word. In Rayner and Raney's study, within the text, critical word pairs were inserted. Pair members were matched for length and meaning, but differed on frequency (e.g., *ancient–archaic; sharp–stark*). Eye movements were very different in the two conditions. First, participants were much faster in the search than in the read condition; they made longer and fewer fixations, suggesting that more words were being processed during each fixation. Most importantly, in the reading task, Rayner and Raney found the typical word frequency effect with a higher skip rate for the frequent than for the less frequent pair member. However, this trademark of reading processes was not observed in the search task. Based on those differences, Rayner et al. (2012) concluded that:

Some people might want to argue that results from these different tasks [reading
and searching for a target in a text and reading only] are generalizable to one another.
However, our inclination would be to argue that each involves different strategies and processes on the part of the participant. Thus we might well have a model of proofreading for
misspellings that differs from a model of proofreading (or searching) for a target word [or
letter]. And both types of models would be different from a model of reading in which the
goal is to comprehend the text. (p. 387)

The dissociation between eye movements in pure reading tasks and in pure visual
search tasks is beyond dispute. However, it is important to keep in mind that in the
studies by Rayner and Raney (1996) and Spragins et al. (1976), participants were
asked to scan the text for a target word without also reading it for comprehension.

The research highlighted in this chapter is based on searching for target letters while *reading for comprehension.* The impact of the letter search requirement
on eye movements in a reading task has been investigated in a series of studies
by Inhoff and his colleagues (Greenberg et al. 2006; Inhoff et al. 1993; Vitu et al.
1995). In those experiments, participants read texts for comprehension only or read
it for comprehension while searching for a target letter. At a global level, the pattern
of eye movements is very similar in both reading only and reading and searching
conditions. The distribution of fixation durations, saccade lengths, landing positions
and skipping rates has similar shapes. The main difference being that on average,
fixation durations are longer, saccades are shorter and skipping rate is lower when
the search requirement is added to the reading task. Most importantly, at the local
level, Greenberg et al. (2006) tested the effect of word class and text predictability. They found no interaction between reading conditions (reading only or reading and searching) and word class or text predictability on skipping rate and the
duration of the first fixation. There was however an interaction with gaze and total
durations, but the interaction simply reflects a larger effect of word class and text
predictability when the letter search requirement was added to reading for comprehension. This pattern of results was reproduced by Roy-Charland et al. (2007) who
also tested and found the typical effect of word frequency on eye movements when
readers were searching for a target letter while reading for comprehension.

Put in a nutshell, results of eye movement studies nicely show that although
letter search globally slows down reading speed—by increasing the number and
the duration of fixations—it does not interfere with the oculomotor behaviour as
evidenced by three benchmark effects: word class, word predictability, and word
frequency. Indeed, neuroimaging findings strongly converge with the independence assumption by showing that the pattern of brain activation during reading is
unaffected by adding a searching task (Newman et al. 2013).

6.1 Is the Missing-Letter Effect Caused by Skipping?

Having established the presence of typical eye movements when searching for a
letter while reading, the relationship between reading and searching can be investigated. As mentioned above, very early in the field, it was suggested that the

missing-letter effect is simply a by-product of eye movements (Corcoran 1966; Hadley and Healy 1991). More specifically, under this view, omissions would be due to skips. According to the parafoveal processing hypothesis, when a word is skipped, it has been identified in the parafovea based on its global shape. Because of the lower resolution in the parafovea, it would not be possible to process individual letters. This assumption was subsequently integrated to the Guidance-Organisation (GO) model of the missing-letter effect (Greenberg et al. 2004). More specifically, within the GO model, it is assumed that "whole-word identification of function words is normally achieved when they are in the parafovea, where visual acuity is too low to afford letter-by-letter analysis but can still support fast access to whole-word unitized representations" (p. 430).

In 2001, Saint-Aubin and Klein conducted the first experiments directly testing the parafoveal processing hypothesis. In one experiment, they monitored eye movements while readers searched for a target letter. In this study, participants read one text while searching for the target letter *t* which was embedded in *the* and in three-letter control content words beginning with *t* (e.g., *tax, tea, toe, tie, ton*) and they read another text while searching for the letter *f* which was embedded in the function word *for* and in three-letter control content words beginning with an *f* (e.g., *fit, fan, fun, fat, fog*). Results first revealed *the-skipping effect* discovered and labelled by O'Regan (1979) with 15 % fewer fixations on *the* than on the control content words. Results also showed that the-skipping effect is not limited to the function word *the*. In effect, there were 20 % more skips on the function word *for* than on the control content words. As required by proponents of the parafoveal processing hypothesis, readers missed more target letters when they were embedded in a skipped than in a fixated word (Hadley and Healy 1991). However, results showed equally strongly that omissions were not simply a by-product of eye movements. In effect, when the subset of fixated and skipped words were analysed separately, in each subset there were more omissions for function than for content words (see also, Roy-Charland et al. 2007, 2009).

As Saint-Aubin and Klein (2001) pointed out, a simple alternative to the parafoveal processing hypothesis is to assume that both eye movements and the missing-letter effect are driven by the same cognitive processes. In order to test this possibility participants read a text for comprehension with a rapid serial visual presentation procedure (RSVP). With an RSVP procedure, words appear one at a time at the centre of the computer screen for a fixed amount of time. As shown in 1980 by Potter, Kroll, and Harris not only reading is possible with an RSVP procedure, but it could even be more efficient than normal reading. Obviously the RSVP procedure distorts the usual pattern of eye movements, by, among other things, preventing parafoveal processing and imposing the same viewing time for all words. In addition, with an RSVP procedure, participants fixate each word in the passage for its entire presentation duration, be it a function or a content word (Saint-Aubin et al. 2010). It is worth noting that a large missing-letter effect has been consistently observed (Saint-Aubin and Klein 2001; Saint-Aubin et al. 2003, 2010) so long as presentation durations are close to those usually seen during reading (varying from 200 to 350 ms), but not with longer presentation durations

(500 ms and more) for which a ceiling effect is obtained with virtually no omission (Healy et al. 1987). Consequently, the missing-letter effect cannot be considered merely a by-product of skipping or parafoveal preview.

In order to further explore the relationship between the missing-letter effect and eye movements, Saint-Aubin and Klein (2004) compared the pattern of omissions obtained with the paper and pencil and the RSVP procedure. As a reminder, contrary to the RSVP procedure, the typical pattern of eye movements is available with the paper and pencil procedure. Using exactly the same text with both procedures, results revealed that the size of the missing-letter effect was virtually the same with a difference in omissions of 16.5 % between function and content words with the paper and pencil procedure and of 17 % with the RSVP procedure. Saint-Aubin and Klein further investigated the relationship between both procedures with item-based correlations. Results revealed correlations between omissions with the paper and pencil and the RSVP procedures as high as the reliability estimate of each procedure. Once corrected for attenuation due to the reliability of each procedure, the correlation was nearly perfect with a value of 0.95.

6.2 The Missing-Letter Effect Is Clearly Not Caused by Skipping

The studies reviewed, so far, nicely show that the letter detection task does not distort the typical pattern of eye movements in reading connected texts. In addition, results with the RSVP procedure further suggest that the missing-letter effect is not a by-product of eye movements. Considered together, these findings pave the way to combining both procedures for generating new data. The power of combining both procedures is illustrated below with two very different research questions.

6.3 Assessing the Effect of Letter Position

It is well acknowledged that letter identification is mandatory for word reading, even for the five most common three-letter English words (Pelli et al. 2003). While the importance of letters for word identification is acknowledged, their relative importance as a function of their position within the word is debated. This debate reached the general public when at the fall of 2003, the following email was widely circulated:

> Aoccdrnig to a rscheearch at Cmabrigde Uinervtisy, it deosn't mttaer in waht oredr the ltteers in a wrod are, the olny iprmoatnt tihng is taht the frist and lsat ltteers be at the rghit pclae. The rset can be a toatl mses and you can sitll raed it wouthit porbelm. Tihs is bcuseae the huamn mnid deos not raed ervey lteter by istlef, but the wrod as a wlohe.

The statement was a hoax as it did not originate from the University of Cambridge. To date, we don't know the real author(s) of this statement, but it nicely illustrates findings showing that the first and last letters of the word play a more important role than interior letters in Roman script (see, e.g., Jordan et al. 2003). However, other studies have shown that only the first letter has a special or critical role (see, e.g., Briihl and Inhoff 1995).

To understand those diverging findings, it is necessary to overview their methodology. Briihl and Inhoff (1995) used an eye-contingent paradigm and manipulated the availability of letters in the parafovea. That is to say, when readers fixated word n, some letters of word $n + 1$ were replaced by xs. The available letters could be the two exterior letters, the first letter or the initial bigram. The presence of the two exterior letters did not produce a larger preview benefit (shorter fixation duration on word $n + 1$) than the presence of the first letter or of the beginning bigram.

Alternatively, with eye monitoring techniques, the impact of letter position can be investigated by assessing the impact of disrupting words' integrity at some letter positions. One way of achieving this degradation is through transposed letters. For instance, White et al. (2008) transposed adjacent letters in some words. The transpositions could involve beginning letters (oslve instead of solve), ending letters (solev instead of solve) or internal letters (sovle or slove instead of solve). Fixation durations of these disrupted words were longer when beginning letters were transposed than when ending letters were transposed, which in turn were longer than when internal letters were transposed. Jordan et al. (2003) also investigated the impact of letter position by degrading selected letters through digital filtering. Their results revealed that degrading exterior letters (first and last) slowed reading rate more than degrading interior letters or degrading only the first two letters.

Despite the creativity of these eye monitoring studies, the question could benefit from the combination of eye monitoring and letter detection. In effect, investigating the impact of letter position with eye monitoring only, either implies manipulating parafoveal preview or words' integrity. In contrast, with a letter detection task, it is possible to assess the importance of letter position without disturbing the integrity of the material being read. Guérard et al. (2012) conducted such a study. As shown in Fig. 6.1, their results demonstrate that irrespective of the distance between the location of the closest fixation that preceded fixation on the critical word and fixation on the critical word, the first letter was better and faster detected than the letter in the middle or last position which did not differ. What is more, in their third experiment, Guérard et al. (2012) included a transposed letter condition. Results reproduced in Fig. 6.2 show that when words were intact, the first letter was better detected than the last letter. However, the effect of letter position was greatly reduced with transposed letters. Consequently, although both initial and final letters assume a special role in word identification, there may be different reasons for the first and last letter special importance.

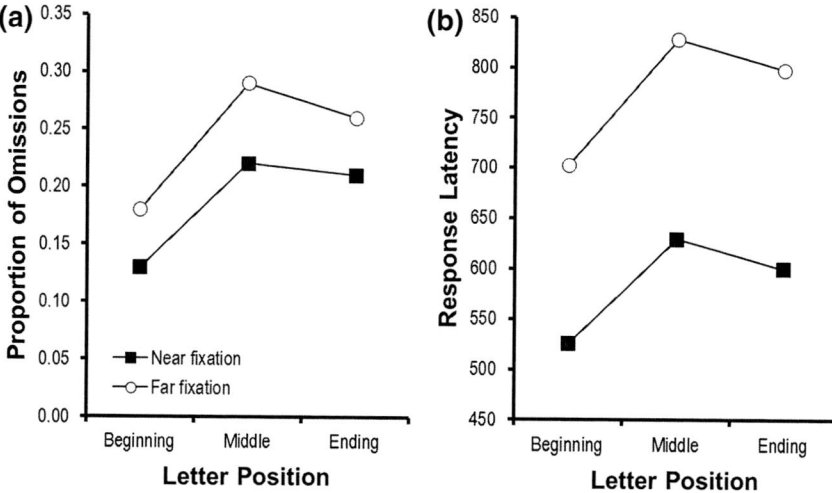

Fig. 6.1 Proportion of omissions (**a**) and response latency (**b**) as a function of letter position within the word and eccentricity of pre-target fixation in Experiment 2 of Guérard et al. (2012)

Fig. 6.2 Proportion of omissions as a function of letter position within the word and writing in Experiment 3 of Guérard et al. (2012). Data from the two texts used in Experiment 3 are combined in the figure, because they produced the same pattern of results

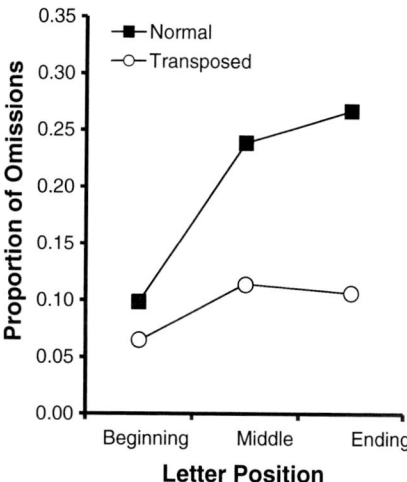

6.4 Parafoveal Postview Processing

The missing-letter effect has also been successfully used to complement eye monitoring for investigating parafoveal postview processing. At each fixation, the available information can be split into three regions as a function of eccentricity from the fixation point: the foveal region, with a radius of one degree centred on fixation, the parafoveal regions extending about five degrees on both sides of fixation, and outside the parafovea, the peripheral region. There has been a lot of work on information processing in the parafovea. However, almost all the work has been carried out in the parafoveal region in the direction of reading and is referred to as the parafoveal preview. Very little is known about parafoveal postview processing, that is information processing in the parafoveal region opposite the direction of reading. Because the studies we describe were conducted in French and English, for which reading proceeds from left to right, we will refer to parafoveal preview as the region to the right of fixation and parafoveal postview as the region to the left of fixation. The type and the amount of information processed in the parafovea to the right of the fixation point is typically investigated by using an eye-contingent paradigm in which the display for word $n + 1$ changes as soon as it is fixated. The impact of parafoveal preview is expressed as the difference in fixation duration between the parafoveal preview conditions.

Parafoveal processing of the word to the left is more difficult to investigate because of the need to prevent both parafoveal processing when the previous word is fixated and fixation on the word itself. Using an eye-contingent procedure, Binder et al. (1999) developed a creative solution to this challenge. In their experiment, once the eyes left the word, a postview display change occurred. More specifically, the word was replaced for only one fixation. In other words, as soon as readers made their next saccade, the original word reappeared. With this procedure, readers could not fixate the word used for the postview change. When the postview word was inconsistent with the presented word, readers made more regressions. This study is very informative about semantic processing in the parafovea to the left of the fixated word, but many questions remain unanswered. The possibility of processing letters in postview is one of them.

Roy-Charland et al. (2012) investigated letter processing in postview by combining the letter detection task with eye movement monitoring techniques. More specifically, as shown in Fig. 6.3, the letters of all words were replaced by *x*s, until the eyes landed on the word itself. If a word was skipped, the letters of the skipped word appeared as soon as the eyes landed on the next word. In addition, readers were asked to detect all instances of a target letter which was embedded in content and function words. Results revealed that readers were able to detect target letters embedded in skipped words, that is to say, in words that were never fixated. This finding is not due to guessing strategies, because false alarms were a rarity, and even among skipped words, readers made more omissions when the target letter was embedded in function than in content words. Because function words are more predictable than content words, a guessing strategy would have produced the opposite pattern of results (Saint-Aubin et al. 2005). The presence of a missing-letter effect among skipped words suggests that letter processing is available in the parafoveal region to the left of the fixated word and that letter processing in this region is sensitive to syntactic factors just as parafoveal processing to the right. This finding nicely extends previous findings using only eye monitoring techniques which showed that readers can extract phonological and semantic information in postview (Binder et al. 1999; Wang et al. 2009).

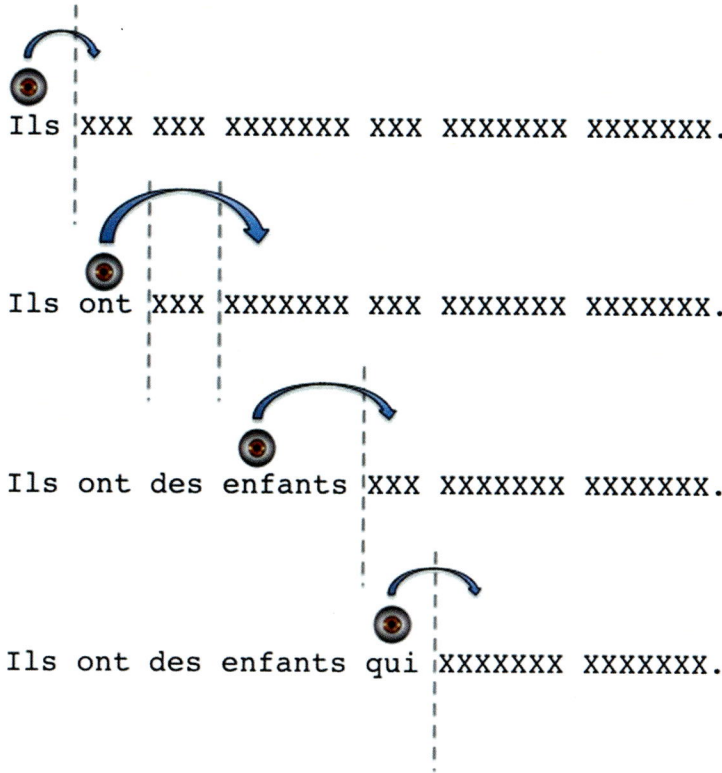

Fig. 6.3 Example of the gaze contingent display procedure in which the critical word *des* is not fixated

6.5 Concluding Remarks

In sum, combining a letter detection task does not distort the pattern of eye movements as long as participants are required to read for comprehension. The higher omission rate for target letters embedded in function than in content words mimics eye movements pattern, but can be observed independently of eye movements. Studies overviewed in this chapter illustrate the added value of combining eye monitoring with letter detection to answer questions that could not be answered otherwise. As such, as suggested by Healy (1994), the letter detection task offers a unique window on the cognitive processes involved in reading.

References

Assink, E. H., Van Well, S., & Knuijt, P. A. (2003). Contrasting effects of age of acquisition in lexical decision and letter detection. *The American Journal of Psychology, 116*, 367–387. doi:10.2307/1423499.

Balota, D. A., & Chumbley, J. I. (1984). Are lexical decisions a good measure of lexical access? The role of word frequency in the neglected decision stage. *Journal of Experimental Psychology: Human Perception and Performance, 10*, 340–357. doi:10.1037/0096-1523.10.3.340.

Binder, K. S., Pollatsek, A., & Rayner, K. (1999). Extraction of information to the left of the fixated word in reading. *Journal of Experimental Psychology: Human Perception and Performance, 25*, 1162–1172. doi:10.1037/0096-1523.25.4.1162.

Briihl, D., & Inhoff, A. (1995). Integrating information across fixations during reading: The use of orthographic bodies and of exterior letters. *Journal of Experimental Psychology. Learning, Memory, and Cognition, 21*, 55–67. doi:10.1037/0278-7393.21.1.55.

Carpenter, P. A., & Just, M. A. (1983). What your eyes do while your mind is reading. In K. Rayner (Ed.), *Eye movements in reading: Perceptual and language processes* (pp. 275–307). New York: Academic Press.

Chamberland, C., Saint-Aubin, J., & Légère, M. (2013). The impact of text repetition on content and function words during reading: Further evidence from eye movements. *Canadian Journal of Experimental Psychology, 67*, 94–99. doi:10.1037/a0028288.

Corcoran, D. W. J. (1966). An acoustic factor in letter cancellation. *Nature, 210*, 658.

Gautier, V., O'Regan, J. K., & Le Gargasson, J. F. (2000). "The-skipping" revisited in French: Programming saccades to skip the article "les". *Vision Research, 40*, 2517–2531.

Greenberg, S. N., Inhoff, A. W., & Weger, U. W. (2006). The impact of letter detection on eye movement patterns during reading: Reconsidering lexical analysis in connected text as a function of task. *Quarterly Journal of Experimental Psychology, 59*, 987–995. doi:10.1080/17470210600654776.

Greenberg, S. N., Koriat, A., & Vellutino, F. R. (1998). Age changes in the missing-letter effect reflect the reader's growing ability to extract the structure from text. *Journal of Experimental Child Psychology, 69*, 175–198. doi:10.1006/jecp.1998.2441.

Greenberg, S. N., Healy, A. F., Koriat, A., & Kreiner, H. (2004). The GO model: A reconsideration of the role of structural units in guiding and organizing text on line. *Psychonomic Bulletin & Review, 11*, 428–433. doi:10.3758/BF03196590.

Guérard, K., Saint-Aubin, J., Poirier, M., & Demetriou, C. (2012). Assessing the influence of letter position in reading normal and transposed texts using a letter detection task. *Canadian Journal of Experimental Psychology, 66*, 227–238. doi:10.1037/a0028494.

Hadley, J. A., & Healy, A. F. (1991). When are reading units larger than the letter? Refinement of the unitization reading model. *Journal of Experimental Psychology. Learning, Memory, and Cognition, 17*, 1062–1073. doi:10.1037/0278-7393.17.6.1062.

Healy, A. F. (1976). Detection errors on the word the: Evidence for reading units larger than letters. *Journal of Experimental Psychology: Human Perception and Performance, 2*, 235–242. doi:10.1037/0096-1523.2.2.235.

Healy, A. F., Oliver, W. L., & McNamara, T. P. (1987). Detecting letters in continuous text: Effects of display size. *Journal of Experimental Psychology: Human Perception and Performance, 13*, 279–290. doi:10.1037/0096-1523.13.2.279.

Healy, A. F. (1994). Letter detection: A window to unitization and other cognitive processes in reading text. *Psychonomic Bulletin & Review, 1*, 333–344.

Hyönä, J., Vainio, S., & Laine, M. (2002). A morphological effect obtains for isolated words but not for words in sentence context. *European Journal of Cognitive Psychology, 14*, 417–433. doi:10.1080/09541440143000131.

Inhoff, A. W., Topolski, R., Vitu, F., & O'Regan, J. (1993). Attention demands during reading and the occurrence of brief (express) fixations. *Perception and Psychophysics, 54*, 814–823.

Jordan, T. R., Thomas, S. M., Patching, G. R., & Scott-Brown, K. C. (2003). Assessing the importance of letter pairs in initial, exterior, and interior positions in reading. *Journal of Experimental Psychology. Learning, Memory, and Cognition, 29*, 883–893. doi:10.1037/0278-7393.29.5.883.

Kambe, G. (2004). Parafoveal processing of prefixed words during eye fixations in reading: Evidence against morphological influences on parafoveal preprocessing. *Perception and Psychophysics, 66*, 279–292. doi:10.3758/BF03194879.

Koriat, A., & Greenberg, S. N. (1991). Syntactic control of letter detection: Evidence from English and Hebrew nonwords. *Journal of Experimental Psychology. Learning, Memory, and Cognition, 17*, 1035–1050. doi:10.1037/0278-7393.17.6.1035.

Koriat, A., Greenberg, S. N., & Goldshmid, Y. (1991). The missing-letter effect in Hebrew: Word frequency or word function? *Journal of Experimental Psychology. Learning, Memory, and Cognition, 17*, 66–80. doi:10.1037/0278-7393.17.1.66.

Minkoff, S. B., & Raney, G. E. (2000). Letter-detection errors in the word the: Word frequency versus syntactic structure. *Scientific Studies of Reading, 4*, 55–76. doi:10.1207/S1532799XSSR0401_5.

Newman, A. J., Kenny, S., Saint-Aubin, J., & Klein, R. M. (2013). Can skilled readers perform a second task in parallel? A functional connectivity MRI study. *Brain and Language, 124*, 84–95. doi:10.1016/j.bandl.2012.11.009.

O'Regan, K. (1979). Saccade size control in reading: Evidence for the linguistic control hypothesis. *Perception and Psychophysics, 25*, 501–509. doi:10.3758/BF03213829.

Pelli, D. G., Farell, B., & Moore, D. C. (2003). The remarkable inefficiency of word recognition. *Nature, 423*, 752–756. doi:10.1038/nature01516.

Pollatsek, A., & Hyönä, J. (2005). The role of semantic transparency in the processing of Finnish compound words. *Language and Cognitive Processes, 20*, 261–290. doi:10.1080/01690960444000098.

Rayner, K. (1999). What have we learned about eye movements during reading? In R. M. Klein & P. A. McMullen (Eds.), *Converging methods for understanding reading and dyslexia* (pp. 23–56). Cambridge: The MIT Press.

Rayner, K., & Pollatsek, A. (1989). *The psychology of reading*. Englewood Cliffs: Prentice Hall.

Rayner, K., Pollatsek, A., Ashby, J., & Clifton, C. R. (2012). *Psychology of reading* (2nd ed.). New York: Psychology Press.

Rayner, K., & Raney, G. E. (1996). Eye movement control in reading and visual search: Effects of word frequency. *Psychonomic Bulletin & Review, 3*, 245–248. doi:10.3758/BF03212426.

Read, J. D. (1983). Detection of Fs in a single statement: The role of phonetic recoding. *Memory & cognition, 11*, 390–399.

Roy-Charland, A., Saint-Aubin, J., Klein, R. M., & Lawrence, M. (2007). Eye movements as direct tests of the GO model for the missing-letter effect. *Perception and Psychophysics, 69*, 324–337.

Roy-Charland, A., Saint-Aubin, J., Klein, R. M., MacLean, G. H., Lalande, A., & Bélanger, A. (2012). Eye movements when reading: The importance of the word to the left of fixation. *Visual Cognition, 20*, 328–355. doi:10.1080/13506285.2012.667457.

Roy-Charland, A., Saint-Aubin, J., Lawrence, M. A., & Klein, R. M. (2009). Solving the chicken-and-egg problem of letter detection and fixation duration in reading. *Attention, Perception, & Psychophysics, 71*, 1553–1562. doi:10.3758/APP.71.7.1553.

Saint-Aubin, J., Kenny, S., & Roy-Charland, A. (2010). The role of eye movements in the missing-letter effect revisited with the rapid serial visual presentation procedure. *Canadian Journal of Experimental Psychology, 64*, 47–52. doi:10.1037/a0016850.

Saint-Aubin, J., & Klein, R. M. (2001). Influence of parafoveal processing on the missing-letter effect. *Journal of Experimental Psychology: Human Perception and Performance, 27*, 318–334. doi:10.1037/0096-1523.27.2.318.

Saint-Aubin, J., & Klein, R. M. (2004). One missing-letter effect: Two methods of assessment. *Canadian Journal of Experimental Psychology, 58*, 61–66. doi:10.1037/h0087440.

Saint-Aubin, J., Klein, R. M., & Landry, T. (2005). Age changes in the missing-letter effect revisited. *Journal of Experimental Child Psychology, 91*, 158–182. doi:10.1016/j.jecp.2005.01.007.

Saint-Aubin, J., Klein, R. M., & Roy-Charland, A. (2003). Direct assessments of the processing time hypothesis for the missing-letter effect. *Journal of Experimental Psychology: Human Perception and Performance, 29*, 1191–1210. doi:10.1037/0096-1523.29.6.1191.

Saint-Aubin, J., & Poirier, M. (1997). The influence of the word function in the missing-letter effect: Further evidence from French. *Memory & Cognition, 25*, 666–676. doi:10.3758 /BF03211308.

Smith, Philip T., & Pattison, H. M. (1982). Models for letter cancellation performance and their implications for models of reading. *The Quarterly Journal of Experimental Psychology, 34A*, 95–116.

Spragins, A. B., Lefton, L. A., & Fisher, D. F. (1976). Eye movements while reading and searching spatially transformed text: A developmental examination. *Memory & Cognition, 4*, 36–42. doi:10.3758/BF03213252.

Vitu, F., O'Regan, J., Inhoff, A. W., & Topolski, R. (1995). Mindless reading: Eye-movement characteristics are similar in scanning letter strings and reading texts. *Perception and Psychophysics, 57*, 352–364. doi:10.3758/BF03213060.

Wang, C., Tsai, J., Inhoff, A. W., & Tzeng, O. L. (2009). Acquisition of linguistic information to the left of fixation during the reading of Chinese text. *Language and Cognitive Processes, 24*, 1097–1123. doi:10.1080/01690960802525392.

White, S. J., Johnson, R. L., Liversedge, S. P., & Rayner, K. (2008). Eye movements when reading transposed text: The importance of word-beginning letters. *Journal of Experimental Psychology: Human Perception and Performance, 34*, 1261–1276. doi:10.1037/0096-1523.34.5.1261.

Chapter 7
Reading in Thai: Visual and Attentional Processes

Heather Winskel

7.1 Introduction

Reading is a highly complex cognitive process, which serves the fundamental purpose of constructing a meaningful cognitive text representation through decoding various visually complex symbols written on the page or screen. The process also involves mapping the phonology of the particular language of the reader onto these orthographic symbols. Different writing systems present quite distinct demands and challenges to the reader. Thus, although the general goal of reading is to form a mental representation of text from decoding these visual symbols, the processes involved in attaining this goal substantially differ as they are dependent on the characteristics of the particular orthography.

Traditionally, reading research has focused on Roman script and a small number of European languages, in particular English. However, more recently a growing interest in investigating a broader range of languages and scripts has emerged, which is essential if we are to delineate between universal and orthography-specific processes as well as build more comprehensive and representative universal models of reading (see Frost 2012, for a recent review). This cross-linguistic research also challenges various assumptions that have been made based on a very limited and unrepresentative group of languages and scripts. Current models of reading and visual word recognition are notoriously anglocentric, as they have been primarily constructed based on English, which can be considered an "outlier" orthographic system (Frost 2012; Share 2008).

H. Winskel (✉)
Psychology, School of Health and Human Sciences, Southern Cross University,
Coffs Harbour Campus, Coffs Harbour, NSW 2450, Australia
e-mail: heather.winskel@scu.edu.au

© Springer India 2015
R.K. Mishra et al. (eds.), *Attention and Vision
in Language Processing*, DOI 10.1007/978-81-322-2443-3_7

Thai with its distinctive script offers fruitful opportunities to investigate the
visual and attentional mechanisms and processes involved in reading and to what
extent these processes are universal or shaped by the characteristics of the particular orthography. It makes particularly useful comparisons with the extensively
studied Roman script, as it is also alphabetic. In the current chapter, some recent
research that has utilised the distinctive features of this script will be examined in
the following four sections: (1) reading without interword spaces, (2) prominence
of initial letter position and transposed-letter effects, (3) parafoveal-on-foveal
effects, and (4) processing of lexical tone. In the final section of the chapter, future
research directions will be discussed. However, first it is important to understand
the characteristics of the Thai language and its script, prior to discussing these different areas of research.

7.2 Characteristics of the Thai Language and Its Script

Thai has an alphabetic script with syllabic characteristics as it has inherent vowels
for some consonants. Consonants are written in a linear order, but vowels can have
a non-linear configuration; they can be written above, below, or to either side of the
consonant as full letters or diacritics, and commonly combine across the syllable to
produce a single vowel or diphthong. Several vowels precede the consonant in writing but phonologically follow it in speech (e.g., แบน <ɛ:bn> 'flat' is spoken as /bɛ:n/),
whereas other vowels are spoken in the order that they are written, as occurs in
English (e.g., บาท <ba:t> 'Baht' is spoken as /ba:t/). This non-alignment of vowels is a
characteristic shared by other Brahmi-derived scripts (e.g., Devanagari, Kannada
and Burmese). However, in contrast to the South Asian languages, Thai is a tonal
language, which is a characteristic it shares with other regional neighbours (e.g.,
Chinese, Burmese, Lao and Vietnamese) (for further discussion refer to Winskel
2014; Winskel et al. 2014).

Thai has five tones (i.e., five different F0 contours) conceptualised as
high, mid, falling, rising, low and four tone markers
(*maj3 e:k1* 'ˋ', *maj3 tho:0* 'ˊ', *maj3 tri:0* 'ˊ', and *maj3 tçat1ta1wa:0* 'ˊ')[1] that orthographically occur above the consonant. An example in
Thai is ขาว /k^{h}a:w4/ 'white', ข่าว /k^{h}a:w1/ 'news', and ข้าว /k^{h}a:w2/ 'rice'. In Thai, consonant letters are divided into three classes (11 high, 9 middle, 24 low), which
reflects old voicing distinctions that have been neutralised in modern Thai
(Gandour 2013; Hudak 1990). These particular classifications of the initial consonant (high, medium, low) in conjunction with the tone marker and syllable structure contribute to phonological tone realisation in written Thai (see Winskel 2014;
Winskel and Iemwanthong 2010, for greater detail).

---

[1]Tones are marked in the Thai examples cited in this paper as follows; 0 = mid, 1 = low,
2 = falling, 3 = high, 4 = rising. This is based on the system that was developed at the
Linguistics Research Unit (LRU) of Chulalongkorn University (Luksaneeyanawin 1993). IPA
transcription is used for the transcription of all other Thai text.

An additional distinctive feature of Thai is that it does not normally have interword spaces (similar in this respect with Chinese, Japanese, Lao, Khmer, Tibetan and Burmese), hence when reading, words have to be segmented using other cues besides spaces. The lack of these salient visual word segmentation cues implies that during normal reading, there is a degree of ambiguity in relation to which word a given letter belongs to (an example to illustrate this difficulty: คุณพ่อของฉันชอบรับประทานอาหารที่มีรสจัด).

7.2.1 Reading Without Interword Spaces

Eye-movement tracking is a method that is increasingly being employed to study reading across different languages. Eye movements provide a window into the underlying cognitive processes and mechanisms involved in reading (Rayner 1998). The different eye-movement measures also give a picture of how word processing and reading unfolds over time (Juhasz et al. 2005).

From research, predominantly conducted on Roman script, it has generally been assumed that interword spaces serve a common facilitatory function because when spaces are removed, eye movement control and word identification are substantially disrupted (Morris et al. 1990; Rayner et al. 1998; Spragins et al. 1976). Removing spaces in English typically slows reading by 30–50 %, disrupting both the way the eyes move through the text and the word identification process. Rayner et al. (1998) observed that the masking or removal of interword spaces was more deleterious to the reading of (relatively unfamiliar) low-frequency words than when reading length-matched, (relatively familiar) high-frequency words. They interpreted these results as indicating that removal of spaces interferes with word identification. Visuomotor control was also disrupted as indicated by substantial changes in the spatial distribution of incoming saccades or landing site distributions over target words. When interword spaces were present, these investigators found that readers tended to land a bit to the left of the middle of the word, whereas when spaces were removed they tended to land closer to the beginning.

However, one problem in investigating the function of spaces in English or other European languages is the fact that readers are not familiar with reading unspaced text; hence, it is hard to disentangle lack of habitual prior experience from the real advantages of spatial segmentation. Thai offers an ideal opportunity to further empirically test the function of interword spaces, as Thai script does not normally have interword spaces to indicate word or sentence boundaries. With this aim in mind, Winskel et al. (2009) examined the eye movements of Thai-English bilinguals when reading both Thai and English with and without interword spaces, and compared their eye movements when reading English to those of English monolinguals. The frequency of critical target words in the sentences was manipulated, as word frequency is considered to be a major determiner of the ease or difficulty of word identification and lexical access (Rayner 1998; Radach and Kennedy 2004). The reason that space information and word frequency were manipulated was so that information could be gained about the effect of spacing on word identification.

Several findings in this study (Winskel et al. 2009) suggested that spacing facilitates later word processing rather than word targeting or early lexical segmentation. The refixation measures (gaze duration and total fixation time) were significantly shorter in duration on the target words in the spaced than unspaced sentences, but notably first fixation durations were not different. First fixation landing positions and landing site distributions were also not influenced by the spacing manipulation. First fixation landing positions in both the spaced and unspaced condition were just left of word centre or what is termed the Optimal Viewing Position (OVP) (O'Reagan 1990). Thus, these results give qualified support for the view that interword spaces have a facilitatory function, as word processing was found to be facilitated, but on the other hand eye guidance (word targeting and lexical segmentation) was neither facilitated nor disrupted by the insertion of interword spaces. Similar findings were found in a subsequent study, in which initial and internal letter transpositions of target words as well as interword spacing were manipulated (Winskel et al. 2012).

If we consider the different demands of reading scripts without interword spaces with those that do, somewhat different processes emerge. Interword spaces serve an important function as they form clear segmentation or word boundary cues in the parafovea prior to word fixation, so that initial word processing can be readily instigated with the end goal of forming a coherent mental representation of the text. In contrast, when an alphabetic writing system provides no spatial segmentation cues, determining the extent of the letter cluster that forms a word becomes an intrinsic part of the initial stage of word processing. Thus, there is an additional in-built process or step involved in reading an unspaced alphabetic script, which involves demarcating where words begin and end using other segmentation cues besides salient interword spaces. Skilled Thai readers have presumably acquired knowledge of the language- or script-specific word segmentation patterns or cues (Bertram et al. 2004). Potential language-specific candidates for word or sylla ble segmentation in Thai are, for example, the misaligned vowels that occur prior to the consonant at the beginning of the syllable (e.g. โรค written as /oːrk/ but spoken as /roːk/ *disease*), as they possibly form salient syllabic segmentation cues to the reader. In addition, tone markers that occur above the syllable or lexeme (e.g. หน้าต่าง /naː2taːŋ1/ *window*) may form effective segmentation cues to the skilled reader. Support for this idea comes from the finding that when the tone markers for a target word were viewed in the parafovea prior to fixating that word, subsequent fixation durations on the target word were shorter (Winskel et al. 2009).

7.2.2 Prominence of Initial Letter Position and Transposed-Letter Effects

Research using transposition letter effects across different orthographies indicates that there is quite a degree of flexibility in the coding of letter position (e.g., *jugde* is readily read as *judge*) (O'Connor and Forster 1981; Schoonbaert and Grainger 2004; Perea and Carreiras 2006; Perea and Lupker 2004, on Roman script [English, French, Basque, and Spanish, respectively]; Perea et al. 2011b, on Japanese Kana script; Velan and Frost 2011, on Hebrew script; Perea et al. 2011a, on Arabic script; Lee and Taft 2009, on Korean Hangul script). In Roman script, letter position coding is particularly noisy in middle positions, but not in the initial letter position, as an illustration of this, *jugde* closely resembles *judge* while *ujdge* does not. The commonly held view that has emerged from this research and related research on Roman script is that initial letter position has a privileged role for word recognition in comparison to internal letters (e.g., Chambers 1979; Estes et al. 1976; Gómez et al. 2008; Jordan et al. 2003; Perea 1998; Rayner and Kaiser 1975; White et al. 2008). Consistent with the importance of the initial letter in Indo-European languages, research on Roman script has consistently failed to find a masked transposed-letter priming effect when the initial letter is involved (e.g., Perea and Lupker 2007).

We were interested in examining whether the importance of initial letter position in word recognition is a universal or a more script-specific phenomenon. Thai makes an interesting candidate to examine this further as it may be particularly flexible with respect to letter position coding, as it does not have interword spaces, which implies that during normal reading there is a degree of ambiguity in relation to which word a given letter belongs to and it also has misaligned vowels, whereby the orthographic and phonological order of vowels does not necessarily correspond. This again implies that position coding in Thai needs to be flexible enough so that readers can appropriately encode the letter positions of words with or without these misaligned vowels.

We utilised the masked priming paradigm with a lexical decision task (Forster and Davis 1984) to investigate the importance of initial letter position in Thai. In the masked priming paradigm a stimulus (the prime) is presented for a very short duration, which is then closely followed by the target. Participants are generally not aware of the briefly presented prime. In this case, the participants had to decide whether the target was a word or not. This technique allows researchers to investigate the effect that different primes have on the subsequent processing of the target stimulus through measuring response latencies. We found a significant masked transposed-letter priming effect when the initial letter was transposed even in short words (e.g., นน-บน was faster than มะน-บน [transposed-letter condition versus replacement-letter condition]) (Perea et al. 2012). This suggests that the role played by the initial letter in Thai is not as critical as in other languages.

In a follow-up study (Winskel et al. 2012), we extended this line of research by examining if initial letters have a privileged position in comparison to internal letters in Thai during normal silent reading. We monitored participants' eye movements while they read sentences with target words with internal [e.g., *porblem*] and external (e.g., *rpoblem*) transposed letters. We were interested in how readily those words could be read when interword spacing and demarcation of word boundaries (using alternating **bold** text) was manipulated. Results revealed that there was no apparent difference in degree of disruption caused when reading internal and initial transposed-letter nonwords. This is in marked contrast with results found in Roman script where, consistent with prior evidence from other paradigms in Indo-European languages, there was greater disruption caused by initial than internal transpositions (White et al. 2008). Therefore, these findings on Thai give further support to the view that letter position encoding in Thai is quite flexible, even for the initial letter position, and that actual identity of the letter is more critical than letter position. Moreover, this flexible encoding strategy is in line with the characteristics of Thai, that is, the lack of interword spaces and the misaligned vowels. These findings point to orthography-specific effects operating in letter encoding in visual word recognition.

The modified receptive field (MRF) theory (Tydgat and Grainger 2009) has been formulated to account for the initial letter advantage found in Roman script. It has been proposed that as children learn to read, they develop a specialised system that is custom-built to handle the very specific nature of letters (Tydgat and Grainger 2009). This is an adaptive mechanism that has developed to optimise processing in crowded conditions associated with reading words or numbers. According to the MRF account, there is a change or expansion in the shape of receptive fields of initial letters to optimise processing at the first position in strings of letters (Tydgat and Grainger 2009, see Fig. 12; see also Grainger and van Heuven 2003), which gives an initial position advantage. However, in Thai we did not find a significant difference between initial and internal transposition effects in the spaced condition—in which theoretically there is less lateral masking on initial letters than on internal letters.

In order to explain these disparate results, we can envisage that a similar elongation of receptive field for initial letter position has not occurred in unspaced Thai; instead, the receptive fields for initial and internal letter positions are similar in shape and size. With experience of reading Thai, presumably, smaller receptive field sizes develop as reading skills become more honed in this extremely crowded letter environment. This parallel processing model is compatible with the view that letter position encoding in Thai is quite flexible, even for the initial letter position, and actual identity of the letter is more critical than letter position.

In sum, research indicates that the Thai orthographic system allows a very flexible process of letter position coding and that the initial letter position is not as critical as in Roman script. Possibly the relative importance of both initial and internal letter positions and not just initial letter varies across languages. Further experiments are required to verify and extend this line of research in Thai and in other orthographies that do not have interword spaces.

7.2.3 Parafoveal-on-Foveal Effects

One controversial question in the field of eye movements and reading is whether there is evidence of parafoveal-on-foveal effects, or in other words, whether there is an effect of the lexical or sub-lexical characteristics of the adjacent nonfixated parafoveal word (n + 1) on the currently fixated word (n) when reading (see Drieghe 2011, for a comprehensive review). These parafoveal-on-foveal effects are of particular theoretical interest as they can potentially support either a serial or parallel processing view of lexical processing when reading (e.g., E-Z Reader versus SWIFT models). According to the E-Z Reader model (Reichle et al. 1998; 2003), words are sequentially attended to one at a time when reading. Hence, the lexical-semantic properties of the adjacent nonfixated word do not affect the processing of the fixated word. In contrast, the SWIFT model (Engbert et al. 2002; Nuthmann et al. 2005) assumes that lexical processing is spatially distributed across words with a competition for processing resources. Thus, the fixated and the nonfixated word can be processed simultaneously. Thus, empirical evidence of parafoveal-on-foveal effects would support this parallel processing model over the serial, E-Z Reader model.

Word frequency is one of the main lexical characteristics that has been investigated in terms of parafoveal-on-foveal effects, but with contradictory findings. Several experimental studies in Roman script have found no evidence of parafoveal-on-foveal effects of word frequency (Calvo and Meseguer 2002; Henderson and Ferreira 1993; Perea and Acha 2009; Rayner et al. 1998; Schroyens et al. 1999; White 2008), whereas other studies have found mixed results (Hyönä and Bertram 2004), and yet, other large corpus studies have found effects of word frequency (Kennedy and Pynte 2005; Kliegl et al. 2006; Pynte and Kennedy 2006; Wotschack and Kliegl 2013).

Thai is particularly suitable for further examining if there is evidence of parafoveal-on-foveal effects due to it not having interword spaces and having misaligned vowels. These characteristics are associated with a level of ambiguity in relation to where a word starts and ends, and as the fixated word and the parafoveal word are adjoining they are, thus, closer to the fovea, which may potentially lead to more parallel processing of adjacent words occurring when reading Thai than in Indo-European languages.

In order to investigate the possible occurrence of parafoveal-on-foveal effects when reading Thai, we manipulated word frequency (high and low) of the word to the right of the currently fixated word to see if it would influence processing of the fixated word (Winskel and Perea 2014b). The experimental sentences were constructed so that the sentence frames were identical for each high- and low-frequency target word. Thus, the foveal word was identical for each matched pair of parafoveal words. The participants read the single sentences with the critical target words while having their eye movements monitored. There was no evidence of the effect of word frequency of the parafoveal word on fixation duration measures of the foveal word, except for a marginal effect in the skipping rates. Thus, the data were in line with previous studies with spaced Indo-European languages, which have found small or no results for parafoveal effects of word frequency during one-line sentence reading. These results are also in agreement with a recent study (Winskel et al. 2012), where we also failed to find parafoveal-on-foveal effects when reading Thai. These results appear to favour models such as the E-Z reading model where lexical processing is considered to be a sequential process. However, there was a modest skipping rate, which may indicate some support for parafo-veal-on-foveal effects, so we cannot rule out these effects entirely and the possibil-ity that fixated and non-fixated words are processed in parallel in Thai.

It is important to note that these lexical frequency effects when they are found are relatively small and the detection of parafoveal-on-foveal effects appear to be limited to instances where the eyes are very close to the parafoveal preview where visual acuity is adequate for parafoveal processing to occur (Drieghe 2011; White 2008; White and Liversedge 2004). Moreover, Wotschack and Kliegl (2013) have shown recently that individual age-related differences and experimental manipula-tion of task demand (manipulation of comprehension question difficulty), can influ-ence the reading strategies adopted by readers, namely the skipping rate on first-pass reading and regressive eye movements, which in turn can affect whether parafoveal-on-foveal effects are found or not. Clearly, additional research is needed to further investigate this phenomenon in Thai and additional writing systems.

7.2.4 Processing of Lexical Tone

In many languages (e.g., Thai, Chinese, Vietnamese, Burmese), tone information (i.e., the pitch of a syllable) forms an integral element in lexical identification as it serves an essential function in distinguishing between lexical entities with a simi-lar phonological structure. However, tone is a much-understudied area of psycho-linguistics. One important research question is whether tonal information plays a critical role in the early stages of lexical access in tonal languages as segmental information (i.e., consonantal and vowel information) does, or whether its effect occurs at a later processing stage, after lexical retrieval.

Previous studies in Chinese have failed to find an effect of tonal information during the early stages of visual word processing using a masked priming para-digm technique. In a series of word naming experiments, Chen et al. (2003) found faster response times on a bisyllabic target word when a briefly presented word prime shared the initial syllable with the target regardless of whether the sylla-ble had the same tone or not as the target (e.g., the prime 爸 /ba4/ 'father' facil-itated the processing of 拔营 /ba2.ying2/ 'break up camp' more than the prime 败 /bai4/ 'failure', where 2 represents the rising, second tone and 4 represents the falling, fourth tone). The presence of an atonal effect of the syllable in Chinese suggests that "the syllable (lacking the tone) is a stored phonological chunk" (Chen et al. 2003, p. 116) and that the tone does not play a special role early in visual word processing. Thus, at the phonological level, segmental metric (i.e., the syllable) seems to be more important than metrical encoding (i.e., the tone) in Chinese (You et al. 2012). However, the tone is not explicitly written in Chinese (e.g., /da1/, /da2/, /da3/, and /da4/ would correspond to 搭,答, 打, and 大, respectively) , whereas in Thai script it is explicitly written. Thus, Thai is particularly suitable for investigating the role of tone during the early stages of visual word recognition.

Initially, Winskel (2011, Experiment 3) investigated if parafoveal lexi-cal tone information contributed to the subsequent processing of the target word when reading Thai. The tone marker of the parafoveal preview was manipulated, so that it was either identical or different from the target word (e.g., identity: ท้องฟ้า /tʰɔ:ŋ3fa:3/ 'sky' or control: ท้องฟ้า /tʰɔ:ŋ2fa:2/). The assumption was that if useful information is obtained from the parafoveal input of the tone markers, then the identical preview would have a greater facilitatory effect on processing of the target word than the incorrect tone marker preview (phonologically and orthographically different). As there was a facilitatory effect of the identical tone marker in comparison to the incorrect tone marker preview, it was concluded that tone information plays a key role in the early processing of Thai words. However, phonological controls were not included in this study, and thus, limiting the conclusions that can be made.

In a more recent study, Winskel and Perea (2014a) further investigated the contribution of orthographic and phonological features to lexical tone processing in Thai using a rapid naming task and a lexical decision task in conjunction with the masked priming paradigm. The masked priming technique is a paradigm that taps into early processing (Forster and Davis 1984; see Grainger 2008, for a review). Given that the rapid naming task explicitly requires an articulatory response, we also used the same materials in a lexical decision task, where phonological effects are not inherent (Carreiras et al. 2005; New et al. 2008). The rationale here was that if a phonological effect occurs in both tasks, this would provide support for the view that these phonological effects reflect core or task-independent rather than task-specific processes.

In this masked priming study, five different primes for a given target word (e.g., ห้อง /hɔ:ŋ2/ 'room') were created: (1) identity (e.g., ห้อง /hɔ:ŋ2/ C+T+, where C represents the consonant and T, the tone marker), (2) same initial consonant, but with a different tone marker (e.g., ห่อง /hɔ:ŋ1/ C+T-), (3) different initial consonant, but with the same tone marker (e.g., ซ้อง /sɔ:ŋ2/ C-T+), (4) orthographic control [different initial consonant, different tone marker C-T-] (e.g., ซ่อง /sɔ:ŋ1/), and (5) same tone homophony, but with a different initial consonant and different tone marker (e.g., ช่อง /tʰɔ:ŋ2/ C-T-+). In relation to the latter prime, an orthographically different consonant was combined with an orthographically different tone marker to produce a phonologically equivalent tone for the rime of the syllable.

Results from these two experiments revealed that segmental information (i.e., consonantal information) appears to be more important than tone information (i.e., tone marker) in the early stages of visual word processing in Thai. In other words, the identity of the initial consonant is more relevant in the initial stages of word processing than the identity of the tone marker. The lack of a purely phonological effect of tone occurred both when the tone in the prime had the same orthographic tone marker (ส้อง /sɔ:ŋ2/- ห้อง /hɔ:ŋ2/ C-T++) and when the tone had the same phonological tone (ช้อง /tʰɔ:ŋ2/ - ห้อง /hɔ:ŋ2/ C-T-+) as in the target word.

Furthermore, the data suggested that there is an additive orthographic facilitative effect when the identical initial consonant is paired with the identical tone marker (e.g., ห้) in Thai, as response times on the target words were faster when preceded by the identity prime that had the same initial consonant with the same tone marker (e.g., ห้อง /hɔ:ŋ2/ - ห้อง /hɔ:ŋ2/C+T+) than when the prime had the same initial consonant but had a different tone marker (ห่อง /hɔ:ŋ1/ - ห้อง /hɔ:ŋ2/ C+T-). This orthographic effect of the tone marker was similar to that found by Winskel (2011) when investigating parafoveal previews when reading continuous text in Thai.

It was inferred that tonal information is having an effect at an orthographic rather than phonological level, as there was an advantage of the identity condition over the priming condition that only differed in the tone marker. Moreover, signs of a purely phonological effect due to tone did not result from either of the two comparisons that were made—one in which prime and target were relatively similar (e.g., ห้อง /sɔːŋ2/ C-T++ - ห้อง /hɔːŋ2/ C+T+) and the other in which the prime and target were graphemically more different (e.g., ถ้อง C-T-+ /tʰɔːŋ2/ - ห้อง /hɔːŋ2/ C+T+). The pattern of data in the lexical decision and naming tasks was quite similar, which suggests that the observed data reflect central processes of lexical access rather than task-specific processes. Thus, the most parsimonious account of the data is that segmental information (i.e., consonantal information) is more important than tone information (i.e., tone marker) in the early stages of visual word processing in Thai. In other words, the data suggested that access to phonological tone information during the process of visual word recognition occurs relatively late.

In sum, findings on tone processing in Thai are consistent with the data in Chinese visual word recognition with the masked priming technique, in which robust effects of syllable priming are obtained even when the phonological syllables of primes and targets had different tonal information (Chen et al. 2003; You et al. 2012). Taken together, these findings suggest that segmental information plays a greater role than tonal information during the early stages of visual word recognition in tonal languages.

Additional research is necessary to examine in further detail the extent and time course of phonological processes in Thai and other tonal languages using different tasks. It is likely that tonal information will play a more relevant role in spoken-word recognition due to its inherent characteristics than in visual word recognition. In Chinese, Lee (2007), for example, found that monosyllabic words differing only in tone (i.e. segmentally identical, but tonally distinct) failed to cause the speeded responses typical of segmental form priming. Facilitation of direct priming was found only when the prime and target were identical in both tonal and segmental structure (i.e., hearing *lou2* 'hall' speeded identification of the identical word *lou2* whereas *lou3* 'hug,' did not). This indicates that tone information is playing a more critical role in spoken-word recognition in comparison to visual word recognition. Future research needs to investigate if there are common underlying processing mechanisms for tone across the spoken and written modalities in Thai and other tonal languages that mark tone orthographically.

7.3 Concluding Comments and Future Research Directions

In the current chapter, research on Thai has been used to illustrate how the distinctive features of orthography can influence the visual and attentional processes involved in visual word recognition and reading. The general goal of reading is to form a mental representation of text from decoding the visual symbols of a script; however, the processes involved in attaining this goal substantially differ as they are shaped by the characteristics of the particular orthography. Different orthographies exert different processing demands and challenges to the reader. In order to effectively read a script, readers need to attend to the distinctive features of the visual symbols of the script and how they interface with the particular language of the speaker. Attention needs to be focused on the critical and salient features of the orthography that are vital in forming such a mental representation. Thus, attentional resources need to be differentially allocated dependent on the specific characteristics of the orthography and the role that they play in forming a coherent mental representation of the words or text. For example, in scripts with interword spaces, these salient visual-word segmentation cues form distinct perceptual markers for word boundaries, whereas in unspaced script, other orthography-specific cues presumably need to be identified and utilised.

From investigating the function of interword spaces in Thai, a script that does not have such salient visual segmentation cues, we have found qualified support for the facilitatory function of interword spaces, as word processing was facilitated but eye guidance was neither facilitated nor disrupted by the insertion of spaces. Thus, comprehending words was facilitated by insertion of the spaces, but the movement of the eyes through the text was not affected. These results form interesting comparisons with studies conducted on other unspaced scripts, namely Chinese and Japanese. In Chinese, sentences with an unfamiliar word spaced format were as easy to read as visually familiar unspaced text (Bai et al. 2008). A more complex picture emerged for Japanese with its mixed script. When reading Japanese Hiragana-only script, Sainio et al. (2007) found similar results to English, as spaces facilitated both eye guidance and word identification to some extent. However, for mixed Kanji-Hiragana text, a tendency was found for spaced text to be read slower than unspaced text, although this difference did not reach significance. Similar to Thai, initial saccade landing positions for Kanji-Hiragana were not affected by the spacing manipulation. However, the Preferred Viewing Location (PVL) for Thai and Japanese were not the same. In Japanese, the PVL was found to be at the word beginning, which is typically occupied by a perceptually salient Kanji character, whereas for Thai the PVL was observed to be just left of mid-word position. Thus, there appear to be script-specific differences emerging, whereby different locations of the word are initially preferentially attended when reading these unspaced scripts.

A much debated question is whether there is sequential or parallel processing occurring while reading. The research examining parafoveal-on-foveal effects in Thai highlights the need to investigate this phenomenon further in a broader range of orthographies, as these effects may be more likely to be found in some orthographies rather than others. Scripts without interword spaces and/or scripts with a nonlinear configuration of letters and diacritics may be good candidates for further investigation. Currently, the limited research that has been reviewed here on Thai is favouring a serial processing model, but this may be overturned by subsequent research.

In Roman script, the initial letter plays a critical role in lexical processing whereas this might not be as apparent in other scripts such as Thai, where there appears to be more flexible encoding of letter position, including initial letter position. Lexical tone also plays a critical role in many languages in the world, as it differentiates between phonologically similar syllables and words. Thus, when reading in those languages, lexical tone needs to be attended to. In some scripts, such as Thai, tone is visually represented in the script, so readers can attend to these visual cues when reading Thai. This feature also enables us to investigate the time course of orthographic and phonological processing of lexical tone in these types of scripts.

It is essential to investigate a broader range of languages and scripts if we are to delineate between universal and orthography-specific processes as well as build more comprehensive and representative universal models of reading. The findings described here challenge current computational models of reading. For example, currently, there are no computational models of visual word recognition and reading that accounts for tonal orthographies (e.g., Thai, Lao, Vietnamese, Burmese) or allows for flexibility in letter position coding. The feature and letter levels of current computational models of visual word recognition do not convey any diacritical marking, which is used to represent tone information in these scripts or that incorporates a flexible parameter that modulates the role of initial letter position.

In summary, to build a more comprehensive and universal model of reading, it is essential to investigate reading in diverse languages and their orthographies. We can see from this review of research conducted on visual word recognition and reading in Thai that there are differences, albeit often small, in the visual and attentional processes involved when reading different orthographies. The implications are that differences in the visual characteristics of scripts and how they interface with the particular language shapes how attention is allocated during the reading process. The lesser studied scripts of South and Southeast Asia with their distinctive characteristics offer extremely interesting opportunities to gain further insights into these common and orthography-specific reading processes and mechanisms.

References

Bai, X., Yan, G., Liversedge, S. P., Zang, C., & Rayner, K. (2008). Reading spaced and unspaced Chinese text: Evidence from eye movements. *Journal of Experimental Psychology: Human Perception and Performance, 34*, 1277–1287.

Bertram, R., Pollatsek, A., & Hyönä, J. (2004). Morphological parsing and the use of segmentation cues in reading Finnish compounds. *Journal of Memory and Language, 51*, 325–345.

Calvo, M. G., & Meseguer, E. (2002). Eye movements and processing stages in reading: Relative contribution of visual, lexical, and contextual factors. *Spanish Journal of Psychology, 5*, 66–77.

Carreiras, M., Ferrand, L., Grainger, J., & Perea, M. (2005). Sequential effects of phonological priming in visual word recognition. *Psychological Science, 16*, 585–589.

Chambers, S. M. (1979). Letter and order information in lexical access. *Journal of Verbal Learning and Verbal Behavior, 18*, 225–241.

Chen, J.-Y., Lin, W.-C., & Ferrand, L. (2003). Masked priming of the syllable in Mandarin Chinese speech production. *Chinese Journal of Psychology, 45*, 107–120.

Drieghe, D. (2011). Parafoveal-on-foveal effects on eye movements during reading. In S. Liversedge, I. Gilchrist, & S. Everling (Eds.), *Oxford handbook on eye movements* (pp. 839–855). Oxford: Oxford University Press.

Engbert, R., Longtin, A., & Kliegl, R. (2002). A dynamical model of saccade generation in reading based on spatially distributed lexical processing. *Vision Research, 42*, 621–636.

Estes, W. K., Allmeyer, D. H., & Reder, S. M. (1976). Serial position functions for letter identification at brief and extended exposure durations. *Perception and Psychophysics, 19*, 1–15.

Forster, K. I., & Davis, C. (1984). Repetition priming and frequency attenuation in lexical access. *Journal of Experimental Psychology. Learning, Memory, and Cognition, 10*, 680–698.

Frost, R. (2012). Towards a universal model of reading. *Behavioral and Brain Sciences, 35*, 263–279.

Gandour, J. T. (2013). A functional deficit in the sensorimotor interface component as revealed by oral reading in Thai conduction aphasia. *Journal of Neurolinguistics, 26*, 337–347.

Gómez, P., Ratcliff, R., & Perea, M. (2008). The overlap model: A model of letter position coding. *Psychological Review, 115*, 577–601.

Grainger, J. (2008). Cracking the orthographic code: An introduction. *Language and Cognitive Processes, 23*, 1–35.

Grainger, J., & van Heuven, W. (2003). Modeling letter position coding in printed word perception. In P. Bonin (Ed.), The mental lexicon (pp. 1–24). New York: Nova Science.

Henderson, J. M., & Ferreira, F. (1993). Eye movement control during reading: Fixation measures reflect foveal but not parafoveal processing difficulty. *Canadian Journal of Experimental Psychology, 47*, 201–221.

Hudak, T. J. (1990). Thai. In B. Comrie (Ed.), *The major languages of East and South-East Asia* (pp. 757–773). London: Routledge.

Hyönä, J., & Bertram, R. (2004). Do frequency characteristics of nonfixated words influence the processing of fixated words during reading? *European Journal of Cognitive Psychology, 16*, 104–127.

Jordan, T. R., Patching, G. R., & Thomas, S. M. (2003). Assessing the role of hemispheric specialization, serial-position processing and retinal eccentricity in lateralized word perception. *Cognitive Neuropsychology, 20*, 49–71.

Juhasz, B. J., Inhoff, A. W., & Rayner, K. (2005). The role of interword spaces in the processing of English compound words. *Language and Cognitive Processes, 20*, 291–316.

Kennedy, A., & Pynte, J. (2005). Parafoveal-on-foveal effects in normal reading. *Vision Research, 45*, 153–168.

Kliegl, R., Nuthmann, A., & Engbert, R. (2006). Tracking the mind during reading: The influence of past, present, and future words on fixation durations. *Journal of Experimental Psychology: General, 135*, 12–35.

Lee, C.-Y. (2007). Does horse activate mother? Processing lexical tone in form priming. *Language and Speech, 50*, 101–123.

Lee, C. H., & Taft, M. (2009). Are onsets and codas important in processing letter position? A comparison of TL effects in English and Korean. *Journal of Memory and Language, 60*, 530–542.

Morris, R. K., Rayner, K., & Pollatsek, A. (1990). Eye movement guidance in reading: The role of parafoveal letter and space information. *Journal of Experimental Psychology: Human Perception and Performance, 16*, 268–281.

New, B., Araujo, V., & Nazzi, T. (2008). Differential processing of consonants and vowels in lexical access through reading. *Psychological Science, 19*(12), 1223–1227.

Nuthmann, A., Engbert, R., & Kliegl, R. (2005). Mislocated fixations during reading and the inverted optimal viewing position effect. *Vision Research, 45*, 2201–2217.

O'Connor, R. E., & Forster, K. I. (1981). Criterion bias and search sequence bias in word recognition. *Memory and Cognition, 9*, 78–92.

O'Reagan, J. K. (1990). Eye movements and reading. In E. Kowler (Ed.), *Reviews of oculomotor research* (Vol. 4, pp. 395–453)., Eye movements and their role in visual and cognitive processes Amsterdam: Elsevier.

Perea, M. (1998). Orthographic neighbours are not all equal: Evidence using an identification technique. *Language and Cognitive Processes, 13*, 77–90.

Perea, M., & Acha, J. (2009). Space information is important for reading. *Vision Research, 49*, 1994–2000.

Perea, M., & Carreiras, M. (2006). Do transposed-letter similarity effects occur at a prelexical phonological level? *Quarterly Journal of Experimental Psychology, 59*, 1600–1613.

Perea, M., & Lupker, S. J. (2004). Can CANISO activate CASINO? Transposed-letter similarity effects with nonadjacent letter positions. *Journal of Memory and Language, 51*, 231–246.

Perea, M., & Lupker, S. J. (2007). La posición de las letras externas en el reconocimiento visual de palabras. *Psicothema, 19*, 559–564.

Perea, M., Abu Mallouh, R., García-Orza, J., & Carreiras, M. (2011a). Masked priming effects are modulated by expertise in the script. *Quarterly Journal of Experimental Psychology, 64*, 902–919.

Perea, M., Nakatani, C., & van Leeuwen, C. (2011b). Transposition effects in reading Japanese Kana: Are they orthographic in nature? *Memory and Cognition, 39*, 700–707.

Perea, M., Winskel, H., & Ratitamkul, T. (2012). On the flexibility of letter position coding during lexical processing: The case of Thai. *Experimental Psychology., 59*(2), 68–73.

Pynte, J., & Kennedy, A. (2006). An influence over eye movements in reading exerted from beyond the level of the word: Evidence from reading English and French. *Vision Research, 46*, 3786–3801.

Radach, R., & Kennedy, A. (2004). Theoretical perspectives on eye movements in reading. Past controversies, current deficits and an agenda for future research. *European Journal of Cognitive Psychology, 16*, 3–26.

Rayner, K. (1998). Eye movements in reading and information processing: 20 years of research. *Psychological Bulletin, 124*, 372–422.

Rayner, K., & Kaiser, J. S. (1975). Reading mutilated text. *Journal of Educational Psychology, 67*, 301–306.

Rayner, K., Fischer, M. H., & Pollatsek, A. (1998). Unspaced text interferes with both word identification and eye movement control. *Vision Research, 38*, 1129–1144.

Reichle, E. D., Pollatsek, A., Fisher, D. L., & Rayner, K. (1998). Toward a model of eye movement control in reading. *Psychological Review, 105*, 125–157.

Reichle, E. D., Rayner, K., & Pollatsek, A. (2003). The E-Z reader model of eye movement control in reading: Comparisons to other models. *Behavioral and Brain Sciences, 26*, 445–476.

Sainio, M., Hyönä, J., Bingushi, K., & Bertram, R. (2007). The role of interword spacing in reading Japanese: An eye movement study. *Vision Research, 47*, 2575–2584.

Schoonbaert, S., & Grainger, J. (2004). Letter position coding in printed word perception: Effects of repeated and transposed letters. Language and Cognitive Processes, 19, 333–367.

Schroyens, W., Vitu, F., Brysbaert, M., & d'Ydewalle, G. (1999). Eye movement control during reading. Foveal load and parafoveal processing. Quarterly Journal of Experimental Psychology: Human Experimental Psychology, 52(A), 1021–1046.

Share, D. L. (2008). On the Anglocentricities of current reading research and practice: The perils of overreliance on an "outlier" orthography. *Psychological Bulletin, 134*, 584–615.

Spragins, A. B., Lefton, L. A., & Fischer, D. F. (1976). Eye movements while reading and searching spatially transformed text: A developmental perspective. *Memory and Cognition, 4*, 36–42.

Tydgat, I., & Grainger, J. (2009). Serial position effects in the identification of letters, digits and symbols. *Journal of Experimental Psychology: Human Perception and Performance, 35*, 480–498.

Velan, H., & Frost, R. (2011). Words with and without internal structure: what determines the nature of orthographic and morphological processing? *Cognition, 118*, 141–156.

White, S. J. (2008). Eye movement control during reading: Effects of word frequency and orthographic familiarity. *Journal of Experimental Psychology: Human Perception and Performance, 34*, 205–223.

White, S. J., & Liversedge, S. P. (2004). Orthographic familiarity influences initial eye fixation positions in reading. *European Journal of Cognitive Psychology, 16*, 52–78.

White, S. J., Johnson, R. L., Liversedge, S. P., & Rayner, K. (2008). Eye movements when reading transposed text: The importance of word-beginning letters. *Journal of Experimental Psychology: Human Perception and Performance, 34*, 1261–1276.

Winskel, H. (2011). Orthographic and phonological parafoveal processing of consonants, vowels, and tones when reading Thai. *Applied Psycholinguistics, 32*(4), 739–759.

Winskel, H. (2014). Learning to read and write in Thai. In H. Winskel & P. Padakannaya (Eds.). South and Southeast Asian Psycholinguistics (pp. 171–178). Cambridge: Cambridge University Press.

Winskel, H., & Iemwanthong, K. (2010). Reading and spelling acquisition in Thai children. *Reading and Writing: An Interdisciplinary Journal, 23*, 1021–1053.

Winskel, H., & Perea, M. (2014a). Does tonal information affect the early stages of visual-word processing in Thai? *Quarterly Journal of Experimental Psychology, 67*(2), 209–219.

Winskel, H., & Perea, M. (2014b). Can parafoveal-on-foveal effects be obtained when reading an unspaced alphasyllabic script (Thai)? *Writing Systems Research, 6*, 94–104.

Winskel, H., Radach, R., & Luksaneeyanawin, S. (2009). Eye movements when reading spaced and unspaced Thai and English: A comparison of Thai-English bilinguals and English monolinguals. *Journal of Memory and Language, 61*, 339–351.

Winskel, H., Perea, M., & Ratitamkul, T. (2012). On the flexibility of letter position coding during lexical processing: Evidence from eye movements when reading Thai. *Quarterly Journal of Experimental Psychology, 65*(8), 1522–1536.

Winskel, H., Padakannaya, P., & Pandey, A. (2014). Eye movements and reading in the alphasyllabic scripts of South and Southeast Asia. In H. Winskel & P. Padakannaya (Eds.). South and Southeast Asian Psycholinguistics (pp. 315–328). Cambridge: Cambridge University Press.

Wotschack, C., & Kliegl, R. (2013). Reading strategy modulates parafoveal-on-foveal effects in sentence reading. *Quarterly Journal of Experimental Psychology, 66*, 548–562.

You, W.-P., Zhang, Q.-F., & Verdonschot, R. G. (2012). Masked syllable priming effects in word and picture naming in Chinese. *PLoS ONE, 7*(10), e46595.

Part III
Attention and Vision in Bilingual Language Processing

Chapter 8
Visual Cues for Language Selection in Bilinguals

Robert J. Hartsuiker

8.1 Introduction

As an exchange student in the US, I once shared an apartment with a German-English bilingual; we consistently spoke English with each other. One day, however (in a state of considerable excitement about something), my roommate seemed to have forgotten which language we normally used, and produced a rather lengthy speech in German (until he was finally stopped by the look of surprise on my face). Such occurrences of language misselection seem to be rare however; we normally know exactly what language to speak at the very moment we see a familiar person. The question addressed in this chapter is whether bilingual speakers use information from the visual environment to help select the right language to speak or comprehend in. To set the stage, I first briefly review studies that have demonstrated parallel language activation in bilinguals and studies that have considered whether such parallel language activation can be modulated by linguistic cues.

8.2 Bilingual Language Processing Is Language Non-selective

Being able to restrict language processing to only the target language would seem to be very useful, given that there is a considerable amount of evidence that in lexical access, words from both a bilingual's languages become active (for a recent

R.J. Hartsuiker (✉)
Department of Experimental Psychology, Ghent University, Henri Dunantlaan 2,
9000 Ghent, Belgium
e-mail: Robert.Hartsuiker@ugent.be

© Springer India 2015
R.K. Mishra et al. (eds.), *Attention and Vision
in Language Processing*, DOI 10.1007/978-81-322-2443-3_8

review see Kroll and Bialystok 2013). In the domain of *visual word recognition*, for instance, many studies have shown differences in the processing of words that are identical or similar in a bilingual's two languages (e.g., cognates such as Dutch and English *ring*, and interlingual homographs such as *list*, meaning trick in Dutch), as compared to words without any overlap in form. For instance, in a seminal study Dijkstra et al. (2000) showed that Dutch-English bilinguals were much slower to respond that a string of letters was a Dutch word when it was an interlingual homograph between Dutch and English (as compared to a Dutch control word). What is more, interlingual homographs like *tree* that are high-frequent in English but low-frequent in Dutch were often not even accepted as Dutch words. Similar findings were obtained when the task was run in the subjects' second language, English. Similarly, studies with cognates, words that overlap both in form and meaning, have shown a cognate advantage in visual word recognition over control words. This cognate advantage does not only occur in subjects' second language, but also in their first language (Van Hell and Dijkstra 2002). This advantage is even larger when multilinguals have a third language for which the word is also a cognate (e.g., *echo* is a word in Dutch, English and German, Lemhöfer et al. 2004).

One might argue that such evidence is restricted to "special words" that belong to more than one language. But is it also the case that upon reading a language-unique word, bilinguals automatically activate the translation of that word in another language? Thierry and Wu (2007) recently provided evidence for the latter view. They asked monolingual speakers of English, monolingual speakers of Chinese, and Chinese-English bilinguals to judge the semantic relatedness of English word pairs such as *wife–husband* or *train–ham* (the Chinese monolinguals saw the Chinese translations of these pairs). These pairs were constructed so that in half of the experimental trials there was a shared character in the Chinese translations of the word pairs. For instance, the Chinese translation of *train* has the same initial character as that of *ham*. While participants conducted this task, EEG was measured. As is to be expected, all groups showed a different brain potential as a function of whether the words were semantically related or not (i.e., an N400). But importantly, both the Chinese monolinguals (who saw the Chinese characters with or without orthographic overlap in between pair members) and the bilinguals (who only saw the words in English), showed differential brain potentials as a function of orthographic overlap (also in the N400 window, as well as in an earlier window) in Chinese (the English monolinguals did not show this component). These findings strongly suggest that upon reading a word in English, these bilinguals automatically activate the Chinese translation of that word up to the level of the orthographic code.

Evidence for language non-selective lexical access has also been found in other domains of language processing. In auditory word recognition, Spivey and Marian (1999) found that Russian-English bilinguals, immersed in an English-speaking environment, were sensitive to form similarity between a Russian word and the English name of an object. This was shown in a visual world eye-tracking experiment, in which subjects' eye movements to a visual scene were monitored as they listened to speech. Upon hearing a Russian instruction to move a stamp (*marku*), subjects were more likely to fixate a marker (related in phonological form) than an unrelated control object. Thus, even though the task was exclusively conducted in the subjects' native language (Russian), form-related words in their second language (English) became active, and did so to such an extent that it influenced looking behaviour in a visual display.

Similarly, in spoken word production evidence for language non-selectivity has also been obtained. For instance, Colomè (2001) asked subjects to engage in a so-called phoneme monitoring task. On each trial, they were assigned a target phoneme (e.g., /m/) and saw a picture (e.g., of a table), and the task was to determine whether the Catalan name of the picture (*taula*) contained the target phoneme. The Spanish name (*mesa)* was an irrelevant dimension for the task, but nevertheless Catalan-Spanish bilinguals were slower to make a no-decision when the phoneme occurred in the Spanish name of the object (e.g., /m/ for *mesa*) compared to a phoneme that occurred in neither the Catalan nor Spanish name. This suggests that when producing the phonological code in Catalan, bilinguals also activate the phonological code in the non-target language, Spanish.

Summarising, these and many other findings constitute clear evidence that bilinguals activate words from both of their languages during language processing and that this is the case irrespective of target language. One consequence is that bilinguals have more words to choose from, which may lead to a processing disadvantage. Indeed, a picture naming study (Ivanova and Costa 2008) showed that monolingual speakers of Spanish were somewhat faster to name pictures of common objects than were Spanish-Catalan bilinguals, even though the bilinguals were using their first and dominant language. It might therefore be beneficial for bilinguals to restrict lexical access to the target language. This leads to the question of whether bilinguals can exploit cues, inherent in the linguistic signal or in the context in which that signal occurs, to "zoom into" (as Elston-Güttler et al. 2005, called it) the right language. One might argue that in Ivanova and Costa's study such cues were weak (as the stimuli to be named were not associated with a particular language and each word was produced as an isolated response, unaffected by any sentence context). We will now turn to the question of whether stronger language cues do affect the extent of language non-selectivity.

8.3 Do Linguistic Cues Allow Bilinguals to Zoom into the Right Language?

The studies reviewed in the previous section have typically studied lexical access for single words that were read, or produced, without the larger context of a sentence or a discourse. One exception is the visual world study of Spivey and Marian, but in that experiment, the same sentence frame "now pick up the <object>" was repeated over and over again, rendering this different from more naturalistic sentence processing. It is very much conceivable that in the latter case, the language of the sentence provides an important cue about the language of each upcoming word, so that words from the other language no longer need to be considered. Consistent with this, De Bruijn et al. (2001) gave example (1), which—to a Dutch-English bilingual—appears to be a perfectly good sentence in Dutch (although one with a rather unusual content). What is not obvious right away is that in fact every word of the sentence is an interlingual homograph with English.

(1)   Door spot leek die brave, dove arts rover met pet (because of mockery, that good, deaf doctor resembled robber with hat)

So does a sentence context help to rule out the irrelevant language? Duyck et al. (2007) argued that if it does, effects of cross-linguistic overlap (i.e., cognate status) should disappear once cognates are embedded in a sentence context (also see Schwartz and Kroll 2006; Van Hell and De Groot 2008). Duyck et al. first presented their subjects, Dutch-English bilinguals, with English-Dutch cognates and English control words in an English lexical decision experiment. They replicated the cognate effect (shorter reaction times for cognates than matched control words). Next, they embedded the cognates and control words in a sentence context; the last word of each sentence was always the cognate/control word, and participants made a lexical decision on the sentence-final word. Importantly, the cognate effect survived this manipulation. Interestingly, the cognate effect was stronger for a subset of the items that were completely identical in form between English and Dutch (*ring–ring*) than items that were similar, but not identical in form (*ship–schip*). A final experiment presented versions of the sentences (but now with critical items in an earlier sentence position, to avoid any effects of sentence wrap-up) and monitored subject's eye movements. Both on relatively early measures (first fixation duration) and late measures (go-past time), there was an effect of cognate status, but this was the case only for the subset of identical cognates. Thus, in this experiment sentence context turned out to be insufficient to "turn off" the other language, but whether there is language non-selectivity under these conditions does seem to be modulated by degree of orthographic overlap.

Importantly, the Duyck et al. (2007) study was conducted in L2 English, and the subjects were clearly dominant in their L1 Dutch. One might argue that whereas one can never turn off a dominant L1 while processing L2, it should be possible to render L1 language non-selective. Van Assche et al. (2009) therefore conducted an L1 version of the Duyck et al. study. They first established a cognate advantage with words presented in isolation (replicating Van Hell and Dijkstra 2002). Importantly, in a sentence reading eye-tracking experiment, there was also cognate facilitation, in the sense that the more similar a Dutch target word (e.g., *oven*) was to its English translation equivalent in orthographic and phonological form, the shorter various eye-movement measures were. A follow-up experiment replicated this finding with a further set of stimuli. Thus, Van Assche et al. concluded that learning a second language has a profound influence on how one reads text in the first language: if a bilingual reads her local newspaper in her native language, she does so differently from a monolingual.

The conclusion that language non-selectivity survives contextual cues is supported by studies in the domain of bilingual auditory word recognition. A language-ambiguous written word (e.g., *ring*) is completely identical in the two languages because the letters are identical in English and Dutch. In contrast, spoken words consist of a much richer signal that includes subphonemic (and perhaps prosodic) language information, which a listener might, in principle, exploit to restrict lexical access to the target language. For instance, Dutch and English use different allophones to realise the phone /r/; Spanish and English notoriously differ in the boundary between voiced and unvoiced consonants. Lagrou et al. (2011) therefore reasoned that if listeners can exploit such cues, and can zoom into the correct language, there should be no difference in the time to recognise an interlingual homophone like /beI/ (Bay in English—Bij [bee] in Dutch) as compared to a monolingual control word. In contrast, lexical decision times to such interlingual homophones were longer than to control words, and this was true both in tasks conducted in the first and in the second language. Additionally, the effect occurred both when the *talker* (either one with L1 Dutch and L2 English or vice versa), produced speech in their L1 or L2 (note though that overall, reaction times were shorter when the talker used their L1). Importantly, monolingual English control listeners did not show the interlingual homophone effect, ruling out that the effects were due to an accidental confound in the stimuli. Finally, Lagrou et al. (2013) embedded the homophones in sentences, and found that even a spoken sentence context does not suffice to render lexical access language-selective.

Interestingly, some studies did show a modulation of cross-linguistic effects by a sentence-level variable, namely semantic constraint, although the results are far from unequivocal. For instance, in the sentence "The handsome man in the white suit is the X" it is not so predictable what X is; but in "The best cabin of the ship belongs to the X", it is perfectly predictable that X is "captain" (examples taken from Van Hell and De Groot 2008). In a sentence reading task in L2, Van Assche et al. (2011) found that semantic predictability did not modulate cognate effects on reading measures. In contrast, other eye-tracking studies (Libben and Titone 2009; Titone et al. (2011) did find modulations of semantic constraint, and so did studies using tasks like lexical decision or translation (Schwartz and Kroll 2006; Van Hell and De Groot 2008). However, also in those studies, sentence contraint did not always modulate cross-linguistic effects, and in the eye-tracking studies this modulation was restricted to late measures such as total reading time.

Finally, the only study that suggested some influence of linguistic cues is Elston-Güttler et al. (2005). In this study, the language cues were extrinsic to the target stimuli themselves, in contrast to the previous ones in which the sentence context in which the stimuli occurred provided the cue. Specifically, the authors manipulated the language of the intertitles in a silent film (i.e., an episode of Louis Feuillade's 1915–1916 film "Les Vampires"). The subjects watched this film while they were being prepared to take part in the EEG experiment and saw a version of it with either L1 German or L2 English intertitles (note that any cues from the actors' lip movements would have cued French and not the languages of interest here, German and English). After exposure to either the German or English version of the film, the subjects saw sentences followed by target words and conducted a lexical decision on each word. Crucially, in experimental trials the L2 English sentence ended in a word that was a homograph between English and German (e.g., *gift*; German *Gift* means poison), and the target word was related (e.g., the English word *poison*) or unrelated to the German reading of the homograph. Both reaction times (i.e., faster lexical decision times) and event-related potentials (i.e., a reduction of the N400 component) showed that the L1 German reading of the target words was activated. But importantly, these effects were only observed when the subjects had prior seen the German-language version of the film, and only in the first block. Thus, these findings indicate that extrinsic cues such as the language that is used in a (task-irrelevant) film can influence the extent to which readers zoom into a language. That the effect did not extend to the second block of the experiment, however, indicates that such an effect is short-lived.

Summarising, studies that embedded words with cross-linguistic overlap, such as interlingual homographs, interlingual homophones and cognates in a sentence context found little evidence that the language of the sentence exerted strong constraints on whether lexical selection is language-selective or not (with the possible exception of words that are highly predictable in the sentence context). Additionally, although the speech signal is very rich and conveys much information about the speaker, including age, gender, social status, dialect and native language (e.g., Van Berkum et al. 2008) it seems that cues about the language that is spoken are not enough to rule out the activation of the other-language reading of interlingual homophones (Lagrou et al. 2011, 2013). Note finally that a more indepth review of this literature is provided in Van Assche et al. (2012).

8.4 Do Visual Language Cues Help Bilinguals to Zoom into the Target Language?

A number of studies have considered the question of whether visual cues for language affect language activation. These share with the Elston-Güttler et al. (2005) study discussed in the previous section that they are extrinsic to the stimuli that are processed. On the other hand, while Elston-Güttler tried to cue a language "mode" that was, in principle, irrelevant for the task involving the critical stimuli, visual stimuli can sometimes be more directly linked to language. This is so because people's visual appearances inform us about who they are, allowing us often to infer which language we can expect them to use. Imagine for instance seeing the face of Mr. Lee. Perhaps Mr. Lee is a good friend with whom you often interact (say in English). One possibility then is that seeing Lee's face provides a strong cue about the language you typically use with him. It is also possible that you're introduced to Mr. Lee for the first time. In that case, more general properties of Mr. Lee's appearance might provide language cues even before the conversation has begun—if Mr. Lee looks Asian, you might expect him to use an Asian language such as Chinese, but if he looks Caucasian, his features might lead you to expect him to speak English. Another possibility is that Mr. Lee is in fact the late Bruce Lee, who was a famous actor in Kung Fu films. In that case, Mr. Lee's appearance might cue you to expect English (if you typically watch the English versions of his films); but if you typically watch Bruce Lee films in Cantonese, Lee's face might cue you to expect that language.

One study that considered the language associated with famous individuals was reported by Hartsuiker and Declerck (2009). These authors elicited language intrusion errors (e.g., producing Dutch *en* instead of its English translation equivalent *and*; for a different paradigm that induces such intrusions see Gollan et al. 2014). To do so, the authors presented their subjects with triplets of pictures of famous people's faces (e.g., Elvis Presley, Eddie Murphy and Jennifer Aniston; Fig. 8.1). On each trial, there was an animation, so that for instance two pictures moved in a downward direction while the third picture stayed put. The subjects, Dutch-English-French trilinguals, described these animations either in their first language Dutch or in one of their non-native languages (English or French), for instance with (2) and (3).

(2) *Elvis **and** Eddie Murphy move down, but Jennifer Aniston stays put*
(3) *Tom Boonen **and** Kim Clijsters move down, but King Albert stays put*

Importantly, this paradigm creates a context around the conjunction *and* (in bold-face in 2–3) in which the language of use and the language associated with the famous people "sandwiching" *and* is either congruent (2; Elvis and Eddie Murphy are associated with English) or *incongruent* (3; at least for the subjects tested, students in the Flemish region of Belgium, the famous cyclist Tom Boonen and tennis player Kim Clijsters are associated with Dutch). Of course, in Dutch-language versions of these sentences congruency is flipped: the individuals mentioned in (2) are then language-incongruent and in (3) language-congruent.

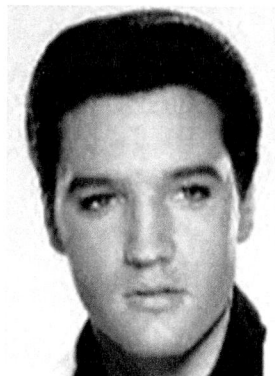 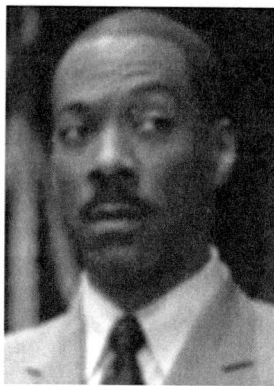 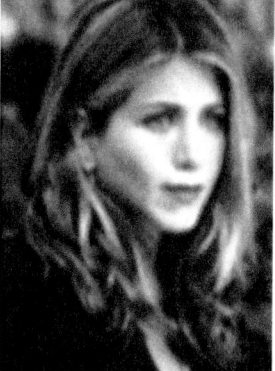

Fig. 8.1 Example of the displays used in Hartsuiker and Declerck (2009). In the actual experiment, two of the pictures would move, for instance the *left* and *middle* picture could move downwards

In their first experiment, Hartsuiker and Declerck (2009) observed that indeed, language intrusions happened from time to time in this paradigm. Such intrusions were more likely in the incongruent than the congruent condition and more likely when the target language was L2 than when it was L1. Because the authors were concerned that English *and* and Dutch *en* are near-homophones, making any language-intrusion errors difficult to detect in speech, this experiment used written production. But follow-up experiments with phonologically distinct conjunctions (i.e., Dutch *en* and French *et*) generalised the language-congruency effect to spoken language as well as written language. Further experiments also generalised the findings to a different type of connective (both "or" and "and"). Interestingly, and in agreement with Gollan et al.'s (2014) findings, a final experiment showed that language intrusions occurred more often with function words (e.g., *and*) than with content words (e.g., *cat*). One possible reason is that function words are more likely to be ignored by the processing systems that check our speech and writing for accuracy (i.e., our self-monitoring systems), just as function words are more likely to be skipped than content words during reading (Rayner 1998). At this point though, this account remains speculative.

The results of this study are suggestive that language-information associated with famous people's faces is activated during language production. However, the study does not allow us to determine whether it is specifically the famous person's face that activates the language, or whether (alternatively or additionally) there is an effect of the person's *name*. That is, one might argue that someone using a name in a different language from the language of the sentence is making a temporary switch to a different language, and it may be difficult to switch back. It is important to note that Gollan et al.'s (2014) experiment is consistent with an effect of names only: that experiment involved reading a text (hence without any visual cues) and also observed language intrusions in mixed language contexts.

It is possible that the case of famous people is a special one. While we may have seen and heard these people in the media, we usually do not interact with them. But in real life, we often have to select a language to use with new people we meet and interact with. Is a short conversation enough to link a language to a person? Woumans et al. (in press) asked this question in two experiments, one in Barcelona, Spain using Catalan-Spanish speakers and one in Ghent, Belgium using Dutch-French speakers. The experiments had two phases. First, participants saw a video of a person under the pretence that this was a session on Skype (in fact, the video was prerecorded). The person introduced him or herself and spoke about their daily lives and interests, and then invited the subject to likewise make a short speech. The person on the video consistently spoke either Catalan or Spanish (Dutch or French in the second experiment). Next, another person introduced themselves in the same way, so that each participant was acquainted with several Catalan and several Spanish speakers.

The second phase of the experiment was a language production task—given a cue word, provided by the same people previously seen on the video, the participants produced an association as quickly as they could; production latency was measured. Each of the people from the video produced two words in the language they used on the video and two words from the other language. The subjects were instructed to use the language of the cue word. If a short "chat" on a computer-based communication system is enough to create an association between the person and the language they used, one would expect faster production latencies when the language of the cue is congruent with the language of the video. In contrast, there was no overall effect. A closer look at the data, however, suggested a language-congruency effect for the initial trials of the production task. This suggests that while exposure to someone speaking a particular language may lead to an association between that person and the language, such an association can be undone after only a few trials in which that person used another language (i.e., only a few incongruent trials are enough to undo the association that was established before).

In addition to effects of the language associated with specific individuals, it is also possible that, specific *groups* of individuals are associated with particular languages. Two recent studies have recently explored whether the facial features (Asian or Caucasian) of a person whose picture was displayed along with the linguistic stimulus affected processing of a language that was congruent (Chinese) or incongruent (English) with those features. Li et al. (2013) conducted an fMRI experiment in which Chinese-English bilinguals and a control group of English monolinguals named line drawings of objects. The bilinguals named these stimuli using Chinese or English, depending on a colour cue (i.e., a red or blue frame around the picture cued the language to use). Importantly, experimental stimulus displays also showed the face of either Asian or Caucasian persons as well as part of their body; they appeared to be holding the frame with one hand and pointing to it with their other hand (Fig. 8.2). In a control condition, the frame appeared by itself. Thus for the bilinguals, there were 6 naming conditions (3 face conditions and 2 language conditions); for the monolingual group there were only the three face conditions.

Li et al. (2013) observed an interaction between naming condition and language in the analysis of naming latencies, so that participants were fastest when they responded in their L1 (Chinese) and an Asian face accompanied the stimulus. The fMRI data revealed a number of brain areas, mostly in the frontal and temporal lobes that were more active when using L1 than L2. There were also several areas of the brain more active when seeing faces compared to the no-face control condition, mostly in occipital areas and the fusiform gyrus. Importantly, an analysis of language-congruent versus—incongruent conditions showed more activation in more areas of the brain (mostly frontal and temporal areas) for the congruent conditions; the effects were strongest when the language was Chinese and the face was Asian.

Finally, the authors also conducted an analysis of four regions of interest, based on earlier brain imaging work that had mapped language control networks (e.g., Abutalebi 2008). Interestingly, two of these regions (the Medial Frontal Gyrus and Anterior Cingulate Cortex) showed language x face interactions, so that these areas were activated above the no-face baseline in the congruent conditions, and deactivated in the incongruent conditions. The authors interpreted the higher and

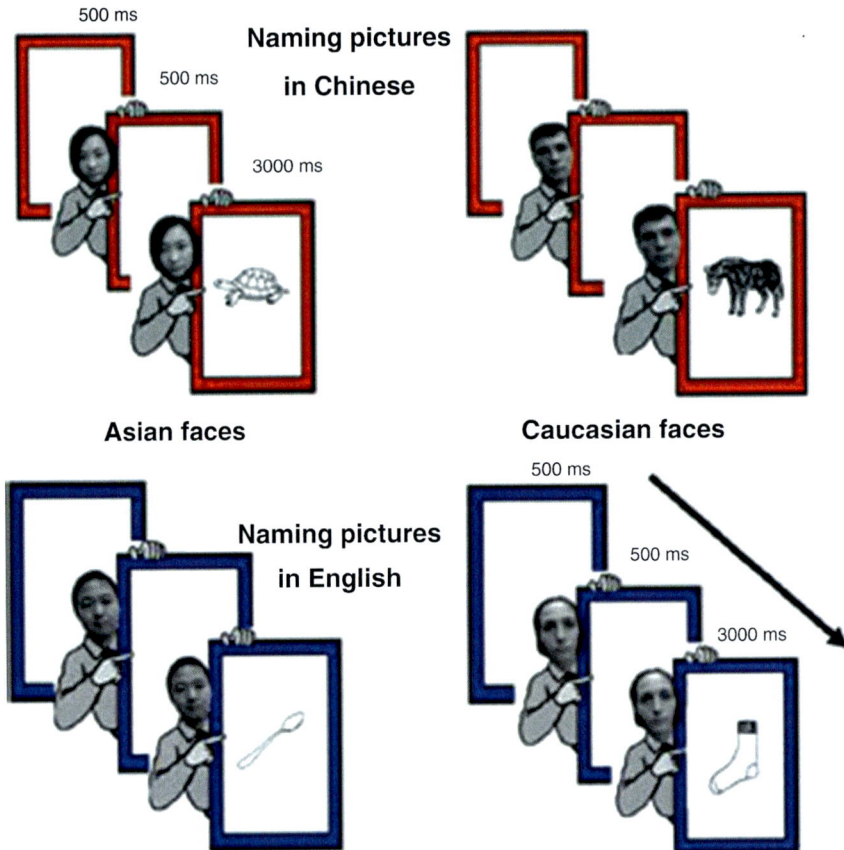

Fig. 8.2 Example of the stimuli used in Li et al. (2013)

more extended activation in the congruent condition as a facilitation effect, in line with the facilitation observed on naming latencies. This is somewhat counterintuitive, as one might expect the language control network to be more highly active when there is a conflict between different cues (i.e., face and colour cue). The authors suggested that this facilitation reflects a successful process of integration of multiple cues.

A priming effect from Chinese versus Caucasian faces was also observed by Zhang et al. (2013). These authors had subjects (Chinese-English bilinguals) engage in a computer-mediated spoken conversation in English with someone introduced as Michael Lee. At the same time, they saw a picture of either a Caucasian or a Chinese male face, and the authors collected two measures of production fluency, namely subjective fluency ratings and a count of fluently spoken words per minute. The authors reported numerically small but statistically

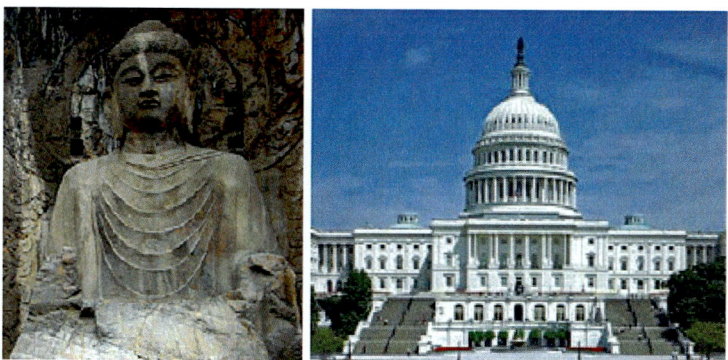

Fig. 8.3 Example of the stimuli used in Zhang et al. (2013)

significant cultural priming effects: when the subjects saw the language-incongruent (Chinese) face, their speech production was less fluent on both the subjective
and objective fluency measures.

Interestingly, Zhang et al.'s (2013) next experiment replaced the faces with
pictures of cultural icons, such as the Great Wall in China or Mount Rushmore
in the United States (Fig. 8.3). The Chinese and American cultural icons were
equally familiar to the subjects. In a first phase of the task, the subjects (23
Chinese-English bilinguals) described the cultural icons; next they described
a set of culture-neutral images. The fascinating result was that in both tasks and
for both fluency measures, the participants who saw Chinese cultural icons were
significantly less fluent than the ones who saw American icons. Further experiments extended these cultural priming effects to a different domain, namely that
of the lexicon. Subjects that were primed with Chinese icons could more quickly
identify a literal Chinese translation (e.g., HAPPY NUT for pistachio) and were
more likely to produce such a literal translation as an undesired intrusion. Thus,
these studies suggest that not only people's faces, but also visual icons of people's cultures can be associated with a language. Some care needs to be taken in
interpreting these results; however, given that some of the experiments were rather
underpowered, the results seemed to be small (unfortunately, no measure of effect
size was reported), and some of the measures (fluency ratings) were subjective.
Additionally, the study did not take into account the proficiency of the participants
and the objective measure of fluency (i.e., speech rate) may not be the best indicator of second language proficiency (see Yang and Yang 2013, for a discussion
of several concerns with the study and Morris and Zhang 2013, for a response to
these concerns; also see Kroll and McClain 2013 for further discussion of this
study).

In agreement with Zhang et al. (2013), Jared et al. (2013) found cultural effects on
picture naming times in a well-controlled study. These authors presented Chinese–
English bilinguals in Canada with objects that either had a Chinese appearance (e.g.,

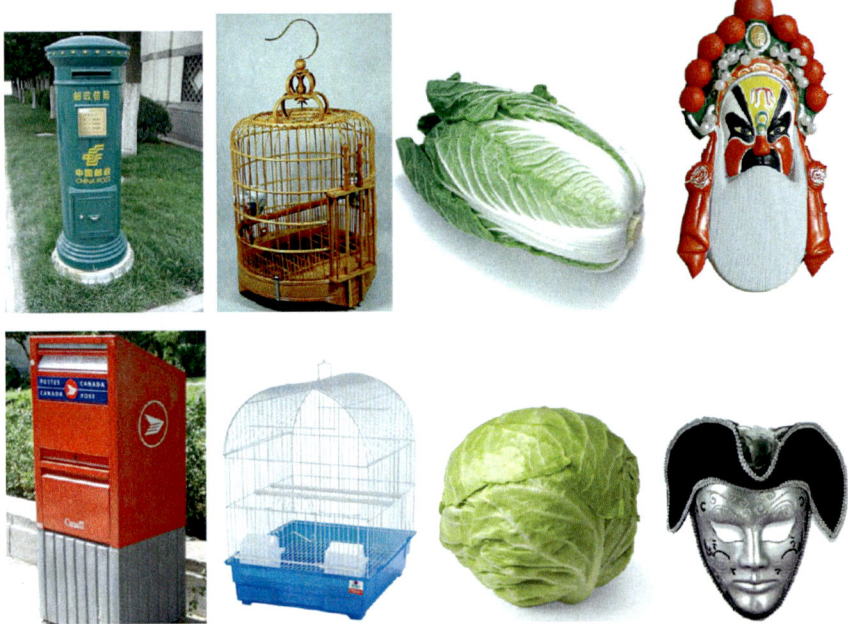

Fig. 8.4 Example of the stimuli used in Jared et al. (2013)

a typical Chinese mailbox or cabbage) or a Canadian appearance (a typical Canadian mailbox or cabbage; Fig. 8.4). The subjects named these objects faster if the language used was congruent with the language of the culture to which the picture belonged than in the incongruent conditions. Importantly, this effect occurred both when the subjects named in their L1 (Chinese) and in their L2 (English).

Summarising, studies in which participants viewed the faces of famous people, of ordinary people they had just interacted with, or with unknown people with either Caucasian or Asian features, converge in showing language-congruency effects. Interestingly, similar effects are also shown with cultural icons as well as with everyday objects that happen to look somewhat different in different cultures.

8.5 Discussion

The work reviewed here demonstrates compellingly that access to lexical representations, both in the written and spoken modality, both in comprehension or production, is language non-selective. Furthermore, studies that have considered lexical access in a linguistic (e.g., sentence) context, have found that the strong language cues provided by such a context are not enough to restrict lexical selection to only the target language; in particular cognate effects, and effects of interlingual homography or homophony still occur in such contexts. This is espe-cially striking in the case of speech, as this signal is very rich and provides many cues about the talker's identity (age, gender, social status; Van Berkum et al. 2008) and crucially about the language the talker is using. For instance, while the name "Bob" may be spelled the same in English and Spanish, the voice onset time of the initial /b/ will differ according to whether one speaks English or Spanish.

At least at first glance, the studies that so far have considered effects of lan-guage-extrinsic cues, such as the visual appearance of people and objects, converge on a rather different conclusion (Hartsuiker and Declerck 2009; Jared et al. 2013; Li et al. 2013; Woumans et al. in press; Zhang et al. 2013). Specifically, these stud-ies found that the language associated with visual representations affected aspects of language production, including naming latencies, language intrusion speech errors, fluency and the network of brain areas activated during picture naming. It is possible perhaps that the visual environment provides cues that more strongly affect representations in the target and non-target language than do linguistic cues. However, before accepting that conclusion it is important to note two major differ-ences between the literatures that considered linguistic and visual cues. First, the literature that considered linguistic cues typically used interlingual effects such as cognate status and homography. No study so far has tested whether such interlin-gual effects are modulated by visual cues. Is it enough, for instance, to see the face of Elvis Presley to reduce the interference that Dutch-English bilinguals experi-ence when processing Dutch-English homographs? It is crucial to test this, because all comparisons between linguistic and visual cues are now confounded by differ-ences in the measures that the cues are hypothesised to affect.

Second, the literature on visual cues has exclusively focused on measures of language production, while most studies looking at sentence cues have looked at language comprehension. An interesting possibility is that the process of language production is more sensitive to language cues than language comprehension. Such a scenario might be the result of the different demands that language processing in each modality places on the language processing system: the comprehender's immediate goal is to understand the sentence they are presented with. For many practical purposes, it may not be relevant in which language that sentence is (pro-vided of course it is a language the comprehender knows well enough). Thus, for the comprehender a cue for language may not be particularly relevant. This is dif-ferent for the speaker who *must* make a selection for language for each and every word they produce, which means that it would be very useful to exploit all lan-guage cues that are available to help this selection, including visual cues.

A further issue concerns the mechanisms that underlie the visual language cue-ing effects we have seen here. One question in particular is whether more fluent production in the context of a language-congruent cue than a language–incongru-ent cue, results from facilitation (i.e., priming of the correct language representa-tions) or interference (priming the incorrect language representations would hinder the selection of correct language representations). Indeed, Zhang et al. (2013) argue for an interference account, based on the conclusions of one experiment (Experiment 3) in which there were Chinese and American primes (cultural icons) but also matched control conditions. The target language was English. While there was a significant interference in the Chinese prime condition relative to its control condition (i.e., on the latency to recognise literal translations), there was no facilitation in the American primes condition (i.e., on the latency to recognise object names) relative to its control condition. However, Zhang et al.'s experiment constitutes very limited evidence for an interference account. As pointed out by Yang and Yang (2013), the literal translation recognition task is far from ideal, as the task trivially requires access to the native language. Furthermore, the conditions that test for interference (involving literal translations) are different from those testing for facilitation (involving object names). Finally, Zhang et al. only tested production in English, with subjects immersed in a context where English was presumably the default (a university in the United States). It is possible that in such a context, exposure to Chinese cultural icons is rather unexpected and draws attention, while exposure to American cultural icons is much more expected. Thus, the addition of a Chinese-language condition would have aided a more reliable assessment of the interference hypothesis.

Fortunately, the picture naming fMRI study reported by Li et al. (2013) contained both a Chinese and an English language condition and had both Chinese and English primes (i.e., faces) and a control condition. The pattern of naming latencies clearly indicated that the effect of face cues is facilitatory in nature. Additionally, the pattern of activation in the brain (i.e., more extensive activation in language control areas in the congruent than incongruent conditions) also suggested a facilitation effect, although it is also possible of course that there is both facilitation *and* interference.

A further issue is how general effects of visual language cues are. For instance, Yang and Yang (2013) suggest that Zhang et al.'s (2013) visual language cueing effects might be restricted to subjects with very low proficiency, based on observations in the literature that grammatical and lexical intrusions of the native language occur more frequently in relatively lower proficiency bilinguals than higher proficiency bilinguals (Poulisse and Bongaerts 1994). Kroll and McClain (2013) similarly suggest that such effects might well be modulated by factors such as age of second language acquisition and whether the bilingual is immersed in their second language or not (also see above). Future research will have to establish what the influence of such factors is, although it is important to note that some of the studies we discussed so far used extremely high-proficient bilinguals (the Spanish-Catalan bilinguals tested by Martin et al.) that typically acquired their second language early, as well as late bilinguals that were immersed in an L1-dominant environment (Hartsuiker and Declerck 2009). Of course, the same question can be asked for effects of linguistic cues too, and as pointed out by Van Assche et al. (2012), those studies also differ in for instance participant characteristics.

Most of the studies discussed so far consider the findings in light of language control, assuming that valid language cues—be they linguistic or visual in nature—can help suppress the irrelevant language. However, the question of which representations in bilingual memory are affected by language cues has so far not been answered conclusively. One possibility is that there are language nodes (e.g., Green

1986; Van Heuven et al. 1998) and that extrinsic language cues directly affect the activation of such nodes. On such an account, if I decide to speak Dutch, but I see a picture of (say) Elvis, this visual cue might activate my language node for L2 English, which would then promote the possibility of interference from English. In Dijkstra and Van Heuven's (2002) BIA+ model, the mechanisms of top-down language suppression by language nodes has been replaced by a so-called task schema, that is sensitive to situational demands (e.g., the specific task the subject has to perform) without directly affecting the activation of representations in the lexicon. A further possibility is then that visual language cues directly affect task schemata, leading for instance to interference when the incorrect task schema is cued.

However, Jared et al. (2013) propose a fascinating alternative account, at least for their findings of a language-congruency effect on the naming of objects with culturally specific looks, such as a Chinese versus a Canadian cabbage. Rather than interpreting this effect in terms of language control mechanisms, they frame the finding in terms of a bilingual dual coding model, which assumes a store of visual conceptual representations (Paivio and Lambert 1981). Importantly, Jared et al. assume that within such a model, there would be asymmetric connections from the visual representations to lexical items in the two languages. Thus, a visual representation for a Canadian cabbage would be more strongly connected to the English word "cabbage" than to its Chinese translation equivalent, while the reverse would be true for a visual representation of a Chinese cabbage. Therefore, naming the Canadian cabbage in English would be easier than naming it in Chinese, with the reverse holding for the Chinese cabbage. In such an account, at least some language-congruency effects can be seen as a direct consequence of the structure of speakers' semantic memory, rather than of language control mechanisms.

In conclusion, bilingual language production is affected by visual cues in the environment that point to one of the two (or more) languages the speaker knows. This is in interesting contrast to the effect of linguistic cues (e.g., sentence context) that has more often been studied in the language comprehension literature. While it may be a while before we understand better when and why such visual language cueing effects occur, the results obtained so far clearly indicate that visual information can directly affect language processing in bilinguals.

Acknowledgments Hans Rutger Bosker is thanked for very insightful comments on an earlier version of this paper.

References

Abutalebi, J. (2008). Neural aspects of second language representation and language control. *Acta Psychologica, 128*, 466–478.

Colomè, A. (2001). Lexical activation in bilinguals' speech production: Language-specific or language-independent? *Journal of Memory and Language, 45*, 721–736.

De Bruijn, E. R. A., Dijkstra, T., Chwilla, D. J., & Schriefers, H. J. (2001). Language context effects on interlingual homograph recognition: Evidence from event-related potentials and response times in semantic priming. *Bilingualism: Language and Cognition, 4*, 155–168.

Dijkstra, T., Timmermans, M., & Schriefers, H. (2000). On being blinded by your other language: Effects of task demands on interlingual homograph recognition. *Journal of Memory and Language, 42*, 445–464.

Dijkstra, T., & Van Heuven, W. J. B. (2002). The architecture of the bilingual word recognition system: From identification to decision. *Bilingualism: Language and Cognition, 5*, 175–197.

Duyck, W., Van Assche, E., Drieghe, D., & Hartsuiker, R. J. (2007). Visual word recognition by bilinguals in a sentence context: Evidence for nonselective lexical access. *Journal of Experimental Psychology: Learning, Memory, and Cognition, 33*, 663–679.

Elston-Güttler, K. E., Gunter, T. C., & Kotz, S. A. (2005). Zooming into L2: Global language context and adjustment affect processing of interlingual homographs in sentences. *Cognitive Brain Research, 25*, 57–70.

Gollan, T. H., Schotter, E. R., Gomez, J., Murillo, M., & Rayner, K. (2014). Multiple levels of bilingual language control: Evidence from language intrusions in reading aloud. *Psychological Science, 25*, 585–595.

Green, D. W. (1986). Control, activation, and resource: A framework for the control of speech in bilinguals. *Brain and Language, 27*, 210–223.

Hartsuiker, R. J. & Declerck, M. (2009, September). *Albert Costa y Julio Iglesias move up but Fidel Castro stays put: Language attraction in bilingual language production.* Paper presented at the AMLaP 2009 conference, Barcelona, Spain.

Ivanova, I., & Costa, A. (2008). Does bilingualism hamper lexical access in speech production? *Acta Psychologica, 127*, 277–288.

Jared, D., Pei Jun Poh, R., & Pavio, A. (2013). L1 and L2 picture naming in Mandarin-English bilinguals: A test of bilingual dual coding theory. *Bilingualism: Language and Cognition, 16*, 383–396.

Kroll, J. F., & Bialystok, E. (2013). Understanding the consequences of Bilingualism for language processing and cognitive control. *Journal of Cognitive Psychology, 25*, 497–514.

Kroll, J. F., & McClain, R. (2013). What bilinguals tell us about culture, cognition, and language. *Proceedings of the National Academy of Sciences of the United States of America, 110*, 11219–11220.

Lagrou, E., Hartsuiker, R. J., & Duyck, W. (2011). Knowledge of a second language influences auditory word recognition in the native language. *Journal of Experimental Psychology: Learning, Memory, and Cognition, 37*, 952–965.

Lagrou, E., Hartsuiker, R. J., & Duyck, W. (2013). The influence of sentence context and accented speech on lexical access in second-language auditory word recognition. *Bilingualism: Language and Cognition, 16*, 508–517.

Lemhöfer, K., Dijkstra, T., & Michel, M. C. (2004). Three languages, one echo: Cognate effects in trilingual word recognition. *Language and Cognitive Processes, 19*, 585–611.

Li, Y., Yang, J., Scherf, K. S., & Li, P. (2013). Two faces, two languages. An fMRI study of bilingual picture naming. *Brain and Language, 127*, 452–462.

Libben, M. R., & Titone, D. A. (2009). Bilingual lexical access in context: Evidence from eye movements during reading. *Journal of Experimental Psychology: Learning, Memory, and Cognition, 35*, 381–390.

Morris, M. W., & Zhang, S. (2013). Reply to Yang and Yang: Culturally primed first-language intrusion into second-language processing is associative spillover, not strategy. *Proceedings of the National Academy of Sciences of the United States of America, 110*.

Poulisse, N., & Bongaerts, T. (1994). 1st Language use in 2nd-language production. *Applied Linguistics, 15*, 36–57.

Paivio, A., & Lambert, W. (1981). Dual coding and bilingual memory. *Journal of Verbal Learning and Verbal Behavior, 20*, 532–539.

Rayner, K. (1998). Eye movements in reading and information processing: 20 years of research. *Psychological Bulletin, 24*, 372–422.

Schwartz, A. I., & Kroll, J. F. (2006). Bilingual lexical activation in sentence context. *Journal of Memory and Language, 55*, 197–212.

Spivey, M. J., & Marian, V. (1999). Cross talk between native and second languages: Partial activation of an irrelevant lexicon. *Psychological Science, 10*, 281–284.

Thierry, G., & Wu, Y. J. (2007). Brain potentials reveal unconscious translation during foreign-language comprehension. *Proceedings of the National Academy of Sciences of the United States of America, 104*, 12530–12535.

Titone, D., Libben, M., Mercier, J., Whitford, V., & Pivneva, I. (2011). Bilingual lexical access during L1 sentence reading: The effects of L2 knowledge, semantic constraint, and L1-L2 intermixing. *Journal of Experimental Psychology: Learning, Memory, and Cognition, 37*, 1412–1431.

Van Assche, E., Duyck, W., Hartsuiker, R. J., & Diependaele, K. (2009). Does bilingualism change native-language reading? Cognate effects in a sentence context. *Psychological Science, 20*, 923–927.

Van Assche, E., Drieghe, D., Duyck, W., Welvaert, M., & Hartsuiker, R. J. (2011). The influence of semantic constraints on bilingual word recognition during sentence reading. *Journal of Memory and Language, 64*, 88–107.

Van Assche, E., Duyck, W., & Hartsuiker, R. J. (2012). Bilingual word recognition in a sentence context. *Frontiers in Psychology, 3*, 174.

Van Berkum, J. J. A., Van den Brink, D., Tesink, C. M. J. Y., Kos, M., & Hagoort, P. (2008). The neural integration of speaker and message. *Journal of Cognitive Neuroscience, 20*, 580–591.

Van Hell, J. G., & De Groot, A. M. B. (2008). Sentence context modulates visual word recognition and translation in bilinguals. *Acta Psychologica, 128*, 431–451.

Van Hell, J. G., & Dijkstra, T. (2002). Foreign language knowledge can influence native language performance in exclusively native contexts. *Psychonomic Bulletin and Review, 9*, 780–789.

Van Heuven, W. J. B., Dijkstra, T., & Grainger, J. (1998). Orthographic neighborhood effects in bilingual word recognition. *Journal of Memory and Language, 39*, 458–483.

Woumans, E., Martin, C. D., Vanden Bulcke, C., Van Assche, E., Costa, A., Hartsuiker, R. J., & Duyck, W. (in press). Can faces prime a language? *Psychological Science*.

Yang, S., & Yang, H. (2013). Does bilingual fluency moderate the disruption effect of cultural cues on second-language processing? *Proceedings of the National Academy of Sciences of the United States of America, 110*.

Zhang, S., Morris, M. W., Cheng, C.-Y., & Yap, A. J. (2013). Heritage-culture images disrupt immigrants' second-language processing through triggering first-language interference. *Proceedings of the National Academy of Sciences of the United States of America, 110*, 11272–11277.

Chapter 9
In the Mind's Eye: Eye-Tracking and Multi-modal Integration During Bilingual Spoken-Language Processing

Sarah Chabal and Viorica Marian

> *Language is a part of our organism and no less complicated*
> *than it. ... The tacit conventions on which the understanding of*
> *everyday language depends are enormously complicated.*
> Ludwig Wittgenstein, May 14, 1915

Language is more than words—it is the amalgamation of sounds and simultaneously co-occurring visual inputs (e.g., facial features, gestures and nearby objects) that combine to mutually influence one another. The human linguistic system[1] is equipped to automatically integrate and process information from multiple modalities and to use this integrated information to enhance processing. Perhaps the most well-known demonstration of the interactivity of the language processing system is the McGurk effect (McGurk and MacDonald 1976), which is a perceptual phenomenon in which competing auditory and visual information lead to the perception of an un-presented sound. For example, if a listener hears the phoneme /ba/ while simultaneously watching a video of a speaker's lips producing /ga/, the combination of the competing inputs often leads listeners to perceive the phoneme /

---

[1]The vocabulary that we use to describe functions such as language, cognition, and perception (e.g., "linguistic system") implicitly identifies entities as distinct from one another. However, language, cognition, and perception are not distinct modules, but rather are part of a highly interactive network. In order to understand how this system operates, we use math symbols (e.g., computational models) or verbal labels (e.g., words) to describe particular functions of the network. The inclusion of these terms does not preclude interactivity, but rather gives us a way to describe functions and refer to concepts either verbally or symbolically.

S. Chabal (✉) · V. Marian
Department of Communication Sciences and Disorders, Northwestern University,
2240 N Campus Dr., Evanston, IL 60208, USA
e-mail: schabal@u.northwestern.edu

© Springer India 2015
R.K. Mishra et al. (eds.), *Attention and Vision in Language Processing*, DOI 10.1007/978-81-322-2443-3_9

da/, even though the sound /da/ was never presented. When one of the modalities is stripped away (i.e., participants receive only auditory or only visual input) participants' perceptions match the input. The McGurk effect holds even when the sources of auditory and visual information are presented with a separation in space (Jones and Munhall 1997; MacDonald et al. 2000) or with a discrepancy in temporal presentation (Van Wassenhove et al. 2007) and therefore do not appear to emanate from the same source (for a demonstration of the McGurk effect see auditory neuroscience.com/McGurkEffect).

The robustness of the McGurk effect and other demonstrations of audio-visual integration (e.g., co-speech hand gestures: Kelly et al. 2004; processing of facial articulatory movements: Van Wassenhove et al. 2005), coupled with evidence that even infants appear able to combine auditory and visual inputs by matching facial movements with their corresponding sounds (Kuhl and Meltzoff 1982), together lend credence to the idea that integration from multiple modalities is important for, and inherent to, language perception and processing (see also the motor theory of speech perception, e.g., Liberman and Mattingly (1985), for an example of integration across motor and auditory domains). This cross-modal integration may be of even greater significance for bilingual speakers, who rely on auditory and visual cues to interpret information from multiple languages.

In the beginning stages of second language learning, visual input can aid in the acquisition of non-native phonemic contrasts (e.g., Hardison 2003; Hazan et al. 2002) and novel vocabulary (Plass et al. 1998). For example, while learning German, native English speakers are better able to remember word translations when they are presented both verbally and with a visual representation (i.e., picture or video clips; Plass et al. 1998). Visual input, in the form of facial cues (e.g., Ronquest and Hernandez 2005; Soto-Faraco et al. 2007) or head movements (e.g., Davis and Kim 2006), can also be used to determine the language of an interlocutor. In fact, bilingual infants are better than monolingual infants at discriminating between languages based on visual input alone (i.e., silent videos of speakers; Sebastián-Gallés et al. 2012; Weikum et al. 2007). The multi-modality of the language system, then, appears to be a crucial part of bilingual language acquisition and perception.

Furthermore, the importance of an interactive language system is not limited to the beginning stages of bilingualism. Even for highly skilled, balanced bilinguals, who use both of their languages on a daily basis, there is a discrepancy between auditory perceptual abilities in their two languages. For example, French-Spanish bilinguals may fail to perceive lexical stress in Spanish (Dupoux et al. 2010), and Catalan-Spanish bilinguals may be unable to recognise certain phonemic contrasts in Catalan in spite of fully developed perceptual abilities in Spanish (Sebastián-Gallés et al. 2005). Such perceptual difficulties in a second language can be overcome by integrating information from the speech stream with visual information provided by facial articulatory gestures (Navarra and Soto-Faraco 2007). Visual input can also aid bilinguals' retrieval of lexical items (Schroeder and Marian, in prep). In speech production, visual and motor input from the use of hand gestures has been linked to better linguistic access (for a review see Krauss and Hadar

1999). In fact, bilinguals often produce more hand gestures than their monolingual peers (see Nicoladis 2007 for a review of bilinguals' use of hand gestures). Together, such findings demonstrate the positive effects of multi-modal processing within a bilingual context.

9.1 Eye-Tracking as an Index of a Multi-Modal Language System

There are a variety of methods that have been developed to explore the interactive nature of the language processing system, including neuroimaging (e.g., Calvert et al. 1997; Campbell et al. 2001) and electrophysiological techniques (e.g., Kelly et al. 2004; Musacchia et al. 2007); computational modelling (e.g., Dupont and Luettin 2000; Shook and Marian 2013); and behavioural methods such as cross-modal priming (e.g., Berry et al. 1997; Loveman et al. 2002) and visual word recognition (e.g., Baron and Strawson 1976). A particularly powerful method is eye-tracking, which can index participants' real-time reactions to simultaneous auditory and visual inputs.

Eye-tracking provides a means of measuring gaze and eye motion around a visual scene by exploiting the reflective properties of the eye. In the most common eye-tracking systems, infrared light, unseen by the participant, illuminates the pupil and cornea. Calculating the angle between the two yields a measure of gaze direction, which can be calibrated to a visual scene.

Current eye-tracking methods are capable of tracking eye movements at sampling rates of up to 2,000 Hz, and provide high temporal resolution that allows for the exploration of real-time language processing.

A popular technique that relies on eye-tracking to study language is the visual world paradigm (e.g., Cooper 1974; Tanenhaus et al. 1995), in which participants carry out spoken instructions to touch, move, or manipulate objects in a visual workspace that is either real or presented on a computer screen (e.g., Tanenhaus and Spivey-Knowlton 1996). Such work has informed our understanding of language processing by illustrating the incremental nature of comprehension. In other words, spoken-language processing occurs over time as auditory information unfolds, and multiple lexical candidates can be partially activated (Marslen-Wilson 1987). For example, the spoken word "candy" will activate words such as "cap," "can," and "candle," as the sounds "c-a-n-d-y" emerge over time. Eye movements are sensitive to these instances of multiple activation, and a participant who is instructed to "Pick up the *candy*" will glance at a *candle* that is also in the visual display (e.g., Allopenna et al. 1998; Tanenhaus et al. 1995). Because participants' eye movements to objects in a visual scene are closely time-locked to the auditory references to those same objects, eye-tracking, by indexing those eye movements, provides an on-line measure of how language comprehension progresses.

By exploiting these temporal dynamics of auditory language processing, eye-tracking research has been able to demonstrate that not only is language processed incrementally and influenced by relationships between linguistic features, but it is also immediately influenced by relevant visual information. For example, when items with phonologically overlapping names are simultaneously present in a search display (e.g., "candy" and "candle") and participants are instructed to interact with one of those objects (e.g., "Click on the candy"), not only do they make eye movements to the phonologically related competitor (e.g., candle), but eye movements are also slower to the target when the competitor is present (e.g., Tanenhaus et al. 1995, 1996). Whereas participants are able to identify the target an average of 55 ms *before* the offset of the target name when no competitor is present, target identification takes place approximately 30 ms *after* word-offset when there is a competitor present (Tanenhaus et al. 1995). Because auditory information is identical across competitor-present and competitor-absent trials and the only variable factor is the visual input, such studies provide evidence that relevant visual context affects the early stages of spoken-language processing.

In addition to providing good temporal correspondence that allows for the indexing of on-line language processing, eye-tracking is also recognised for its ability to be used in natural language contexts. When words are embedded in natural sentence structures, eye movements can be measured without disrupting spoken input. This allows researchers to explore real-time language comprehension (as discussed throughout this chapter) and production (e.g., Griffin and Bock 2000; Meyer et al. 1998).

9.2 Using Eye-Tracking to Explore Bilingual Multi-Modal Language Processing

Because of its ability to index natural language with good temporal correspondence, eye-tracking has found its niche not only in monolingual language processing research but also in the exploration of bilingual language processing. Within bilingualism research, eye-tracking was first introduced to explore whether bilinguals process their two languages in parallel or separately. Parallel processing assumes that both of a bilingual's two languages are activated simultaneously; conversely, separate or sequential processing assumes that a bilingual speaker or listener has selective access only to the language system that is currently in use. While some behavioural evidence suggested that a bilingual's languages were independently activated and that interference did not occur across languages (e.g., Durgunolu and Roediger 1987; Gerard and Scarborough 1989; Kirsner et al. 1980; Ransdell and Fischler 1987; Scarborough et al. 1984; Watkins and Peynircioglu 1983), other studies provided reason to believe that bilingual language processing may occur in parallel, with both languages becoming simultaneously activated and mutually influencing one another (e.g., bilingual Stroop task: Chen and Ho 1986; Preston and Lambert 1969; Tzelgov et al. 1990; cross-linguistic priming: Beauvillain and Grainger 1987).

However, in tasks such as cross-linguistic priming paradigms and the bilingual Stroop (in which participants see printed colour words in one language and are instructed to name the ink colour of those words in another language, i.e., the Spanish word for blue, "azul", written in yellow ink), both of a bilingual's languages are overtly cued. It is therefore not clear whether parallel processing occurs when only one language is intentionally accessed. In the Stroop task, for example, visual input is provided in one language and production happens in the second; in cross-linguistic priming tasks both languages are visually presented. What is needed, then, is a methodology that allows for the activation of two languages to be tested while only requiring input or output in a single language.

Techniques that probe the activation of a language without overt cuing have been used to explore parallel language access in bilingual production (e.g., Colomé 2001; Costa et al. 2000; Hoshino and Kroll 2008; for a review see Kroll et al. 2006), written comprehension (e.g., Midgley et al. 2008; Morford et al. 2011; Thierry and Wu 2007; Van Heuven et al. 1998), and spoken comprehension (Marian and Spivey 2003a, b; Spivey and Marian 1999). Specifically, in spoken comprehension, eye movements are often used to index language processing in bilinguals (but see also Thierry and Wu 2007 for an example of how electrophysiological techniques can be used to explore parallel language access).

Using the visual world paradigm, Spivey and Marian (1999) provided the first eye-tracking evidence of parallel language activation during bilingual language comprehension. They tested Russian-English bilinguals in monolingual Russian sessions in which participants were requested, for example, to pick up the postage stamp ("Poloji marku nije krestika"). In competitor conditions, the target object (e.g., *marka*," Russian for "postage stamp") was accompanied by an object whose English name shared initial phonological features with the target (e.g., "marker"). As the auditory instructions unfolded, incoming phonological information mapped to both of the bilinguals' languages, and participants made looks to the phonologically competing "marker", even though input was only received in Russian (see Fig. 9.1). Moreover, not only do bilinguals experience between-language competition (e.g., "marker" competes with "marka") but, like monolinguals, they also experience within-language competition in each of their two languages (e.g., "candy" competes with "candle" in English, and "spichki" [matches] competes with "spitsy" [knitting needles] in Russian; Marian and Spivey 2003a). Although within-language competition is typically stronger than between-language competition (Marian and Spivey 2003b), bilinguals must still contend with multiple sources of competition—in contrast to monolinguals who only encounter competition within a single language.

Furthermore, to add to these already challenging processing demands, within-language competition and between-language competition can occur simultaneously (Marian and Spivey 2003b). When Russian-English bilinguals were presented with visual world displays that contained a target object (e.g., "speaker") paired with both a within-language competitor (whose English name was phonologically similar to the target, e.g., "spear") and a between-language competitor (whose Russian name was phonologically similar to the target; e.g.,

Fig. 9.1 An illustration of a search display showing a Russian-English bilingual's fixations (crosshairs) on the phonologically competing "marker" (*top left quadrant*) when instructed in Russian to pick up the postage stamp (*marka* in Russian; *bottom right quadrant*). (Adapted from Spivey and Marian 1999, Fig. 1.)

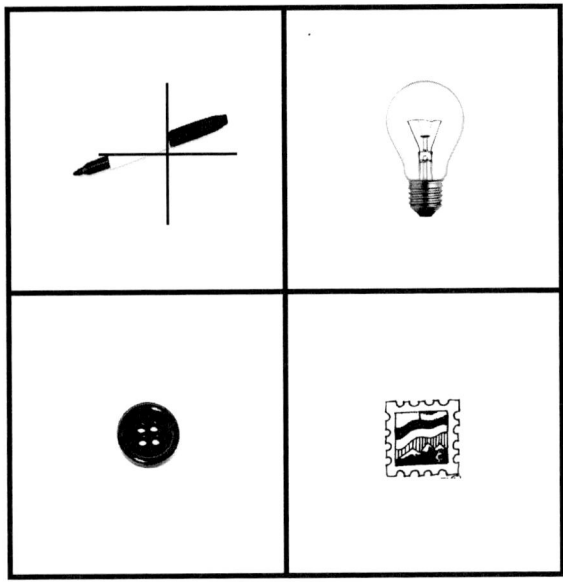

"spichki" [matches]), they made eye movements to both the Russian and the English competitors. This suggests that bilinguals simultaneously experience competing activation from lexical items that overlap phonologically both within and across their two languages. Importantly, these findings are robust and have been replicated in language pairs including Dutch and English (e.g., Lagrou et al. 2013; Weber and Cutler 2004), French and German (e.g., Weber and Paris 2004), Spanish and English (e.g., Canseco-Gonzalez et al. 2010; Ju and Luce 2004), and Japanese and English (e.g., Cutler et al. 2006).

Not only do these eye-tracking studies demonstrate that both of a bilingual's languages are activated in parallel, but they also illustrate how the surrounding visual display interacts in real time with the phonological information being received by the bilingual listener (Marian 2009). This audio-visual integration during spoken-language processing has been explored computationally using the Bilingual Language Interaction Network for Comprehension of Speech (BLINCS; Shook and Marian 2013), which is, to our knowledge, the only model to date that illustrates and predicts bilingual spoken-language activation as it occurs over time (as individual phonemes unfold) within a constraining visual environment (see Fig. 9.2). Specifically, the model receives a word one phoneme at a time and, after each phonemic unit, determines which words (in two languages) best match that input. Lexical units that match the phonemic input receive activation, with activation levels of each unit changing over time as additional phonemes are introduced into the model. Simultaneously, information about visual representations is integrated into the semantic level of linguistic processing, so that words with meanings that map more closely to the semantic information provided by the visual input receive a greater amount of activation. Through direct top-down links

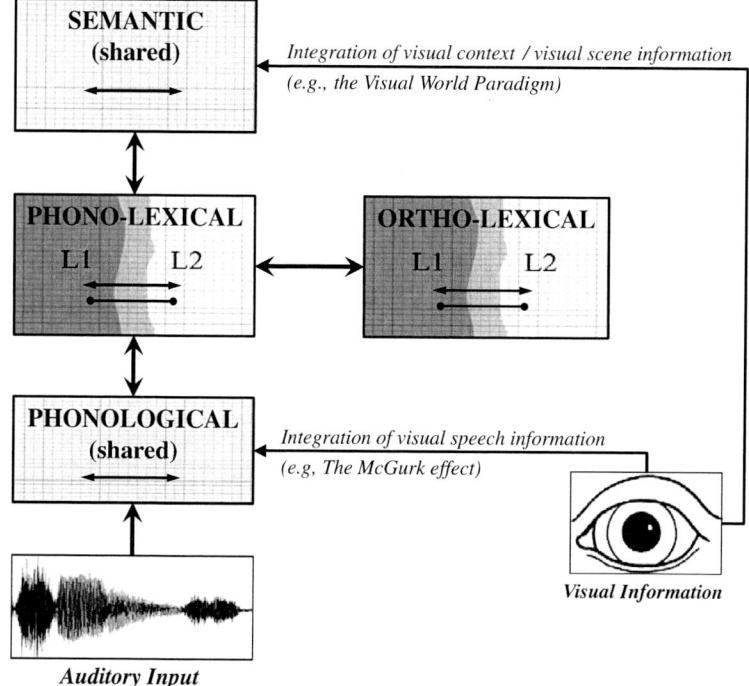

Fig. 9.2 The *Bilingual Language Interactive Network for Comprehension of Speech* (*BLINCS*) is equipped to integrate visual information with unfolding auditory input to model and predict bilingual spoken-language activation as it occurs over time within a constraining visual environment. (From Shook and Marian 2012, Fig. 1.)

between the semantic and phono-lexical levels, BLINCS is able to simulate how objects in a visual scene affect the activation (and eventual selection) of words within the bilingual's lexicon and can make predictions that are supported by behavioural eye-tracking data (see Fig. 9.3).

One prediction made by BLINCS is that competition and dual-language activation in bilinguals can occur both from bottom-up phonological input *and* from top-down connections.

In fact, recent eye-tracking work supports this hypothesis by demonstrating that bimodal bilinguals, who are users of a spoken and a signed language such as English and American Sign Language (ASL), experience competition between their two languages (Shook and Marian 2012). Shook and Marian instructed ASL-English bilinguals to click on a target image, such as "cheese." Embedded in the computerised display was a competitor item whose name overlapped in ASL on three of four phonological parameters—hand-shape, motion, location of the sign in space, and orientation of the palm or hand. For example, the ASL sign for "paper" overlaps with "cheese" in hand-shape, location, and orientation, whereas the pair differs in the motion of the signs. Importantly, none of the target-competitor pairs overlapped in English phonology. Participants were instructed, in

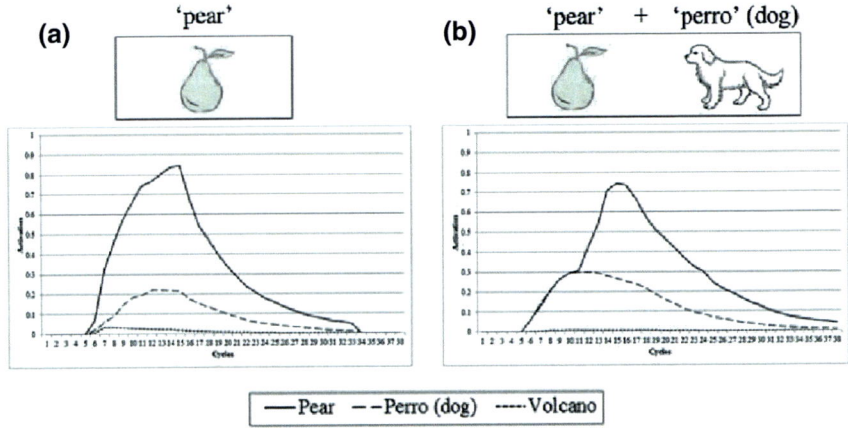

Fig. 9.3 Activation of the BLINCS model during auditory presentation of the word "pear" accompanied by visual presentation of *pear* alone (**a**) and *pear* and *dog* [*perro* in Spanish] (**b**). These figures illustrate how BLINCS allows for interactions between auditory and visual inputs within the bilingual language processing system. (Adapted from Shook and Marian 2013, Fig. 11 Panels A and B.)

English only, to click on the target item (i.e., "Click on the cheese") while their eye movements were recorded. Recall that in the classic visual world paradigm studies, unfolding auditory information leads to competition between items in the non-target language (e.g., "Click on the speaker" leads to looks to the matches, "spichki" in Russian; Marian and Spivey 2003b). However, in Shook and Marian's study, the bilinguals' languages did not share auditory phonology. Nevertheless, despite a lack of unfolding English phonological information that would lead to the activation of "paper" when "cheese" was heard, ASL-English bilinguals gave more looks to the paper than did English monolinguals, and they also gave more looks to the paper than to control items that did not overlap with the target in ASL phonology. This demonstrates that languages are activated in parallel even when bottom-up, featural information is only available for one of the languages, and provides support for a language system that includes top-down or lateral connections (see Fig. 9.4). It also suggests that information in a visual display can affect linguistic processing even if the visual input cannot be mapped directly onto the incoming language stream.

Further support for a highly interactive bilingual language system and the role of visual input in language activation comes from recent research suggesting that bilingual language access can proceed even in the absence of *any* bottom-up linguistic information. Chabal and Marian (2015) presented Spanish-English bilinguals with an image of a target object (e.g., a *clock*, "reloj" in Spanish) and asked them to search for that item in a subsequent visual display. Even though the objects' linguistic forms were never explicitly presented (i.e., there was no auditory input), participants made eye movements to objects whose names overlapped with the target in English (e.g., a *cloud*, "nube" in Spanish) and to objects whose

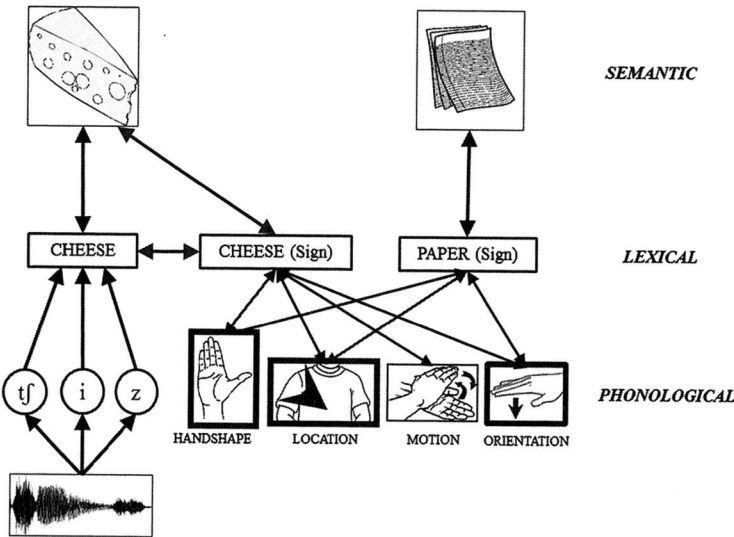

Fig. 9.4 Proposed pathways showing *bottom-up* (e.g., auditory phonological information to the lexical item "cheese"), *lateral* (e.g., the spoken lexical item "cheese" to the sign for cheese), and *top-down* (e.g., the lexical sign for cheese to the phonological feature of handshape) connections between languages. When bimodal bilinguals were instructed in English to find the "cheese," they made eye movements to the "paper," which shares phonological overlap with cheese in American Sign Language but not in English. (From Shook and Marian 2012, Fig. 4.)

names overlapped with the target in Spanish (e.g., a *present*, "regalo" in Spanish). The same image, therefore, was able to lead to access of both of the bilinguals' languages. This demonstrates the ubiquity of multi-modal linguistic processing by showing that visual input alone may be sufficient to spark language access. Moreover, it provides strong evidence for the parallel access of both of a bilingual's languages because the viewing of pictures activated not only English but also Spanish, which was never used within the context of the experiment (all task instructions and experimenter interactions occurred in English only).

9.3 Consequences of an Interactive Bilingual Language System

One consequence of the highly interactive nature of the bilingual language system is that bilinguals must develop strategies to cope with the constant activation of both of their languages. It has been proposed (e.g., Kroll 2008) that as a result of suppressing information from the unneeded language and of attending only to the relevant language, bilinguals have enhanced executive function abilities relative to monolinguals (e.g., Bialystok 2006, 2008; Costa et al. 2008; Martin-Rhee and Bialystok 2008; Prior and Macwhinney 2009). For example, bilingual children have been found to outperform monolingual children on tasks requiring attentional control (e.g., Martin-Rhee and Bialystok 2008), and similar bilingual advantages have been observed across the lifespan (e.g., Bialystok et al. 2004; Bialystok 2008; Costa et al. 2009). It is important to note, however, that the extent of bilinguals' executive function gains and inhibitory abilities may be dependent upon a number of factors including proficiency levels across their two languages (e.g., Khare et al 2013; Singh and Mishra 2013), their amount of experience within a bilingual environment (Bialystok and Barac 2012), and the age at which they became actively exposed to both languages (Luk et al. 2011). Nevertheless, consistent with the multi-modality of the bilingual experience, executive function advantages are seen in the auditory (e.g., Soveri et al. 2010), visual (for a review see Bialystok 2011), and combined audio-visual (e.g., Bialystok et al. 2006; Krizman et al. 2012) domains.

However, the link between bilinguals' need to control interference within and across their languages and their performance on executive tasks remained largely inferential. Bilinguals were known to activate both of their languages and were known to display enhanced cognitive control abilities, but a direct connection between the two had never been empirically demonstrated. In order to explain how the processing of ambiguous auditory information (which could lead to activation of multiple words within the lexicon) can be associated with executive function, Blumenfeld and Marian (2011) tested monolinguals and bilinguals on a visual world paradigm task containing an item whose name overlapped phonologically with the name of a spoken target (e.g., "Click on the plum" while a plug was present in the search display). Following each eye-tracking trial, participants completed a negative priming task to probe residual activation or inhibition of locations that had previously contained competitor items (see Fig. 9.5). Although monolinguals and bilinguals both experienced similar competition between the phonologically overlapping items, as evidenced by eye movements to competitors, the groups differed in how they responded to the negative priming probes. Specifically, bilinguals inhibited the visual location of the auditorily received input, and the strength of this inhibition was correlated with their performance on a non-linguistic executive control task. For the monolingual group, inhibition of phonological competitors did not relate with the group's executive control abilities. By exploiting the tight link between incoming auditory information and the corresponding visual representations, Blumenfeld and Marian provided empirical support for the idea that cognitive control mechanisms can be affected by linguistic experience.

These enhancements in bilinguals' executive function render a number of practical advantages. For example, bilinguals' ability to avoid distraction from irrelevant languages may be one reason that they are better than monolinguals at learning a new language's vocabulary (e.g., Cenoz 2003; Kaushanskaya and Marian 2009; Keshavarz and Astaneh 2004). To test this possibility, Bartolotti and Marian (2012) trained monolinguals and bilinguals to equivalent levels on vocabulary in a made-up language called Colbertian (matching the groups on novel-language proficiency ensured that effects were not due to one group learning better than the other).

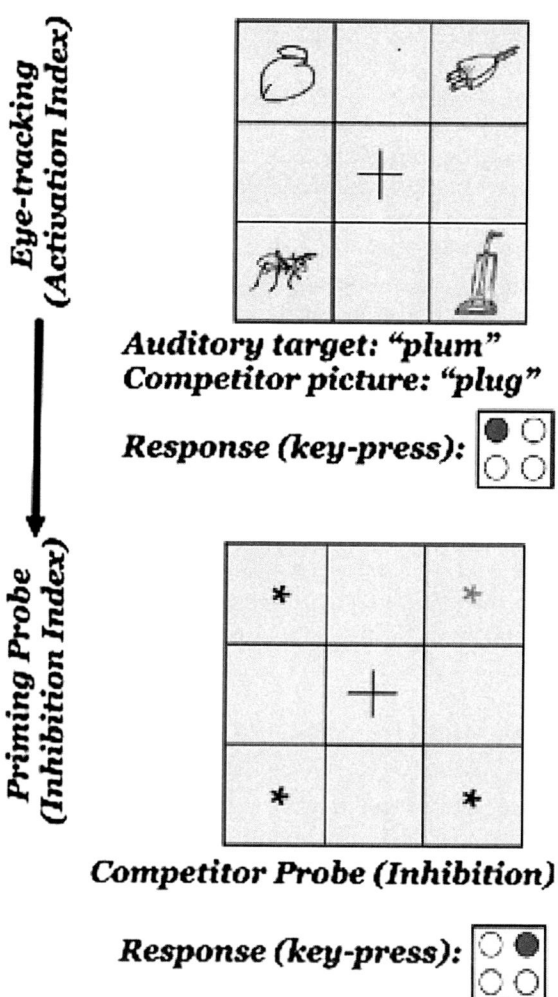

Fig. 9.5 Sample visual display from the eye-tracking and negative priming paradigms. Participants were presented with an eye-tracking trial, in which they were instructed to locate the picture of a spoken object while another object on the display competed phonologically within the same language, English (e.g., *plum-plug*) (*top* of figure). Next, the inhibition of the competitor item was explored by asking participants to quickly locate a shaded asterisk that was positioned where the phonological competitor had been previously (*bottom* of figure). Although both English monolinguals and Spanish–English bilinguals made looks to phonological competitor pictures, bilinguals displayed less residual inhibition of competitor locations than monolinguals, suggesting that their inhibitory processes may be more efficient. Consistent with this interpretation, bilinguals' (but not monolinguals') inhibition on the priming probes was inversely correlated with their performance on a non-linguistic executive control task. (Adapted from Blumenfeld and Marian 2011 Fig. 1 Panel A.)

Interference from participants' previously known language (i.e., English) was then
tested using the visual world paradigm. As in other visual world paradigm studies
we have discussed in this chapter, participants were presented with a target object
(e.g., an acorn, called "shundo" in Colbertian) and a distractor object whose English
name either overlapped (e.g., "shovel") or did not overlap (e.g., "mushroom")
with the newly learned name of the target object. As the phonological information, "shundo," unfolded, bilinguals made fewer looks to competitor items than did
monolinguals. Although both monolinguals and bilinguals experienced competition between items that competed phonologically, Bartolotti and Marian's findings
suggest that the groups differ in how they manage this competition. Specifically,
bilinguals were better able to suppress competition from their previously known languages, which may be a contributing factor to observed language-learning benefits.

Together, Bartolotti and Marian's (2012) and Blumenfeld and Marian's (2011)
studies illustrate how eye-tracking evidence can be combined with knowledge
gleaned from other behavioural, neuroimaging and electrophysiological techniques to explore how and why bilinguals' multi-modal linguistic experiences
shape their cognitive systems. Methods that allow for the integration of auditory
and visual inputs (such as eye-tracking) will advance the field of bilingual research
by facilitating the exploration of higher order cognitive processes such as language, memory, attention, and decision making.

9.4 Constraints of the Visual World Paradigm

Although eye-tracking provides bilingual researchers with an invaluable tool to
index language processing and audio-visual integration within a spoken-word
context, there are a few limitations (as with any behavioral or neuroimaging technique) that must be kept in mind. First, because of constraining study environments, researchers conducting eye-tracking experiments must select only a small
subset of visual objects and auditory tokens when designing their studies. In reality, the human language experience is not confined to utterances concerning only
the objects within our immediate visual scenes. While a number of studies using
the visual world paradigm have included full sentence structures (e.g., Tanenhaus
et al. 1995), and some have investigated eye movements after the relevant visual
scene has been removed (e.g., Altmann 2004), eye-tracking studies continue to
rely primarily on tightly controlled auditory and visual inputs.

Second, effects of phonological competition within the visual world paradigm are
susceptible to subtle task and presentation manipulations. For example, the amount
of time that the visual images are displayed before the onset of an auditory stimulus
affects the types of information that participants are able to access about those pictures
(e.g., shape, semantic, or phonological information; Huettig and McQueen 2007), and
phonological competition effects can be abolished by eliminating or providing only
a short preview of the search display (for a review of how the mechanisms of visual
processing affect language-mediated eye movements, see Dahan et al. 2007).

9.5 Conclusions

> What we learn only through the ears makes less impression upon our minds than what is presented to the trustworthy eye.
>
> Horace

Eye-tracking with the visual world paradigm continues to be a valuable method for researchers interested in both the auditory and visual components of the language system. The use of eye-tracking to examine both the architecture of the bilingual language system and the consequences of bilingualism for broader cognitive functioning has provided crucial insight into the bilingual experience and the multi-modality of language. For example, eye-tracking research has demonstrated that a bilingual's two languages are simultaneously activated (e.g., Ju and Luce 2004; Spivey and Marian 1999; Weber and Cutler 2004) and interact in bottom-up and top-down fashions (Shook and Marian 2012). In fact, both of a bilingual's languages are activated even when neither is being used (Chabal and Marian 2015). As a consequence, bilinguals must contend with competition arising both within and between their two languages (Marian and Spivey 2003a, b), which bolsters their executive functioning abilities (Blumenfeld and Marian 2011). More efficient executive functioning abilities, in turn, manifest in practical benefits such as the ability to more easily learn additional languages (Bartolotti and Marian 2012).

Such advances in the field of bilingual language processing and cognition can, in part, be attributed to the use of eye-tracking. By combining information from auditory and visual sources to closely resemble real-world, multi-modal situations, and by allowing language processing to proceed in a naturalistic context (Huettig et al. 2011), the visual world paradigm provides an ecologically valid methodology for studying language processing. At the intersection of perceptual (e.g., auditory and visual) and higher order processing, eye-tracking techniques can be used to explore how language interacts with other cognitive functions in a highly interconnected, non-modular mind (e.g., Prinz 2006).

Acknowledgments Preparation of this chapter was supported in part by grant NICHD R01HD059858 to Viorica Marian. The authors would like to thank Anthony Shook, Scott Schoeder, James Bartolotti, Jennifer Krizman and Tuan Lam for helpful comments on this work.

References

Allopenna, P., Magnuson, J. S., & Tanenhaus, M. K. (1998). Tracking the time course of spoken word recognition using eye movements: Evidence for continuous mapping models. *Journal of Memory and Language, 38*(4), 419–439. doi:10.1006/jmla.1997.2558.

Altmann, G. T. M. (2004). Language-mediated eye movements in the absence of a visual world: The "blank screen paradigm". *Cognition, 93*(2), B79–B87. doi:10.1016/j.cognition.2004.02.005.

Baron, J., & Strawson, C. (1976). Use of orthographic and word-specific knowledge in reading words aloud. *Journal of Experimental Psychology: Human Perception and Performance, 2*(3), 386–393. doi:10.1037/0096-1523.2.3.386.

Bartolotti, J., & Marian, V. (2012). Language learning and control in monolinguals and bilinguals. *Cognitive Science, 36*, 1129–1147. doi:10:1111/j.1551-6709.2012.01243.x.

Beauvillain, C., & Grainger, J. (1987). Accessing interlexical homographs: Some limitations of a language-selective access. *Journal of Memory and Language, 26*(6), 658–672.

Berry, D. C., Banbury, S., & Henry, L. (1997). Transfer across form and modality in implicit and explicit memory. *The Quarterly Journal of Experimental Psychology A, 50*(1), 1–24. doi:10.1080/027249897392206.

Bialystok, E. (2006). Effect of bilingualism and computer video game experience on the Simon task. *Canadian Journal of Experimental Psychology, 60*(1), 68–79. doi:10.1037/cjep2006008.

Bialystok, E. (2008). Bilingualism: The good, the bad, and the indifferent. *Bilingualism: Language and Cognition, 12*(01), 3. doi:10.1017/S1366728908003477.

Bialystok, E. (2011). Reshaping the mind: The benefits of bilingualism. *Canadian Journal of Experimental Psychology, 65*(4), 229–235. doi:10.1037/a0025406.

Bialystok, E., & Barac, R. (2012). Emerging bilingualism: Dissociating advantages for metalinguistic awareness and executive control. *Cognition, 122*(1), 67–73. doi:10.1016/j.cognition.2011.08.003.

Bialystok, E., Craik, F. I. M., Klein, R., & Viswanathan, M. (2004). Bilingualism, aging, and cognitive control: Evidence from the Simon task. *Psychology and Aging, 19*(2), 290–303. doi:10.1037/0882-7974.19.2.290.

Bialystok, E., Craik, F. I. M., & Ruocco, A. C. (2006). Dual-modality monitoring in a classification task: The effects of bilingualism and ageing. *Quarterly Journal of Experimental Psychology, 59*(11), 1968–1983. doi:10.1080/17470210500482955.

Blumenfeld, H. K., & Marian, V. (2011). Bilingualism influences inhibitory control in auditory comprehension. *Cognition, 118*(2), 245–257. doi:10.1016/j.cognition.2010.10.012.

Calvert, G. A., Bullmore, E. T., Brammer, M. J., Campbell, R., Williams, S. C. R., McGuire, P. K., & David, A. S. et al. (1997). Activation of auditory cortex during silent lipreading. *Science, 276*(5312), 593–596. doi:10.1126/science.276.5312.593.

Campbell, R., MacSweeney, M., Surguladze, S., Calvert, G. A., McGuire, P. K., Suckling, J., & David, A. S. et al. (2001). Cortical substrates for the perception of face actions: An fMRI study of the specificity of activation for seen speech and for meaningless lower-face acts (gurning). *Cognitive Brain Research, 12*(2), 233–243.

Canseco-Gonzalez, E., Brehm, L., Brick, C., Brown-Schmidt, S., Fischer, K., & Wagner, K. (2010). Carpet or carcel: The effect of age of acquisition and language mode on bilingual lexical access. *Language and Cognitive Processes, 25*(5), 669–705. doi:10.1080/01690960903474912.

Cenoz, J. (2003). The additive effect of bilingualism on third language acquisition: A review. *International Journal of Bilingualism, 7*(1), 71–89. doi:10.1177/13670069030070010501.

Chabal, S., & Marian, V. (2015). Speakers of different languages process the visual world differently. *Journal of Experimental Psychology: General, 144*(3).

Chen, H., & Ho, C. (1986). Development of stroop interference in Chinese-English bilinguals. *Journal of Experimental Psychology: Learning, Memory, and Cognition, 12*(3), 397–401. doi:10.1037/0278-7393.12.3.397.

Colomé, À. (2001). Lexical activation in bilinguals' speech production: Language-specific or language-independent? *Journal of Memory and Language, 45*(4), 721–736. doi:10.1006/jmla.2001.2793.

Cooper, R. M. (1974). The control of eye fixation by the meaning of spoken language. *Cognitive Psychology, 107*, 84–107.

Costa, A., Caramazza, A., & Sebastián-Gallés, N. (2000). The cognate facilitation effect: Implications for models of lexical access. *Journal of Experimental Psychology. Learning, Memory, and Cognition, 26*(5), 1283–1296. doi:10.1037/0278-7393.26.5.1283.

Costa, A., Hernández, M., & Sebastián-Gallés, N. (2008). Bilingualism aids conflict resolution: Evidence from the ANT task. *Cognition, 106*(1), 59–86. doi:10.1016/j.cognition.2006.12.013.

Costa, A., Hernández, M., Costa-Faidella, J., & Sebastián-Gallés, N. (2009). On the bilingual advantage in conflict processing: Now you see it, now you don't. *Cognition, 113*(2), 135–149. doi:10.1016/j.cognition.2009.08.001.

Cutler, A., Weber, A., & Otake, T. (2006). Asymmetric mapping from phonetic to lexical representations in second-language listening. *Journal of Phonetics, 34*(2), 269–284. doi:10.1016/j.wocn.2005.06.002.

Dahan, D., Tanenhaus, M. K., & Salverda, A. P. (2007). The influence of visual processing on phonetically driven saccades in the "visual world" paradigm. In R. P. G. van Gompel, H. Fischer, Martin, S. Murray, Wayne, & L. Hill, Robin (Eds.), *Eye movements: A window on mind and brain* (p. 720). Amsterdam, Netherlands: Elsevier.

Davis, C., & Kim, J. (2006). Audio-visual speech perception off the top of the head. *Cognition, 100*(3), B21–B31. doi:10.1016/j.cognition.2005.09.002.

Dupont, S., & Luettin, J. (2000). Audio-visual speech modeling for continuous speech recognition. *IEEE Transactions on Multimedia, 2*(3), 141–151. doi:10.1109/6046.865479.

Dupoux, E., Peperkamp, S., & Sebastián-Gallés, N. (2010). Limits on bilingualism revisited: Stress "deafness" in simultaneous French-Spanish bilinguals. *Cognition, 114*(2), 266–275. doi:10.1016/j.cognition.2009.10.001.

Durgunolu, A. Y., & Roediger, H. L. (1987). Test differences in accessing bilingual memory. *Journal of Memory and Language, 26*(4), 377–391. doi:10.1016/0749-596X(87)90097-0.

Gerard, L. D., & Scarborough, D. L. (1989). Language-specific lexical access of homographs by bilinguals. *Journal of Experimental Psychology. Learning, Memory, and Cognition, 15*(2), 305–315. doi:10.1037/0278-7393.15.2.305.

Griffin, Z. M., & Bock, K. (2000). What the eyes say about speaking. *Psychological Science, 11*(4), 274–279. doi:10.1111/1467-9280.00255.

Hardison, D. M. (2003). Acquisition of second-language speech: Effects of visual cues, context, and talker variability. *Applied Psycholinguistics, 24*(04), 495–522. doi:10.1017/S0142716403000250.

Hazan, V., Sennema, A., & Faulkner, A. (2002). Audiovisual perception in L2 learners. In *Proceedings of ICSLP* (pp. 1685–1688).

Hoshino, N., & Kroll, J. F. (2008). Cognate effects in picture naming: Does cross-language activation survive a change of script? *Cognition, 106*(1), 501–511. doi:10.1016/j.cognition.2007.02.001.

Huettig, F., & McQueen, J. M. (2007). The tug of war between phonological, semantic and shape information in language-mediated visual search. *Journal of Memory and Language, 57*(4), 460–482. doi:10.1016/j.jml.2007.02.001.

Huettig, F., Olivers, C. N. L., & Hartsuiker, R. J. (2011). Looking, language, and memory: Bridging research from the visual world and visual search paradigms. *Acta Psychologica, 137*(2), 138–150. doi:10.1016/j.actpsy.2010.07.013.

Jones, J. A., & Munhall, K. G. (1997). The effects of separating auditory and visual sources on audiovisual integration of speech. *Canadian Acoustics, 25*(519), 13–20.

Ju, M., & Luce, P. A. (2004). Falling on sensitive ears: Constraints on bilingual lexical activation. *Psychological Science, 15*(5), 314–318. doi:10.1111/j.0956-7976.2004.00675.x.

Kaushanskaya, M., & Marian, V. (2009). The bilingual advantage in novel word learning. *Psychonomic Bulletin & Review, 16*(4), 705–710. doi:10.3758/PBR.16.4.705.

Kelly, S. D., Kravitz, C., & Hopkins, M. (2004). Neural correlates of bimodal speech and gesture comprehension. *Brain and Language, 89*(1), 253–260. doi:10.1016/S0093-934X(03)00335-3.

Keshavarz, M. H., & Astaneh, H. (2004). The impact of biliguality on the learning of English vocabulary as a foreign language (L3). *International Journal of Bilingual Education and Bilingualism, 7*(4), 295–302. doi:10.1080/13670050408667814.

Khare, V., Verma, A., Kar, B., Srinivasan, N., & Brysbaert, M. (2013). Bilingualism and the increased attentional blink effect: Evidence that the difference between bilinguals and monolinguals generalizes to different levels of second language proficiency. *Psychological Research, 77*(6), 728–737. doi:10.1007/s00426-012-0466-4.

Kirsner, K., Brown, H. L., Abrol, S., Chadha, N. K., & Sharma, N. K. (1980). Bilingualism and lexical representation. *The Quarterly Journal of Experimental Psychology, 32*(4), 585–594. doi:10.1080/14640748008401847.

Krauss, R. M., & Hadar, U. (1999). The role of speech-related arm/hand gestures in word retrieval. In R. Campbell & L. Messing (Eds.), *Gesture, speech, and sign* (pp. 93–116). Oxford: Oxford University Press.

Krizman, J., Marian, V., Shook, A., Skoe, E., & Kraus, N. (2012). Subcortical encoding of sound is enhanced in bilinguals and relates to executive function advantages. *Proceedings of the National Academy of Sciences of the United States of America, 109*(20), 7877–7881. doi:10.1 073/pnas.1201575109.

Kroll, J. F. (2008). *Juggling two languages in one mind.* Psychological Science Agenda: American Psychological Association. 22.

Kroll, J. F., Bobb, S. C., & Wodniecka, Z. (2006). Language selectivity is the exception, not the rule: Arguments against a fixed locus of language selection in bilingual speech. *Bilingualism, 9*(02), 119. doi:10.1017/S1366728906002483.

Kuhl, P., & Meltzoff, A. N. (1982). The bimodal perception of speech in infancy. *Science, 218,* 1138–1141.

Lagrou, E., Hartsuiker, R. J., & Duyck, W. (2013). Interlingual lexical competition in a spoken sentence context: Evidence from the visual world paradigm. *Psychonomic Bulletin & Review, 20*(5), 963–972. doi:10.3758/s13423-013-0405-4.

Liberman, A. M., & Mattingly, I. G. (1985). The motor theory of speech perception revised. *Cognition, 21*(1), 1–36.

Loveman, E., Van Hooff, J. C., & Gale, A. (2002). A systematic investigation of same and cross modality priming using written and spoken responses. *Memory, 10*(4), 267–276. doi:10.1080/09658210143000380.

Luk, G., De Sa, E., & Bialystok, E. (2011). Is there a relation between onset age of bilingualism and enhancement of cognitive control? *Bilingualism: Language and Cognition, 14*(4), 1–8. doi:10.1017/S1366728911000010.

MacDonald, J., Andersen, S., & Bachmann, T. (2000). Hearing by eye: How much spatial degradation can be tolerated? *Perception, 29*(10), 1155–1168. doi:10.1068/p3020.

Marian, V. (2009). Audio-visual integration during bilingual language processing. In A. Pavlenko (Ed.), *The bilingual mental lexicon: Interdisciplinary approaches* (pp. 52–78).

Marian, V., & Spivey, M. J. (2003a). Bilingual and monolingual processing of competing lexical items. *Applied Psycholinguistics, 24*(2), 173–193. doi:10.1017/S0142716403000092.

Marian, V., & Spivey, M. J. (2003b). Competing activation in bilingual language processing: Within- and between-language. *Bilingualism: Language and Cognition, 6*(2), 97–115. doi:10.1017/S1366728903001068.

Marslen-Wilson, W. D. (1987). Functional parallelism in spoken word-recognition. *Cognition, 25*(1–2), 71–102.

Martin-Rhee, M. M., & Bialystok, E. (2008). The development of two types of inhibitory control in monolingual and bilingual children. *Bilingualism: Language and Cognition, 11*(01), 81–93. doi:10.1017/S1366728907003227.

McGurk, H., & MacDonald, J. (1976). Hearing lips and seeing voices. *Nature, 264,* 746–748.

Meyer, A. S., Sleiderink, A. M., & Levelt, W. J. M. (1998). Viewing and naming objects: Eye movements during noun phrase production. *Cognition, 66*(2), B25–33.

Midgley, K. J., Holcomb, P. J., VanHeuven, W. J. B., & Grainger, J. (2008). An electrophysiological investigation of cross-language effects of orthographic neighborhood. *Brain Research, 1246,* 123–135. doi:10.1016/j.brainres.2008.09.078.

Morford, J. P., Wilkinson, E., Villwock, A., Piñar, P., & Kroll, J. F. (2011). When deaf signers read English: Do written words activate their sign translations? *Cognition, 118*(2), 286–292. doi:10.1016/j.cognition.2010.11.006.

Musacchia, G., Sams, M., Skoe, E., & Kraus, N. (2007). Musicians have enhanced subcortical auditory and audiovisual processing of speech and music. *Proceedings of the National Academy of Sciences of the United States of America, 104*(40), 15894–15898. doi:10.1073/p nas.0701498104.

Navarra, J., & Soto-Faraco, S. (2007). Hearing lips in a second language: Visual articulatory information enables the perception of second language sounds. *Psychological Research, 71*(1), 4–12. doi:10.1007/s00426-005-0031-5.

Nicoladis, E. (2007). The effect of bilingualism on the use of manual gestures. *Applied Psycholinguistics, 28*(03), 441–454. doi:10.1017/S0142716407070245.

Plass, J. L., Chun, D. M., Mayer, R. E., & Leutner, D. (1998). Supporting visual and verbal learning preferences in a second-language multimedia learning environment. *Journal of Educational Psychology, 90*(1), 25–36. doi:10.1037//0022-0663.90.1.25.

Preston, M. S., & Lambert, W. E. (1969). Interlingual interference in a bilingual version of the stroop color-word task. *Journal of Verbal Learning and Verbal Behavior, 8*(2), 295–301. doi:10.1016/S0022-5371(69)80079-4.

Prinz, J. J. (2006). Is the mind really modular? In R. Stainton (Ed.), *Contemporary debates in cognitive science* (pp. 22–36). Oxford: Blackwell.

Prior, A., & MacWhinney, B. (2009). A bilingual advantage in task switching. *Bilingualism: Language and Cognition, 13*(2), 253. doi:10.1017/S1366728909990526.

Ransdell, S. E., & Fischler, I. (1987). Memory in a monolingual mode: When are bilinguals at a disadvantage? *Journal of Memory and Language, 26*(4), 392–405. doi:10.1016/0749-596X(87)90098-2.

Ronquest, R., & Hernandez, L. (2005). *Lip-reading skills in bilinguals: Some effects of L1 on visual-only language identification. Research on Spoken Language Processing, Progress Report No. 27* (pp. 219–226). Bloominton, Indiana.

Scarborough, D. L., Gerard, L. D., & Cortese, C. (1984). Independence of lexical access in bilingual word recognition. *Journal of Verbal Learning and Verbal Behavior, 23*(1), 84–99. doi:10.1016/S0022-5371(84)90519-X.

Schroeder, S. R., & Marian, V. (in preparation). Audio-visual interactions during memory encoding in monolinguals and bilinguals.

Sebastián-Gallés, N., Echeverría, S., & Bosch, L. (2005). The influence of initial exposure on lexical representation: Comparing early and simultaneous bilinguals. *Journal of Memory and Language, 52*(2), 240–255. doi:10.1016/j.jml.2004.11.001.

Sebastián-Gallés, N., Albareda-Castellot, B., Weikum, W. M., & Werker, J. F. (2012). A bilingual advantage in visual language discrimination in infancy. *Psychological Science, 23*(9), 994–999. doi:10.1177/0956797612436817.

Shook, A., & Marian, V. (2012). Bimodal bilinguals co-activate both languages during spoken comprehension. *Cognition, 124*(3), 314–324. doi:10.1016/j.cognition.2012.05.014.

Shook, A., & Marian, V. (2013). The bilingual language interaction network for comprehension of speech (BLINCS). *Bilingualism: Language and Cognition, 16*, 304–324. doi:10.1017/S1366728912000466.

Singh, N., & Mishra, R. K. (2013). Second language proficiency modulates conflict-monitoring in an oculomotor stroop task: Evidence from Hindi-English bilinguals. *Frontiers in Psychology, 4*, 322. doi:10.3389/fpsyg.2013.00322.

Soto-Faraco, S., Navarra, J., Weikum, W. M., Vouloumanos, A., Sebastián-Gallés, N., & Werker, J. F. (2007). Discriminating languages by speech-reading. *Perception and Psychophysics, 69*(2), 218–231. doi:10.3758/BF03193744.

Soveri, A., Laine, M., Hämäläinen, H., & Hugdahl, K. (2010). Bilingual advantage in attentional control: Evidence from the forced-attention dichotic listening paradigm. *Bilingualism: Language and Cognition, 14*(03), 371–378. doi:10.1017/S1366728910000118.

Spivey, M. J., & Marian, V. (1999). Cross talk between native and second languages: Partial activation of an irrelevant lexicon. *Psychological Science, 10*(3), 281. doi:10.1111/1467-9280.00151.

Tanenhaus, M. K., & Spivey-Knowlton, M. (1996). Eye-tracking. *Language and Cognitive Processes, 11*(6), 583–588.

Tanenhaus, M. K., Spivey-Knowlton, M., Eberhard, K. M., & Sedivy, J. C. (1995). Integration of visual and linguistic information in spoken language comprehension. *Science, 268*(5217), 1632–1634. doi:10.1126/science.7777863.

Tanenhaus, M. K., Spivey-Knowlton, M., Eberhard, K. M., & Sedivy, J. C. (1996). Using eye movements to study spoken language comprehension: Evidence for visually mediated incremental interpretation. In *Attention and performance XVI: Information integration in perception and communication* (pp. 457–478). Boston: The MIT Press.

Thierry, G., & Wu, Y. J. (2007). Brain potentials reveal unconscious translation during foreign-language comprehension. *Proceedings of the National Academy of Sciences of the United States of America, 104*(30), 12530–12535. doi:10.1073/pnas.0609927104.

Tzelgov, J., Henik, A., & Leiser, D. (1990). Controlling stroop interference: Evidence from a bilingual task. *Journal of Experimental Psychology: Learning, Memory, and Cognition, 16*(5), 760–771. doi:10.1037/0278-7393.16.5.760.

Van Heuven, W. J. B., Dijkstra, T., & Grainger, J. (1998). Orthographic neighborhood effects in bilingual word recognition. *Journal of Memory and Language, 39*(3), 458–483. doi:10.1006/jmla.1998.2584.

Van Wassenhove, V., Grant, K. W., & Poeppel, D. (2005). Visual speech speeds up the neural processing of auditory speech. *Proceedings of the National Academy of Sciences of the United States of America, 102*(4), 1181. doi:10.1073/pnas.0408949102.

Van Wassenhove, V., Grant, K. W., & Poeppel, D. (2007). Temporal window of integration in auditory-visual speech perception. *Neuropsychologia, 45*(3), 598–607. doi:10.1016/j.neuropsychologia.2006.01.001.

Watkins, M. J., & Peynircioglu, Z. F. (1983). On the nature of word recall: Evidence for linguistic specificity. *Journal of Verbal Learning and Verbal Behavior, 22*(4), 385–394. doi:10.1016/S0022-5371(83)90246-3.

Weber, A., & Cutler, A. (2004). Lexical competition in non-native spoken-word recognition. *Journal of Memory and Language, 50*(1), 1–25. doi:10.1016/S0749-596X(03)00105-0.

Weber, A., & Paris, G. (2004). The origin of the linguistic gender effect in spoken-word recognition: Evidence from non-native listening. In *Proceedings of the 26th Annual Meeting of the Cognitive Science Society*, 1446–1451.

Weikum, W. M., Vouloumanos, A., Navarra, J., Soto-faraco, S., Sebastián-gallés, N., & Werker, J. F. (2007). Visual language discrimination in infancy. *Science, 316*, 1159.

Chapter 10
Spoken Word Mediated Interference in a Visual Task: Eye Tracking Evidence from Bilinguals

Ramesh Kumar Mishra and Niharika Singh

10.1 Introduction

Recent developments in the analysis of how language interacts with other cognitive systems like attention and memory has led to the emergence of newer questions. Mapping shifts in the visual attention during comprehension of spoken language (see Mishra 2009; Huettig et al. 2012 for reviews) has shown the dynamic links between language and vision. Listening and looking seem to be time bound, at least given the a particular task. Recently it was proposed that listening to words leads to activation of stored representations and such traces remain active in working memory which leads to patterns of looking behaviour (Huettig and Altmann 2005, 2011). There is also a good deal of indication that spoken language affects the oculomotor system very rapidly, propelling it towards visual targets that are related (Huettig and Altmann 2005; Huettig and McQueen 2007; Huettig and Hartsuiker 2008). Many have explored how such listening and looking behaviour can lead to better understanding of psycholinguistic issues, pertaining to sentence comprehension (Altmann and Kamide 2004; Huettig and Altmann 2004, 2007; Kamide et al. 2003; Nation et al. 2003). Given a visual display and matching language, human subjects engage in anticipatory processing (Kamide and Altmann 2004) which seems arising from the nature of language itself. However, not much is currently known related to the task irrelevant effect of spoken words on visual processing. It is an everyday observation that often we look at things

R.K. Mishra (✉)
Center for Neural and Cognitive Sciences, University of Hyderabad, Hyderabad, India
e-mail: rkmishra@uohyd.ac.in

R.K. Mishra · N. Singh
Center for Behavioural and Cognitive Sciences, University of Allahabad, Allahabad, India

© Springer India 2015
R.K. Mishra et al. (eds.), *Attention and Vision in Language Processing*, DOI 10.1007/978-81-322-2443-3_10

when what we hear is not directly related to it. How can this happen given the enormous influence of top-down goals one sees in cognition? We first review findings from the research areas where speech has been shown to cause interference during cognitive processing. We particularly review reporting the so called irrelevant speech effects and also the working memory effects. Then, we present data from an eye tracking study on bilinguals where we observe interference in a visual task.

10.2 Interference from Speech and Memory

Early studies on the nature of working memory had explored interference from speech stimuli on recall. Unattended speech has the ability to penetrate into processing modules and cause interference. Speech has both phonological as well as conceptual properties. What one hears may resemble something in the real world or may simply be a sequence of sounds. In a task that involves immediate recall of visually presented digits, one sees interference from unattended spoken words (Saalame and Baddeley 1982). It appears that resemblance at the level of form disrupts memory performance while semantics of this material does not. However, it is not clear if one can ignore the activation of semantic material from spoken words willfully, even when one is given demanding tasks. Speech seems to enter into the working memory buffer even when it is to be ignored thus causing a resource crunch. A likely explanation could be that verbal material will cause interference with a memory task, if the retrieval depends on access of verbal material. When there is a match at the level of phonology, there is some sort of confusion and delay. Unattended speech leads to interference during reading comprehension while unattended music does not (Martin et al. 1988). Again the argument has been that verbal material causes interference if there is a match at the level of the code. It appears that changing patterns of the speech stimuli have greater power to cause disruption in the memory task, than speech that is unchanging (Jones et al. 1992). What seems to be causing the disruption is the match between the serial orders of the phonological information with the visual sign. Since visual signs have phonological codes, there is a competition for retrieval. These data do suggest that irrelevant speech leads to some kind of disruption with selective attention tasks, which may include working memory tasks of different types. Many such experiments have used meaningless syllables as speech stimuli and short-term memory tasks, while either the timing of retention or order of presentation has been manipulated. Speech, when meaningful, disrupts immediate memory recall performances more than meaningless speech (LeCompte et al. 1997). The issue of semantic interference in these demonstrations of irrelevant speech effects on tasks of attention and memory is not very clear. For example, Buchner (1996) did not find any effect of phonologically related speech on the recall of digits. On the other hand, Neely and LeCompte (1999) observed that semantically related words offered maximum interference. Studies with reading comprehension in the presence of both meaningful as well as meaningless speech show disruption but qualitative difference (Oswald et al. 2000). If speech is meaningful, it causes greater disruption even when it is not relevant for the task at hand. This inconsistency in results could be an artifact of the paradigm or its limitations.

10.3 Attention, Unattended Speech and Distraction

Attention is at the heart of selection and goal-directed action. The above discussed examples of studies that asked participants to recall items from short term memory in the presence of unattained speech involve selective attention. However, it is not clear how speech disrupts selective attention and causes changes in action plans. Can one ignore speech completely so as to deploy selective attention on task irrelevant stimuli? There seems to be evidence which suggests that spoken words are processed automatically even when there is no intention to do so (Parmentier et al. 2013). One can think of processing the distractors in the Stroop like interference tasks which show automaticity and capture selective attention. In these tasks, some dimension of the stimuli gets processed which causes delay in response. The distractors compete with the targets and bias attention. Speech on the other hand attracts attention reflexively as it is a significant biological stimulus. Sudden onset of speech disrupts selective attention. It is very similar to the way sudden onset of visual distractors summon attention bias its focus (Yantis and Jonides 1984; Irwin et al. 2000). Interference results when attention resource is shared by competing stimuli. In order to ignore or inhibit, one requires executive control. Sudden onset also leads to capture of attention exogenously which is difficult to resist (Chua 2013). However, listeners often do not report this distraction consciously. What is not yet clear if such distractions are caused by conceptual access which is automatic during listening to speech. It is likely that the ability to resist distraction to speech is linked to cognitive control. Higher cognitive control leads to less distraction by speech stimuli. In an interesting study, Tun et al. (2002) examined the effect of cognitive control in speech related distraction in younger and older adults. Participants listened to speech either meaningful speech or non-meaningful speech playing in the background. The results showed that older participants were more distracted by meaningful speech in a task of later recall while the younger adults were distracted by meaningless speech. This shows a connection between decreasing cognitive control and distraction caused by speech. These results also show that meaningful speech and meaningless speech require different types of cognitive control. However, it is not very clear from this demonstration if there is a precise link between conceptual access and cognitive control in situations when one has to recognise stimuli in spite of distractors.

An attentional role in speech-induced distraction can be examined by manipulating the speech stimuli. It may be a possibility that the frequency of distractor words can affect the magnitude of the interference observed. It has been demonstrated that high- and low-frequency words lead to different types of interference during recall task (Buchner and Erdfelder 2005). An effect of frequency suggests that the attentional system is selective to the speech stimuli's statistical properties and not much with content. However, others have found an effect of content on the size of distraction produced (Marsh et al. 2008). Speech that is salient in meaning or in valence can cause higher distraction during a selective attention task (Buchner et al. 2004). Most of these studies have examined a role of working memory (indirectly selective attention) on recall during interference. These studies thus do not examine attentional engagements directly. Furthermore, many of the tasks have dual load. While one set of tasks have looked at how meaning in speech interferes with ongoing cognitive processing, others have looked at working memory effects. For example, it is often very difficult to pinpoint the exact nature of interference caused by background speech since the signal can be contaminated by attention demanding task. Recently, use of the eye tracking visual world paradigm has opened up ways to study cognitive processing in multi-modal scenario. It is possible to study interference from spoken words while participants attend to visual information. In this paradigm, eye movements are measured as someone is doing some type of change detection task in the visual domain. Such a task also does not cost the working memory a lot; at least working memory related effects are not directly examined. Participants are not asked to remember or report anything and this can give a high level of ecological validity to the task. Thus it is possible to directly examine how cognitive control maintains goals during distractions. Further, these studies do not show how distractions caused in one modality can lead to interference in another modality. Below we describe a study where we show interference caused by spoken words can lead to distraction in a visual task. This study reports data from an original study where we observed interference in a visual task where spoken words were task irrelevant. Below we briefly review the recent findings in this area.

10.4 Bilingual Translation and Interference

Words, be they in the spoken or in the auditory form, often automatically summon attention in many everyday task situations (Salverda and Altmann 2011). For example, we immediately orient our attention towards some location when someone calls our name. Similarly, verbal warnings and noise can as well capture attention in a reflexive manner and cause interference with ongoing tasks (Ljungberg et al. 2012). In the written modality, classic studies using the colour word Stroop task have shown the automaticity of semantic access in word recognition. This semantic activation often leads to attention capture and conflict with another task. However, much more recently, researchers have been studying how spoken words or speech in general can induce interference in the visual domain when these auditory inputs are task-irrelevant. Many past studies have suggested that stimuli from different modalities can interact and lead to shifts in spatial attention in a cross-modal situation (Driver and Spence 1998). On the other hand task irrelevant speech can induce interference in memory and attention tasks suggesting automatic processing (LeCompte et al. 1997; see also Elliott and Briganti 2012). More recently, studies with cross-modal stimuli have shown that attention capture through irrelevant spoken words is automatic in the sense that participants are unable to ignore these task irrelevant stimuli (Salverda and Altman 2011). Some other studies have shown that spoken words can have facilitative effect on visual processing (Zeelenberg and Bocanegra 2010). Similarly, emotional content of words has been shown to capture attention (Bertels et al. 2011). However, it is still not very clear if it is the activation of semantics of task-irrelevant spoken words that captures attention in a cross-modal situation causing disruption with the goal oriented visual processing. Further, it is also not clear, how bilingual subjects behave in this sort of situation. In this study, we addressed these issues to further understand how task-irrelevant spoken words capture attention in a cross-modal situation and lead to interference with saccadic eye-movements. We examine this issue with a bilingual population that has been shown to automatically activate words from the irrelevant non-target language, i.e. language currently not in use during word processing in a variety of situations. Thus, our goal is to see if spoken words that are irrelevant to the current goal, receive rich semantic processing and this captures attention in a task which otherwise requires a response in the visual modality. Since we use a visual world eye tracking paradigm, below we briefly review findings in this domain as relevant for understanding activation semantics during spoken word processing in the presence of visual referents.

Several visual world eye tracking studies have shown that listeners activate a range of conceptual and semantic information within moments of the auditory onset of spoken words and immediately orient attention towards suitable visual referents (Allopenna et al. 1998; Cooper 1974; Huettig and Altmann 2007; Yee et al. 2009). Huettig and Altmann (2005) showed that listeners immediately activate semantics of spoken words and move their eyes towards related visual objects with the auditory onsets. Importantly, participants also seem to move their eyes towards objects whose names have phonological resemblance with the semantic associates of spoken words (Yee and Sedivy 2006). For example, listening to the word "dog" it is much more likely that participants will move their eyes towards the picture of a "cat" or even "cap" among unrelated distractors. One possible explanation is that related words get activated in a spreading activation manner and affect oculomotor processing leading to attention capture. This is crucial to our design in this study, since we explore if bilingual subjects activate phonological cohorts of translation equivalents during spoken word processing leading to attention capture. However, it is only recently that researchers have started to explore if such language-mediated eye movements seen in visual world studies are automatic. Language-mediated eye movements can be considered automatic if the spoken words drive attention towards task irrelevant distractors when selective attention is engaged in a visual task.

Salverda and Altmann (2011) presented participants with line drawings and asked them to make an eye movement towards one target object that underwent a colour change. However, just before this colour change, participants heard a spoken word which either referred to a distractor or referred to an object that was not in the display. Salverda and Altmann (2011) observed that saccades towards the object that changed colour were slow when the spoken word referred to one of the other distractor objects present than when it was not so. Listeners were slow in detecting a location change of a target visual object in the presence of a spoken word which was not directly relevant for the task. Participants were however faster in their response when the spoken words directly mentioned the object that underwent the colour or the location change. This data indicates both facilitation as well as interference with visual search in the presence of spoken word. Most importantly, spoken words that referred to a distractor caused disruption with the primary visual task. The authors interpreted their findings suggesting that, like Stroop interference seen with written words, spoken words are processed automatically and this leads to attention capture. It might be difficult to deploy selective attention to targets in the visual modality while ignoring spoken words. Taken together, this research implies that it is the semantics of spoken words whose automatic activation creates some kind of attentional bottleneck and reorients saccadic programming which is goal driven. Thus, spoken words act more or less like exogenous cues that capture attention and disrupt goal-driven processing in a cross-modal scenario. The results suggest automatic processing of spoken words that affected oculomotor programming.

Other researches have shown that processing spoken words unintentionally can facilitate visual search. Lupyan and Swingley (2011) asked participants to name objects during a visual search task. It was found that search was more efficient when the spoken verbal label matched the search target and there was higher interference when the name was different from the search target. This indicates that spoken words processed unintentionally narrow down search when the extracted semantics matches with the search target. Visual referents that are related to the spoken words compete with the target for selection and bias attention causing interference. Verbal labels even have been shown to guide attention automatically during visual search in a top-down manner (Soto and Humhreys 2007). Cleland et al. (2012) asked participants to make response to a visual stimulus (a word, face or a shape) in the presence of a spoken word. Response times were higher when the spoken word's uniqueness point was closer to the appearance of the visual stimulus and also effects were stronger as the gap between the spoken word and the visual stimulus decreased. Further, response interference was higher when the visual stimulus was a word compared to a shape and a picture. These data suggest that spoken words automatically receive rich phonological as well as semantic processing and thus create attentional bottleneck during search for visual targets. Even unintentional processing of spoken words can lead to shifts in attentional states which in turn may lead to changes in goal planning and action selection. Previous studies have shown that visual and spoken words that are semantically related to the targets or distractors influence saccadic behaviour by driving eye movements towards these task irrelevant referents (Moores et al. 2003; Telling et al. 2010). It is quite possible that spoken words enter into short-term memory and thus capture attention (Klatte et al. 2010). Attention capture due to spoken words can happen even when subjects are not explicitly instructed to keep verbal information in working memory (Downing 2000). Neurobiological studies on speech processing suggest that spoken words can activate important brain circuits even when listeners do not pay any attention to them. Shtyrov et al. (2010) found that despite explicit instruction to ignore the spoken words, the results showed that within 120 ms of the spoken word onset the negative going potentials were modulated by the frequency and lexicality of the words. This suggests that words can affect neuronal processing without attentional engagement.

Recently, Mishra et al. (2012) reviewed studies from visual world and visual search paradigms and observed that in order to establish automaticity of language mediated eye movements one has to either control attention or increase search difficulty with higher set sizes as has been done traditionally with many visual search tasks. Interestingly the notion of automaticity still remains contested (Logan 1998; Jonides et al. 1985). Automatic processes are not under one's voluntary control and occur unintentionally. The most crucial test perhaps is if they still occur when attention is controlled. Recently, De Houwer and Moors (2006) have argued that it might not be enough just to suggest that some mental process is automatic unless we identify what component of automaticity that process recruits. For example, under this compositional view of automaticity, while activation of semantics in a colour word Stroop task could be unintentional, it also demands selective attention. If attention is not paid to the written word, one may probably not see Stroop interference. Further, it is crucial to examine if automaticity holds under task demands or when attention is strictly controlled. The load theory of attention (Lavie 2005) argues that one may not see any automatic interference with a visual task caused by auditory stimuli when the visual task demands excessive amount of selective attention. These issues have not been examined with language mediated eye movements with the manipulation of visual search complexity or with memory load. Therefore, further studies are required to understand under what empirical circumstances automaticity of spoken word processing holds. We have approached this problem with a completely different angle by examining a group of bilinguals who nevertheless activate cross-language competitors of words when the task may not demand so. In this case, it's not just the activation of semantics of the spoken word that seems unintentional but also the activation of translation equivalent and further words related to it. This can provide useful information about automatic and covert activation of semantics causing disruption in an oculomotor visual task.

We kept our experimental design close to that of Salverda and Altmann (2011) with some crucial changes. For example, we presented the spoken words and the visual colour change events at different temporal gaps to see if the activation of semantics is fast and unintentional. We increased the search set by using four line drawings. Importantly, in our design the task irrelevant spoken word never directly referred to the target object that underwent colour change and to which a saccadic response had to be made. Crucially, to see if semantic activation is automatic and covert, our critical trials contained an object in the display which was a phonological cohort of the translation equivalent of the spoken word. It is important to note that Hindi and English do not share orthography and therefore do not have common cognate words. Many past studies have shown that bilinguals process cognate words faster because of their shared phonology and semantics (Dijkastra et al. 2010). However, not many studies have shown if bi-scriptal bilinguals activate cross-language semantics in a cross-modal task situation when they process visual objects and listen to spoken words. Broadly, our goal was to see if we can replicate the main findings of Salverda and Altmann (2011) with a bilingual population who speak two different languages. We wanted to examine if access of semantics of irrelevant spoken words is automatic in such a population. Previous eye tracking studies have shown that bilinguals covertly activate cross-language information rapidly and automatically (Marian and Spivey 2003a, b; Spivey and Marian 1999; Weber and Cutler 2004). Relevant to our study, bilinguals have been shown to activate translation equivalents of words automatically (see Sundermann and Priya 2012; Guo et al. 2012). We exploited this typical bilingual behaviour to further probe the automaticity of spoken words leading to interference in a visual task. The participants listened to a spoken word and saw four line drawings. On critical trials, one of the objects was a phonological neighbour of the translation equivalent of the spoken word. Participants always listened to the words in English, their L2. For example, if the spoken word was 'gun', the display contained a picture of 'bandar' which was the phonological neighbour of the translation equivalent 'bandook'. On other trials, the spoken word had a direct referent in the display. Participants were asked to move their eyes towards the object that changed colour.

We hypothesised that if spoken words unintentionally lead to the activation of the translation equivalents and they in turn activate the phonologically related words, participants were going to be slow with their visual search task. Such objects will compete for selective attention with the target and thus will bias saccades towards them. We also manipulated the temporal gap between the appearance of spoken words and colour change in order to examine how this might modulate interference. In experiment one, the target object changed colour after the offset of the spoken words while in experiment two these events were simultaneous. We included this to replicate Salverda and Altmann (2011) and we predicted that in this condition participants will suffer maximum interference. In the baseline condition, where spoken words were not related to any visual referent we predicted minimal interference with the goal-directed saccades towards the object that changed colour. With this design, we aimed at testing the hypothesis that language-driven eye movements are automatic in a bilingual context and are driven by activation of semantics.

Twenty high proficient Hindi-English bilinguals (Mean age = 21.1 years, SD = 2.4 years) from the University of Allahabad took part in the experiment. They were all native speakers of Hindi (L1) and had acquired English as their second language in school. The formal age of acquisition of L2 was 3.6 years (SD = 0.82. Participants also indicated their proficiency in writing, reading, speaking, and listening abilities in L1 and L2 on a five-point scale ranging from *poor* (1) to *excellent* (5). There were 135 displays and each display consisted of four equal sized (300 × 300 pixel) line drawings of common objects. The distance between the central fixation and centre of each object was 8.5°. One of the four drawings turned into green which was the target to which participants had to make a saccade. A spoken word was presented in English (L2). Depending upon the relationship between task-irrelevant spoken input and one of the three distracters, three conditions were created: (i) Translation cohort condition: when the cohort of the spoken word's translation equivalent (TE) was presented as a competitor (ex. If the spoken word was "gun" (*bandook*), then "*bandar*" as TE cohort was present as competitor while other two distractors were completely unrelated to the spoken input (ii) Referent present condition: when the referent of the spoken input was presented as competitor among two distractors and the target (ex. If spoken word was "apple" then line drawing of an apple was in the display as competitor) and (iii) Control condition: when all the three distracters were unrelated to the spoken input. The mean durations of spoken words in the translation cohort, referent present, and control condition were 819 ms (SD = 96.3), 776.7 ms (SD = 111.9) and 745 ms (SD = 87.2) respectively. There were 45 trials in each condition making total of 135 trials.

Participants were seated at a distance of 60 cm from a 17′ LCD colour monitor with 1024 × 768 pixel resolution. Eye movements were recorded with a SMI High speed eye–tracking system (Sensomotoric Instruments, Berlin) running with a sampling rate of 1250 Hz. Participants' eye movements were calibrated at 13 different points at the beginning of the experiment. Each trial began with the presentation of the fixation cross (+) at the centre of the screen for 1000 ms followed by a display containing line drawings of four objects. After 500 ms, one of the object changed colour to green and simultaneously a spoken word was presented to the participants. The display continued till 2000 ms after colour change. After this animacy judgment (on 40 % of trials) task was presented followed by blank screen for 2000 ms. Trials were randomised for each participant. The participants were instructed to move their eyes towards the object that turned green in colour as soon possible. Participants were asked not to move their eyes before the colour change and were required to fixate at the centre. Participants were informed that the spoken word was irrelevant to the task and they should make eye movements in response to the colour change and not to the spoken input.

The data from each participant's right eye were extracted using the Begaze analysis software (SMI, Berlin). Saccade latency to the target was calculated, that is, the time gap between the colour change and the first correct saccade made towards it. Saccade latencies less than 80 ms (anticipatory) and higher than 1000 ms were excluded from further analysis. We only analysed those trials where participants responded correctly by making an appropriate eye movement towards the target. A repeated measure of variance analysis was conducted to see mean saccadic latencies to the target in the presence of different competitors (TE cohort, referent present and unrelated). A significant main effect of competitor type on latency to the target was found, $F(2, 38) = 5.7$, MSE $= 7111.52$, $p = 0.006$, $\eta_p^2 = 0.23$. The mean saccadic latency to the target in the unrelated condition (519.82 ms, SD = 74.89) was significantly faster than in the TE cohort competitor condition (545.2 ms, SD = 65.42) and the referent present condition (556.65 ms,

SD = 69.95). Participants were slower in making a saccade towards the object that changed colour in the presence of the cross-language translation distractor as well as the direct referent.

We considered first saccades landing on any object other than the target after colour change as errors. The main effect of competitor type on errors was found to be significant, $F(2, 38) = 3.1$, MSE = 17.0, $p = 0.05$, $\eta_p^2 = 0.14$, showing higher error rates in referent present (18.6, SD = 7.4) and unrelated condition (18.6, SD = 7.0) than TE cohort condition (17.0, SD = 7.3).

10.5 Conceptual Activation and Distraction

In this study we examined if task irrelevant spoken words capture attention in bilingual subjects and cause interference with a visual task. Our results suggest two important findings. First, task irrelevant spoken words receive rich semantic processing and slow down goal-directed saccades in a visual task and second, bilinguals' obligatorily activate translations of words leading to interference. We thus replicate and advance Salverda and Altmann's (2011) findings with a bilingual population and show that listeners automatically activate semantics of the spoken words which causes attention capture and diverts goal directed search in a cross-modal situation. Our results are thus in agreement with previous studies (Lupyan and Swingley 2011; Cleland et al. 2012) that have shown words capture attention automatically and interfere with visual processing. Participants were given the explicit task of detecting colour change of a visual object in an array of line drawings. The spoken word was task-irrelevant and never referred directly to the target. However, saccades towards the target were slowest when the spoken word directly referred to a distractor. Crucially, when this word referred to an object which was a cross-linguistic translation competitor, participants were slower in their saccadic response. Interference was highest when the object directly referred to one of the distractors. This result directly replicates the findings of Salverda and Altmann (2011) with four objects. However, errors were similar across the conditions.

Participants were naive as to their bilingual status since all the spoken words were in English, their L2. Participants were given the explicit instruction to detect the colour change of an object. However, they covertly and automatically activated the semantics of the spoken word and oriented their attention towards an object which then competed for attention with the target object. This bias in goal-directed oculomotor control was a result of automaticity of meaning activation of the irrelevant words. Further, our manipulation of the temporal gap between the onset of the spoken word and the colour change did not affect the interference. In sum, we have shown that spoken words, if they are meaningful, can capture attention. Also, in both the experiments latency to the target in the translation cohort and direct referent did not differ from one another. Participants were fastest in the colour discrimination task when the spoken word did not refer to any object in the display either directly or indirectly.

The results suggest that listeners quickly activate semantics from ignored spoken words that capture attention and lead to interference in oculomotor tasks. Several previous eye-tracking visual world studies have shown that listeners quickly access semantics from spoken words (Dahan et al. 2001; Huettig and Altmann 2005; Mani and Huettig 2012; Yee and Sedivy 2006). The results suggest that spoken words directly act on visual referents (Lupyan and Swingley (2011). In a more applied context, Jones et al. (1990) have shown that task irrelevant speech only affected proofreading only when it was meaningful. Interestingly, Jones et al. (1990) also found that serial recall of visually presented lists got impaired when participants heard speech that was reversed or in a foreign language, demonstrating the powerful effect of speech on action control. It has even been shown that compared to meaningless tones, irrelevant speech can cause disruption in recall (LeCompte et al. 1997). However, compared to these tasks, our task was not a recall task but required participants to make eye movements on detecting a visual colour change. It involved selecting a target for saccade purely based on a visual factor and participants were not asked to remember anything. The task also required them to extract the animacy of the target object and our task was cross-modal in nature.

Is it possible to avoid attentional distraction caused by task-irrelevant stimuli completely? The perceptual load theory (see Lavie 2005 for a review; Lavie and Tsal 1994) predicts that high perceptual load which can engage attentional deployment fully can also lead to complete elimination of distraction from task-irrelevant distractors. Tellinghuisen and Nowak (2003) asked participants to search visual targets with either visual or auditory distractors. Visual distractors influenced search under low load conditions but auditory distractors slowed down search under both high and low load conditions. However, Tellinghusen and Nowak (2003) observed that influence of auditory distracters was less under high visual load condition. Nevertheless in our experiments, the colour change detection task of course demanded a high level of selective attention. We found very high level of semantic processing of task irrelevant auditory presented words on saccadic eye movements. We observed this when the spoken words preceded the visual display as well as when they followed. Our results thus suggest that it is probably impossible to avoid distraction from spoken words and this leads to unwanted attentional shifts and interference with a primary task. It would be further interesting to examine how increasing perceptual or memory load modulates this interference from spoken words during visual search or detection tasks.

Others have shown that irrelevant written words can capture attention in an oculomotor task. Weaver et al. (2011) observed significantly larger saccade trajectory deviations when a taboo word was presented as an irrelevant visual distractor compared to a neutral word. Recently, Cleland et al. (2012) have shown that uniqueness points of spoken words can influence visual processing. In this study, it was observed that response to visual targets was slower when they were preceded by task irrelevant spoken words. Participants were slower in visual object processing when the lag between spoken words and visual targets decreased. Further, the interference was higher when visual targets were words. This suggests that semantics extracted from spoken words cause attentional bottlenecks and impact visual processing. All of these researches suggest that both written and spoken words automatically capture attention and lead to changes in current cognitive goals and action control. It will be interesting to see of application of higher cognitive control leads to suppression of these effects.

There have been claims about automaticity in some other domains of language processing. Pickering and Garrod (2004) suggest that alignment in spoken dialogues is an automatic process. This means that participants in a conversation are more likely to use linguistic structures used by the interlocutors and this happens automatically. This does not mean that speakers cannot monitor their language production. Similarly, semantic access of meaning during speech perception comes from ERP studies that show an MMN effect (Pulvermüller and Shtyrov 2006). The MMN effect is an early component that is evident when participants do not pay attention to the speech stream. Interestingly researchers have noticed this when participants are given some other visual task and thus MMS effects seem to suggest automatic and unconscious access of meaning in speech. Importantly MMN effects for real words have been found to have larger compared to pseudo words. These examples suggest that some aspects of language processing could be automatic, if one follows Bargh's (1994) graded notion of automaticity. Mainly these processes proceed without the engagement of attention and can cause interference with another task. Our finding that subjects automatically activate translations of spoken words adds to these earlier evidences.

Our findings have implications for studies that have shown parallel activation of lexicons in bilinguals. Previous eye-tracking visual world studies on bilinguals have shown that these subjects activate cross-linguistic phonological information automatically during spoken word processing (Weber and Cutler 2004; Blumenfeld and Marian 2007; Ju and Luce 2004). In addition to these studies we have shown that bilingual subjects activate semantics automatically during spoken word processing of the task irrelevant lexicon and they do so when their attention is controlled. Thus, these results show an extreme form of automaticity in bilingual word processing that supports the bilingual interactive models of word processing (Dijkstra and Van Heuven 2002). It's the interactive and spreading activation of semantics from one language to other that caused capture of attention by the object whose name was a cohort of the translation equivalent. Importantly, Hindi–English as language pairs do not have cognates and have different orthographies. We have shown that even bi-scriptal bilinguals automatically activate translation equivalents of spoken words during second language listening (Guo et al. 2012; Sunderman and Priya 2012; Thierry and Wu 2010). They do so even under an attentional demanding task situation. We extend Salverda and Altmann's (2011) observation that language-mediated eye movements are automatic and one can access semantics from spoken words unintentionally. Crucially, we have shown that this access of meaning is rather very fast and is capable of creating interference in a visual task.

In sum, both written (as in the classic colour word Stroop task) and spoken words automatically capture attention in a variety of task situations. In a cross-modal situation, this can lead to re-orientation of oculomotor plan and affect goal-directed action control. Bilingual subjects seem to be particularly vulnerable since they activate not only semantics of spoken words but also their cross-linguistic translations automatically leading to interference. This study thus provides strong evidence of spoken words interfering with visual search during simultaneous processing. Future research should explore the neurobiological nature of this interaction.

10.6 Implications for Bilingual Mental Organisation

We have shown that distraction in the visual saccade task occurred since bilinguals unintentionally translated the spoken words. There have been many arguments in the literature on the issue of translation in bilinguals. One dominant model argues that low proficient bilinguals need to translate words in their L2 since they have a weak conceptual representation in this language. However, there is currently evidence which suggests that even highly proficient bilinguals translate words. In this study our participants were highly proficient Hindi–English speaking bilinguals who lived in an L1 dominant language environment. However, we found that they translated words into the corresponding L1 lexicon and this lead to interference. Another dimension to the bilingual cognitive profile is their increasing cognitive control that arises in demanding situations. We have demonstrated that Hindi-English bilinguals, similar to participants used in this study, show greater cognitive control in Sproop like selective attention tasks (Singh and Mishra 2012, 2013). However, it is not clear why these bilinguals fail to exercise cognitive control in a visual world type task but show interference. It is apparent that these bilinguals could not ignore the spoken words and which could have been possible to exercise of executive control. This disparity is not explained by current studies on bilingual lexical organisation or cognitive control. In a direct examination of this link between bilingual cognitive control and parallel activation of lexicons, Blumenfeld and Marian (2013) found that bilinguals with higher proficiency also show higher parallel activations but show reduced Stroop interference. The paradigm that we used did not explicitly require conceptual access of objects. Participants did not have to search an object with regard to a spoken name, but had to make a saccade towards an object which changed colour. Therefore, this task offered limited scope for parallel lexicon activation. In sum, we have shown that bilinguals activate lexicons more automatically even when task demands are different. Further, we have shown that it is unintentional conceptual access during spoken word listening, which captures attention and causes interference in the main task.

10.7 Conclusion

To conclude, we can say that it is probably very difficult to ignore semantic access from spoken words even in situations where it is not necessary. Using the visual world eye tracking paradigm we have shown that attention capture occurs when the linguistic system extracts meaning from the spoken words and this causes an attentional bottleneck. It is though still not clear, why saccades should be affected because of unintentional linguistic processing in a task like this. It is interesting to further examine if working memory and attentional load influence such interference. We have emphasised the individual difference aspect of cognitive processing which shows language abilities have an interface with attentional control.

Acknowledgments Support for this chapter came from a DST grant awarded to RKM under the Cognitive Science Initiative Scheme.

References

Allopenna, P. D., Magnuson, J. S., & Tanenhaus, M. K. (1998). Tracking the time course ofspoken word recognition using eye movements: Evidence for continuous mapping models. *Journal of Memory and Language, 38*(4), 419–439.

Altmann, G. T. M., & Kamide, Y. (2004). Now you see it, now you don't: Mediating the mapping between language and the visual world. In J. Henderson & F. Ferreira (Eds.), *The integration of language, vision and action* (pp. 347–386). Psychology Press.

Bargh, J. A. (1994). The four horsemen of automaticity. In R. S. Wyer & T. K. Srull (Eds.), *Handbook of social cognition* (pp. 1–40). Hillsdale, NJ: Erlbaum.

Bertels, J., Kolinsky, R., Bernaerts, A., & Morais, J. (2011). Effects of emotional spoken words on exogenous attentional orienting. *Journal of Cognitive Psychology, 23*(4), 435–452.

Blumenfeld, H. K., & Marian, V. (2007). Constraints on parallel activation in bilingual spoken language processing: Examining proficiency and lexical status using eye-tracking. *Language and Cognitive Processes, 22*, 633–660.

Blumenfeld, H. K., & Marian, V. (2013). Parallel language activation and cognitive control during spoken word recognition in bilinguals. *Journal of Cognitive Psychology, 25*(5), 547–567.

Buchner, A., & Erdfelder, E. (2005). Word frequency of irrelevant speech distractors affects serial recall. *Memory and Cognition, 33*, 86–97.

Buchner, A., Rothermund, K., Wentura, D., & Mehl, B. (2004). Valence of distractor words increases the effects of irrelevant speech on serial recall. *Memory and Cognition, 32*, 722–731.

Buchner, A. (1996). On the irrelevance of semantic information for the lIrrelevant speech effect. *The Quarterly Journal of Experimental Psychology: Section A, 49*(3), 765–779.

Chua, F. K. (2013). Attentional capture by onsets and offsets. *Visual Cognition, 21*(5), 569–598.

Cleland, A. A., Tamminen, J., Quinlan, P. T., & Gaskell, M. G. (2012). Spoken word processing creates a lexical bottleneck. *Language and Cognitive Processes, 27*(4), 572–593.

Cooper, R. M. (1974). The control of eye fixation by the meaning of spoken language: A new methodology for the real-time investigation of speech perception, memory, and language processing. *Cognitive Psychology, 6*(1), 84–107.

Dahan, D., Magnuson, J. S., & Tanenhaus, M. K. (2001). Time course of frequency effects in spoken-word recognition: evidence from eye movements. *Cognitive Psychology, 42*, 317–367.

Dijkstra, T., Miwa, K., Brummelhuis, B., Sappelli, M., & Baayen, H. (2010). How crosslanguage similarity and task demands affect cognate recognition. *Journal of Memory and Language, 62*, 284–301.

Dijkstra, A. F. J., & Van Heuven, W. J. B. (2002). The architecture of the bilingual word recognition system: From identification to decision. *Bilingualism: Language and Cognition, 5*(3), 175–197.

Downing, P. E. (2000). Interactions between visual working memory and selective attention. *Psychological Science, 11*, 467–473.

Driver, J., & Spence, C. (1998). Cross-modal links in spatial attention. *Philosophical Transactions of the Royal Society B: Biological Sciences, 353*(1373), 1319.

Elliott, E. M., & Briganti, A. M. (2012). Investigating the role of attentional processes in the irrelevant speech effect. *Acta Psychologica, 140*, 64–74.

Guo, T., Misra, M., Tam, J. W., & Kroll, J. F. (2012). On the time course of accessing meaning in a second language: An electrophysiological investigation of translation recognition. *Journal of Experimental Psychology. Learning, Memory, and Cognition, 38*, 1165–1186. doi:10.1037/a0028076.

Huettig, F., & Altmann, G. T. M. (2004). Language-mediated eye movements and the resolution of lexical ambiguity. In M. Carreiras & C. Clifton (Eds.), *The on-line study of sentence comprehension: Eye-tracking, ERP, and beyond* (pp. 187–207). New York, NY: Psychology Press.

Huettig, F., & Altmann, G. T. M. (2005). Word meaning and the control of eye fixation: semantic competitor effects and the visual world paradigm. *Cognition, 96*(1), 23–32.

Huettig, F., & Altmann, G. T. M. (2007). Visual-shape competition and the control of eye fixation during the processing of unambiguous and ambiguous words. *Visual Cognition, 15*(8), 985–1018.

Huettig, F., & Altmann, G. T. M. (2011). Looking at anything that is green when hearing 'frog'— How object surface colour and stored object colour knowledge influence language-mediated overt attention. *Quarterly Journal of Experimental Psychology, 64*(1), 122–145.

Huettig, F., & Hartsuiker, R. J. (2008). When you name the pizza you look at the coin and the bread: Eye movements reveal semantic activation during word production. *Memory and Cognition, 36*(2), 341–360. doi:10.3758/MC.36.2.341.

Huettig, F., Mishra, R. K., & Olivers, C. N. (2012). On the mechanisms and representations of language-mediated visual attention. *Frontiers in Cognition, 2*, 394.

Huettig, F., & McQueen, J. M. (2007). The tug of war between phonological, semantic and shape information in language-mediated visual search. *Journal of Memory and Language, 57*(4), 460–482. doi:10.1016/j.jml.2007.02.001.

Irwin, D. E., Colcombe, A. M., Kramer, A. F., & Hahn, S. (2000). Attention and oculomotor capture by onset luminance and color singletons. *Vision Research, 40*, 1443–1458.

Jones, D. M., Miles, C., & Page, J. (1990). Disruption of proofreading by irrelevant speech: Effects of attention, arousal or memory? *Applied Cognitive Psychology, 4*(2), 89–108.

Jones, D. M., Madden, C., & Miles, C. (1992). Privileged access by irrelevant speech to short-term memory: The role of changing state. *Quarterly Journal of Experimental Psychology: Human Experimental Psychology, 44*, 645–669.

Jonides, J., Naveh-Benjamin, M., & Palmer, J. (1985). Assessing automaticity. *Acta Psychologica, 60*(2), 157–171.

Ju, M., & Luce, P. A. (2004). Falling on sensitive ears. *Psychological Science, 15*, 314–318.

Kamide, Y., & Altmann, G. T. M. (2004). The time-course of constraint-application during sentence processing in visual contexts: Anticipatory eye-movements in English and Japanese. In M. Tanenhaus & J. Trueswell (Eds.), *World situated language use: Psycholinguistic, linguistic and computational perspectives on bridging the product and action traditions.* Cambridge: MIT Press.

Kamide, Y., Altmann, G. T. M., & Haywood, S. (2003). The time-course of prediction in incremental sentence processing: Evidence from anticipatory eye-movements. *Journal of Memory and Language, 49*, 133–159.

Klatte, M., Lachmann, T., Schlittmeier, S., & Hellbrück, J. (2010). The irrelevant sound effect in short-term memory: Is there developmental change?*European. Journal of Cognitive Psychology, 22*(8), 1168–1191.

Lavie, N. (2005). Distracted and confused? Selective attention under load. *Trends in Cognitive Sciences, 9*, 75–82.

Lavie, N., & Tsal, Y. (1994). Perceptual load as a major determinant of the locus of selection in visual attention. *Perception and Psychophysics, 56*, 183–197.

LeCompte, D. C., Neely, C. B., & Wilson, J. R. (1997). Irrelevant speech and irrelevant tones: The relative importance of speech to the irrelevant speech effect. *Journal of Experimental Psychology: Learning, Memory, and Cognition, 23*, 472–483.

Logan, G. D. (1998). What is learned during automatization? Obligatory encoding of location information. *Journal of Experimental Psychology: Human Perception and Performance, 24*, 1720–1736.

Lupyan, G., & Swingley, D. (2011). Self-directed speech affects visual processing. *Quarterly Journal of Experimental Psychology, 65*(6), 1068–1085.

Ljungberg, J. K., Parmentier, F. B., Hughes, R. W., Macken, W. J., & Jones, D. M. (2012). Listen out! Behavioural and subjective responses to verbal warnings. *Applied Cognitive Psychology, 26*(3), 451–461.

Mani, N., & Huettig, F. (2012). Prediction is a piece of cake—but only for skilled producers. *Journal of Experimental Psychology: Human Perception and Performance, 38*, 843–847.

Marsh, J. E., Hughes, R. W., & Jones, D. M. (2008). Auditory distraction in semantic memory: A process-based approach. *Journal of Memory and Language, 58*(3), 682–700.

Marian, V., & Spivey, M. (2003a). Bilingual and monolingual processing of competing lexical items. *Applied Psycholinguistics, 24*, 173–193.

Marian, V., & Spivey, M. (2003b). Competing activation in bilingual language processing: Within and between-language competition. *Bilingualism: Language and Cognition, 6*, 97–115.

Martin, R. C., Wogalter, M. S., & Forlano, J. G. (1988). Reading comprehension in the presence of unattended speech and music. *Journal of Memory and Language, 27*, 382–398.

Mishra, R. (2009). Interface of language and visual attention: Evidence from production and comprehension. *Progress in Brain Research, 176*, 277–292.

Mishra, R. K., Huettig, F., & Olivers, C. N. (2012). Automaticity and conscious decisions during language-mediated eye gaze in the visual world. In N. Srinivasan & V. S. C. Pammi (Eds.), *Progress in Brain Research: Decision Making: Neural and Behavioral Approaches*. Amsterdam: Elsevier.

Moors, A.., & De Houwer, J. (2006). Automaticity: a theoretical and conceptual analysis. *Psychological bulletin, 132*(2), 297.

Moores, E., Laiti, L., & Chelazzi, L. (2003). Associative knowledge controls deployment of visual selective attention. *Nature Neuroscience, 6*, 182–189.

Nation, K., Marshall, C., & Altmann, G. T. M. (2003). Investigating individual differences in children's real-time sentence comprehension using language-mediated eye movements. *Journal of Experimental Child Psychology, 86*, 314–329.

Neely, C. B., & LeCompte, D. C. (1999). The importance of semantic similarity to the irrelevant speech effect. *Memory and Cognition, 27*, 37–44.

Oswald, C. J. P., Tremblay, S., & Jones, D. M. (2000). Disruption of comprehension by the meaning of irrelevant sound. *Memory, 8*, 345–350. doi:10.1080/09658210050117762.

Parmentier, F. B. R., Turner, J., & Perez, L. (2013). A dual contribution to the involuntary semantic processing of unexpected spoken words. *Journal of Experimental Psychology: General*. doi:10.1037/a0031550.

Pickering, M. J., & Garrod, S. (2004). Toward a mechanistic psychology of dialogue. *Behavioral and Brain Sciences, 27*(2), 169–189.

Pulvermüller, F., & Shtyrov, Y. (2006). Language outside the focus of attention: The mismatch negativity as a tool for studying higher cognitive processes. *Progress in Neurobiology, 79*(1), 49.

Salamé, P., & Baddeley, A. (1982). Disruption of short term memory by unattended speech: Implications for thestructure of working memory. *Journal of Verbal Learning and Verbal Behavior, 21*, 150–164.

Salverda, A. P., & Altmann, G. T. M. (2011). Attentional capture of objects referred to by spoken language. *Journal of Experimental Psychology: Human Perception and Performance, 37*, 1122–1133.

Shtyrov. Y., Kimppa, L., Pulvermüller, F., Kujala, T. (2010). Event-related potentials reflecting the frequency of unattended spoken words: A neuronal index of connection strength in lexical memory circuits? *Neuroimage, 15;55*(2), 658–668.

Singh, N., & Mishra, R. K. (2013). Second language proficiency modulates conflict-monitoring in an oculomotor stroop task: Evidence from Hindi-English Bilinguals. *Frontiers in Psychology,*. doi:10.3389/fpsyg.2013.00322.

Singh, N., & Mishra, R. K. (2012). Does language proficiency modulate oculomotor control? Evidence from Hindi-English bilinguals. *Bilingualism: Language and Cognition, 15*, 771–781.

Soto, D., & Humphreys, G. W. (2007). Automatic guidance of visual attention from verbal working memory. *The Journal of Experimental Psychology: Human Perception and Performance, 33*(3), 730–737.

Spivey, M. J., & Marian, V. (1999). Cross talk between native and second languages: Partial activation of an irrelevant lexicon. *Psychological Science, 10*(3), 281–284.

Sunderman, G., & Priya, K. (2012). Translation recognition in highly proficient Hindi-Englis bilinguals the influence of different scripts but connectable phonologies. *Language and Cognitive Processes, 27*(9), 1265–1285.

Telling, A. L., Kumar, S., Meyer, A. S., & Humphreys, G. W. (2010). Electrophysiological evidence of semantic interference in visual search. *Journal of Cognitive Neuroscience, 22*(10), 2212–2225.

Tellinghuisen, D. J., & Nowak, E. J. (2003). The inability to ignore auditory distractors as a function of visual task perceptual load. *Perception and Psychophysics, 65*, 817–828.

Thierry, G., & Wu, Y. J. (2010). Chinese–English bilinguals reading english hear Chinese. *The Journal of Neuroscience, 30*, 7646–7651.

Tun, P. A., O'Kane, G., & Wingfield, A. (2002). Distraction by competing speech in younger and older listeners. *Psychology and Aging, 17*, 453–467.

Weaver, M. D., Lauwereyns, J., & Theeuwes, J. (2011). The effect of semantic information on saccade trajectory deviations. *Vision Research, 51*, 1124–1128.

Weber, A., & Cutler, A. (2004). Lexical competition in non-native spoken-word recognition. *Journal of Memory and Language, 50*, 1–25.

Yantis, S., & Jonides, J. (1984). Abrupt visual onsets and selective attention: Evidence from visual search. *Journal of Experimental Psychology: Human Perception and Performance, 5*, 625–638.

Yee, E., Overton, E., & Thompson-Schill, S. L. (2009). Looking for meaning: Eye movements are sensitive to overlapping semantic features, not association. *Psychonomic Bulletin and Review, 16*(5), 869–874.

Yee, E., & Sedivy, J. C. (2006). Eye movements to pictures reveal transient semantic activation during spoken word recognition. *Journal of Experimental Psychology: Learning, Memory, and Cognition, 32*, 1–14.

Zeelenberg, R., & Bocanegra, B. R. (2010). Auditory emotional cues enhance visual perception. *Cognition, 115*, 202–206.

Part IV
Language Processing in a Social Context

Chapter 11
Adjusting the Manner of Language Processing to the Social Context: Attention Allocation During Interactions with Non-native Speakers

Shiri Lev-Ari

11.1 Introduction

Models of language processing traditionally assume that we process the language of all speakers similarly, regardless of who they are. Thus, they assume that we will understand the sentence *I just ate two pieces of pie* using the same cues and reaching the same interpretation regardless of whether it was uttered by a young teenager, an elderly woman, our middle-aged neighbour or our non-native-speaking friend. Occasionally, there might be break downs in communication. For example, a language learner might select a suboptimal lexical item, using the sentence above, for example, to describe eating slices of a quiche, a cake or even two brownies. In these cases, we, as listeners, would note the error, and then correct it, inferring the meaning from the context. Importantly, the initial process of constructing a meaning out of the input is implicitly assumed to remain invariable, and the correction takes place after an incompatibility between the linguistic input and the context had been detected. More recent evidence, however, indicates that language processing is not invariable, but, in fact, adjusts to the situation. This evidence shows that the cues that listeners attend to during language processing might change according to the identity of the speaker. This chapter will review such evidence while focusing on evidence that shows that listeners' expectations of non-native speakers lead them to allocate less attention to linguistic cues and greater attention to contextual cues when processing the language of non-native speakers.

S. Lev-Ari (✉)
Nijmegen, Netherlands
e-mail: shiri.lev-ari@mpi.nl

© Springer India 2015
R.K. Mishra et al. (eds.), *Attention and Vision in Language Processing*, DOI 10.1007/978-81-322-2443-3_11

11.1.1 Expectations and Language Processing

When we listen to people, we spontaneously generate expectations for what they might say. In fact, upon hearing the voice of an unfamiliar speaker, we immediately extract from it information about the speaker's gender, age, and socio-economic status, and this information is sufficient to immediately induce certain expectations about what the speaker is likely to say. Therefore, hearing a voice of a child saying *Every evening I drink some wine before I go to sleep* leads to increased N400, an ERP component associated with greater difficulty in semantic integration, that is similar in timing and distribution to the one induced by semantic anomalies (Van Berkum et al. 2008).

In fact, the integration of social information is an integral aspect of language processing. For example, the interpretation of a phoneme as /ʊ/ or /ʌ/ depends on whether we see or imagine a man or a woman speaking, as the boundary between the two vowels is at different formant frequencies for men and women (Johnson et al. 1999). Such integration of social information, however, can sometimes lead us astray and distort our perception. For example, it can lead us to perceive the same vowel as a standard /a/ if we believe the speaker is from a region where standard American English is spoken, but as an /aw/ if we believe the speaker is from Canada, where /a/is produced as the raised diphthong /aw/ (Niedzielski 1999).

The role of expectations is not restricted to the stage of the final interpretation of speech. Recent studies show that expectations can influence the very manner of language processing by shifting the weight we give different cues. Such shifting of weights can lead us to avoid making inferences that we commonly do (Arnold et al. 2007; Grodner and Sedivy 2011). For example, while listeners commonly infer from disfluency in the speech that the speaker is about to describe something hard, they no longer make that inference if they believe the speaker suffers from object agnosia, a difficulty with naming objects (Arnold et al. 2007). Similarly, expecting the input to be noisy and therefore unreliable attenuates our tendency to rely on onset versus offset phonetic information (McQueen and Huettig 2012).

11.2 Processing the Language of Non-native Speakers

One type of situation in which listeners hold specific expectations about the speaker is the case of processing the language of non-native speakers. Non-native speakers often have lower linguistic proficiency. They may make grammatical errors or suboptimal lexical choices, and we as listeners know and expect that (Hanulikova et al. 2012). Non-native speakers' lower proficiency can render their speech less reliable in conveying their intentions. Therefore, one way for listeners to optimise communication is to attend less to the less reliable linguistic input, and instead attend more to contextual information, which is equally reliable with native and non-native speakers. The remainder of this chapter will focus on this case of processing the language of non-native speakers in order to illustrate the manner in which the allocation of attention and resources can adjust to circumstances. It will also survey the consequences of such an adjustment as well as its constraints.

11.2.1 Good-Enough Representations

Suppose your friend who had just referred to the *quiche* as a *pie* tells you about the wonderful dish he is planning to prepare tonight. Your friend may use specific terms, such as a *pie* or a *quiche*, to refer to this dish, but considering his unreliable use of such terms, encoding the message as being about a baked good or a dish might be better, as it would require less effort while potentially increasing accuracy.

Less detailed "good-enough" processing occurs often even when processing the language of native speakers. We often do not process linguistic input in full, but, instead, only process it to a level that is perceived to be sufficient for the situational demands, and then fill-in missing information based on our general knowledge. This can lead us to occasionally not notice anomalies in the input, misrepresent the content of the utterance, or miss content changes in it. Thus we might encode a sentence about a man biting a dog as being about a dog biting a man, because our world knowledge would favour this interpretation of the less-detailed representation we generated (Ferreira et al. 2002). At other times, we might miss changes in story details such as the fact that a story that earlier mentioned cider being drunk at the pub now describes beer (Sturt et al. 2004).

Importantly, this tendency of ours to process and represent language in less detail depends on our expectations regarding speaker reliability. This leads us to attend even less to the details in the linguistic input when we listen to non-native speakers. This was evidenced by a recent study in which participants needed to detect changes in a story told by either a native or a non-native speaker. In this study, participants first listened to either a native or a non-native speaker tell a story about his friend. Later, they received a surprise memory test, in which they read a modified written version of the story, and were asked to detect changes that were made to the story. The changes were always word substitutions to semantically related words. For example, a statement by the speaker that his friend never has the *time* to cook changed to a statement declaring that she never has the *patience* to cook. As predicted, participants who listened to a non-native speaker tell the story detected fewer changes than those who listened to a native speaker (Lev-Ari and Keysar 2012). One may wonder whether it is simply because non-native speakers are harder to understand, and because processing their speech imposes greater cognitive load. The study, however, had two listening conditions that manipulated the relevance of participants' communicative expectations. When participants' goal was to listen for comprehension in anticipation of later answering comprehension questions, participants showed the aforementioned difference in memory for the language of the native compared with the non-native speaker. In the other condition, however, where participants were told to memorise the story they hear, because they will later be asked to detect word changes, participants showed equal performance with the two speakers. This indicates that we are able to process the language of non-native speakers in detail, but choose to attend to the linguistic details less when listening for comprehension.

This study then shows adjustment in the manner of language processing according to the speaker's characteristics. In general, there is evidence that working memory can influence listeners' and readers' ability to integrate different types of information in a timely manner during language processing (Federmeier and Kutas 2005; Just and Carpenter 1992; Traxler et al. 2005). A follow-up study examined whether this better ability at integrating different types of information leads those with higher working memory to be better able to integrate the information about the speaker in order to better adjust their manner of processing according to whether the speaker is a native or a non-native speaker. Using the same word change detection task, the follow-up study showed that above a certain working memory threshold, higher working memory leads to greater engagement in less-detailed processing, and consequently, to poorer performance with the non-native speaker. This finding is particularly striking, as higher working memory is often associated with better performance (Conway et al. 2002).

11.2.2 Attention to Contextual Cues

Other than representing language in less detail, listeners can also potentially improve communication with non-native speakers by attending more to contextual information when processing the language of non-native speakers, as the reliability of contextual information is unaffected by the proficiency of the speaker. Such greater reliance on contextual information can be reflected in at least two manners: by weighing contextual information more heavily than ordinarily, but also by using it earlier in order to predict what a speaker is about to say. After all, we commonly make such use of contextual information—whether it is the linguistic context, the visual context or the context's affordances—to predict the forthcoming input, and such contextual information can influence both syntactic and lexical interpretation of the linguistic input (Chambersa et al. 2004; Duffy et al. 1988; Tanenhaus et al. 1995). The question is then whether we increase this tendency to rely on contextual information when its reliability is relatively high compared with other sources of information.

To understand how such an increase in reliance might be manifested, consider the following example from one of the experiments that tested for increased reliance when processing the language of non-native speakers. Suppose you sit in front of a screen with pictures, and are asked to follow instructions that will indicate which pictures from the set to select. You are further told that all the pictures that you will be asked to select share something in common. You are then told to select the cookie. Once you select it, you are told to select the cheese, and after you do so as well, you are told to select the tortilla. By this stage, you will have likely noted that all the pictures that you had selected were food items. You will therefore expect to next be instructed to select the brownie. If attention to top-down information and reliance on it increase during the processing of non-native language, then you should be more likely to rely on this expectation to be told to click on the brownie if you follow instructions provided by a non-native rather than a native speaker. Such greater reliance on expectations can be indicated, for example, by greater likelihood of fixating on the brownie (the competitor) already at word onset, just before you hear the next instruction.

The next instruction, however, is to select the /paɪ/. One meaning of /paɪ/ is pie, which is semantically related to a brownie, as both are food items. Therefore, if listening to non-native speakers leads listeners to attend less to the linguistic details, then you should be less likely to notice that there is a discrepancy between the label, /paɪ/, and the expected referent, the brownie, if the instructions are provided by a non-native speaker. This would be indicated by lower likelihood of attending to the target object, the symbol π, which relates to the previous selected pictures by the much less dominant theme of the geometry of a circle (as all previously selected items are round).

Additionally, greater reliance on top-down expectations, whether while noticing the discrepancy of the label or not, should lead to greater likelihood of selecting the brownie rather than the symbol π.

To recapitulate, participants in this experiment selected pictures that were semantically related to one another according to instructions provided by either a native or a non-native speaker. On critical trials, the first three pictures participants were instructed to select induced an expectation for a specific fourth object (competitor) to be selected. The following critical instruction, however, was always a homophone, which had one meaning that is semantically related to the expected object, yet inappropriate for it (e.g., pie), and one meaning that fits another object on the screen (π), whose relation to the first three objects is more tenuous. It was tested whether the participants who listened to the non-native speakers were more likely to allocate attention to the contextually expected competitor object earlier, whether they were more likely to eventually select it, and whether they were less likely to attend to the target object.

Results indeed showed all these patterns of adjustment to non-native speakers (Lev-Ari 2015): In terms of final selection, listeners selected the context-appropriate competitor (brownie) rather than the target (π) more often when they followed instructions provided by a non-native speaker than by a native speaker. Listeners were also more likely to look at the contextually appropriate competitor already at word onset and were less likely to look at the target at all if they listened to a non-native rather than a native speaker, but these effects were modulated by working memory. As with the shift to less-detailed representation in the change detection task described earlier, higher working memory led to greater difference between performance with native and non-native speakers, whereas lower working memory led to a more invariable manner of processing that does not depend on speaker.

The study then illustrates the flexibility of our processing mechanisms and their ability to adjust to the social circumstances. It shows that both the type of cues we attend to and the point in time at which we do so can vary according to the expected reliability of the cues. The studies also indicate that this ability to adjust our manner of processing according to the social circumstances is demanding and therefore constrained by our cognitive abilities, such as our working memory.

11.2.3 Consequences for Other Aspects of Language Processing

So far, this chapter described the allocation of attention to different cues as an isolated process. Yet the allocation of attention to a specific cue is a sub-process in a complex language processing mechanism that is composed of multiple inter-related components. Consequently, modifications to one aspect of the mechanism can have consequences for other aspects. Such is the case with the lesser attention to linguistic detail in processing. As will be described below, this adjustment in attention allocation impacts lexical competition and access.

Lexical access is achieved by inhibiting semantic competitors, and the more similar a competitor is, the greater effort that is needed to inhibit it (Anderson et al. 1994). Yet similarity is context-dependent. In the case of listening to a non-native speaker, the lesser attention to linguistic details can lead to greater similarity between items. This is so, because specifying fewer details for each lexical item means that many of the characteristics that distinguish related items from one another are likely to be left unspecified.

One study tested whether the processing of the language of non-native speakers therefore leads to greater lexical competition. The study relied on the Retrieval-Induced Inhibition paradigm, also known as the Retrieval-Induced Forgetting (Anderson et al. 1994; Veling and van Knippenberg 2004). In this task, participants memorise words from a few specific categories. The presentation of these words is blocked by category and the words appear next to their category name. Following the memorisation stage, participants do a cued recall task, in which they receive the category name with the first letter of a word they had memorised, and their task is to retrieve that word. Importantly, in this stage, they practice only half of the words from some of the categories, and no words from other categories. Consequently, there are three types of words: practiced words, words that were not practiced but belong to categories that were practiced, and words that were not practiced and belong to categories from which no word had been practiced. Finally, participants perform a recognition test on all memorised words, together with fillers. Practiced words are naturally recognised faster than non-practiced words in this task. The crucial question though is whether there is a difference between the recognition of the two types of words that were not practiced. The exercise of inhibition during lexical access in the cued recall task should lead to the inhibition of the unpracticed words from the practised categories. This should lead those words to be recognised more slowly than the unpracticed words from the unpracticed categories, and this difference in recognition should be larger the more inhibition was exercised during cued recall.

Returning to the case of processing the language of non-native speakers, if listeners attend less to linguistic details and thus experience greater lexical competition with non-native speakers, then they should show greater difference between the recognition of the two types of unpracticed words. This is what the study found (Lev-Ari et al. 2011). Participants who earlier listened to a story by a non-native speaker showed greater lexical competition than those who listened to a story by a native speaker. This is despite the fact that the lexical items whose competition was measured were not produced by the native and non-native speakers but were presented afterwards. Therefore, the words in the two speaker conditions did not differ in any way nor did they require different amounts of processing. The direction of the difference in inhibition—greater inhibition after listening to non-native speakers—also rules out the option that the difference is due to the greater cognitive load involved in processing the language of non-native speakers, as greater cognitive load should lead to the dwindling of resources, and therefore, to lower, rather than higher inhibition. Still, one may wonder whether the greater inhibition following the processing of the language of non-native speakers is linguistic in nature or whether it is due to some change in the general use of inhibition when processing the language of non-native speakers. To examine that possibility, a non-linguistic version of the task, in which participants memorised and practiced novel difficult-to-label shapes and visual arrays, was run. In contrast to the linguistic version, there were no differences in this case between the level of inhibition that those who listened to the native speaker and those who listened to the non-native speaker exhibited. The changes in the exercise of inhibition, then, are linguistic in nature and restricted to language processing mechanisms. The study then shows how changing the allocation of attention to linguistic detail influences lexical competition. It thus illustrates how adapting one aspect of processing to improve communication can lead to unintended changes in other aspects of the language processing mechanisms.

11.2.4 Consequences for Processing Other Linguistic Input

Our language processing mechanisms, then, are flexible. As I have shown, the way that attention is allocated—which cues are considered, at what point in time, and how much weight they are assigned—varies according to the nature and demands of the situation. One may wonder, however, how flexible our language processing mechanism is in terms of switching between manners of language processing. For example, do we adjust to each speaker in a multi-party interaction? Furthermore, even when interacting solely with one speaker, a non-native one, are we able to use different manners of processing for her language and for ours? This latter question is particularly intriguing considering models that posit that language production mechanisms are engaged during comprehension of others' language

(Pickering and Garrod 2007) and that language comprehension mechanisms monitor our own productions (Levelt 1983).

A recent study tested this question by comparing the level of detail in the representation of one's own language during interactions with non-native versus native speakers. Participants in this study were interviewed by a native or non-native speaking confederate about a short story they had both read. After a short distractor task, participants received a surprise memory test, where they had to identify their responses from a list of possible responses. Those who were interviewed by a non-native speaker performed more poorly in this task (Lev-Ari et al. 2011).

Another interesting aspect of this study was the finding that the degree of adjustment to the non-native speaker in production predicted the degree of adjustment in processing. In general, we adjust our productions to the characteristics of our speakers. A particularly well-studied adaptation is the one towards infants. Yet we adjust our production to non-native speakers as well, and one of the phonetic hallmarks of such adjustment is slower speech rate (Uther et al. 2007). Interestingly, in the aforementioned study, those who adjusted their productions the most towards non-native speakers, as indicated by slower speech rate, also showed the greatest adjustment in processing, as reflected in poorer detection of their own responses. Importantly, there was no relation between speech rate and response detection among those who were interviewed by a native speaker, indicating that it is not simply that those who speak slowly have poorer recall.

This study then shows that our language processing mechanism adjusts as a whole: the degree of adjustment in speaking relates to the degree of adjustment in processing and representation, and adjustment to one speaker modifies the processing of the language of other speakers. Thus, when we adjust the way we allocate attention while listening to one speaker, this modified manner of allocation of attention carries over to the processing of other language, even our own.

11.2.5 Social Consequences

As we have seen so far, social factors, such as speaker characteristics, influence the allocation of attention during language processing. The relation between allocation of attention and social factors, however, is a two ways street. As linguistic interactions are embedded in social interactions, the studies presented so far suggest that the characteristics of our linguistic interaction partner can influence the degree to which we attend to the context of a social situation. Such differential allocation of attention context can have far reaching consequences, as many social phenomena depend on consideration of top-down contextual information. To take one, perspective taking, the ability to take into account the fact that others hold different information from us, depends on an ability to attend to and integrate common ground. Therefore, the findings that we attend more to the context when interacting with non-native speakers suggest, quite counter-intuitively, that we would be better at perspective taking when interacting with non-native speakers.

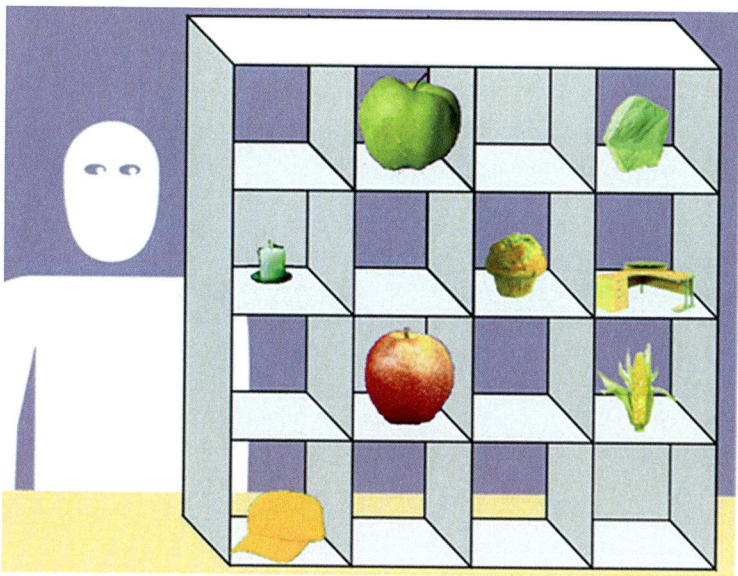

Fig. 11.1   An illustration of a trial in a perspective taking task

One study tested this possibility using a computerised version of the common perspective taking task (Keysar et al. 2000; Dumontheil et al. 2010). In this task, a "director" instructs a participant, sitting on the other side of a grid, to move objects from one cell in the grid into another. Some of the cells of this grid are occluded from the director's point of view but not from the instruction-follower's view (see Fig. 11.1). On experimental trials, the director's instruction, e.g., *Put the apple below the muffin,* could fit both a mutually visible object (the green apple) and an object occluded from the director's view (the red apple), if the director's perspective is not taken into account. Therefore, greater proportion of looks towards the occluded apple in such trials compared with a control trial, where a non-competing object is placed in the occluded cell, indicates failure to take the director's perspective. A comparison of the gaze pattern of participants who listened to a non-native speaker with those who listened to a native speaker revealed that, indeed, participants were more attuned to the perspective of the director when she was a non-native speaker (Lev-Ari, Barr and Keysar, under review). This effect was found despite the fact that listening to non-native speakers imposes a cognitive load, and added cognitive load in general leads to worse perspective taking (Epley et al. 2004). This study thus shows that adjustment in allocation of attention during language processing can have non-linguistic social consequences.

11.3 Summary

Language processing is a complex mechanism where multiple cues must be attended to and integrated. Importantly, this mechanism operates in a social context. Therefore, the traditional study of it in a decontextualized setting obscures some of its characteristics. One such understudied characteristic is the way that social characteristics, such as an interlocutor's identity, can influence the allocation of attention during language processing.

The studies described here provide strong support that listeners process differently the language of non-native speakers. They further illustrate the manner in which the processing mechanism can adjust itself, namely, by changing the time point at which different cues are attended to and the weight that they are given. The studies also show how an adjustment in allocation of attention can influence other aspects of processing because of the interrelated nature of the processing mechanism. Furthermore, the studies show that adjustments in manner of processing can lead to unexpected social consequences. At the same time, the research demonstrates the constraints of the flexibility of our processing mechanism. For example, it shows that flexibility in attention allocation requires cognitive resources, and that we do not easily re-allocate our attention with frequent changes in the source of the input, such as a switch between speakers. This chapter described one specific unintended linguistic consequence and one social consequence to the adjustment in processing. Needless to say, there could be additional linguistic and social consequences to the adjustment in attention allocation when listening to non-native speakers. Similarly, there could be different adaptations in allocation of attention when interacting with other types of speakers, who induce other types of expectations.

The research described here, then, points to the importance of examining language processing, including its sub-processes such as allocation of attention to different cues, under different social conditions and understanding how cognitive processes are socially mediated.

References

Anderson, M. C., Bjork, R. A., & Bjork, E. L. (1994). Remembering can cause forgetting: Retrieval dynamics in long-term memory. *Journal of Experimental Psychology. Learning, Memory, and Cognition, 20*(5), 1063–1087.

Arnold, J. E., Hudson Kam, C. L., & Tanenhaus, M. K. (2007). If you say thee uh—you're describing something hard: The on-line attribution of disfluency during reference comprehension. *The Journal of Experimental Psychology: Learning, Memory and Cognition, 33*, 914–930.

Chambers, C. G., Tanenhaus, M. K., & Magnuson, J. S. (2004). Actions and affordances in syntactic ambiguity resolution. *Journal of Experimental Psychology. Learning, Memory, and Cognition, 30*, 687–696.

Conway, A. R. A., Cowan, N., Bunting, M. F., Therriault, D., & Minkoff, S. (2002). A latent variable analysis of working memory capacity, short term memory capacity, processing speed, and general fluid intelligence. *Intelligence, 30*, 163–183.

Duffy, S. A., Morris, R. K., & Rayner, K. (1988). Lexical ambiguity and fixation times in read-
  ing. *Journal of Memory and Language, 27*, 429–446.
Dumontheil, I., Apperly, I. A., & Blakemore, S. J. (2010). Online use of mental state inferences
  continues to develop in late adolescence. *Developmental Science, 13*(2), 331–338.
Epley, N., van Keysar, B., Boyen, L., & Gilovich, T. (2004). Perspective Taking as Egocentric
  Anchoring and Adjustment. *Journal of Personality and Social Psychology, 87*(3), 327–339.
Federmeier, K. D., & Kutas, M. (2005). Aging in context: Age-related changes in context use
  during language comprehension. *Psychophysiology, 42*, 133–142.
Ferreira, F., Ferraro, V., & Bailey, K. G. D. (2002). Good-enough representations in language
  comprehension. *Current Directions in Psychological Science, 11*, 11–15.
Grodner, D., & Sedivy, J. C. (2011). The effects of speaker-specific information on
  Pragmaticinferences. In N. Pearlmutter & E. Gibson (Eds.), *The processing and acquisition
  of reference* (pp. 239–272). Cambridge: MIT Press.
Hanulikova, A., Van Alphen, P. M., Van Goch, M., & Weber, A. (2012). When one person's mis-
  take is another's standard usage: The effect of foreign accent on syntactic processing. *Journal
  of Cognitive Neuroscience, 24*(4), 878–887.
Johnson, K., Strand, E. A., & D'Imperio, M. (1999). Auditory-visual integration of talker gender
  in vowel perception. *Journal of Phonetics., 27*, 359–384.
Just, M. A., & Carpenter, P. A. (1992). A capacity theory of comprehension: Individual differ-
  ences in working memory. *Psychological Review, 99*, 122–149.
Keysar, B., Barr, D. J., Balin, J. A., & Brauner, J. S. (2000). Taking perspective in conversation:
  The role of mutual knowledge in comprehension. *Psychological Science, 11*, 32–38.
Lev-Ari, S. (2015). Comprehending non-native speakers: Theory and evidence for adjustment in
  manner of processing. *Frontiers in Psychology, 5*, 1546.
Lev-Ari, S., Barr, D., & Keysar, B. (under review). Listeners are better attuned to non-native
  speakers' perspectives.
Lev-Ari, S., Ho, E., & Keysar, B. (2011). Interacting with non-native speakers induces "good-
  enough" representation. *Poster presented at The 24th Annual CUNY Conference on Human
  Sentence Processing*. CA: Stanford.
Lev-Ari, S., & Keysar, B. (2012). Less-detailed representation of non-native language: Why non-
  native speakers' stories seem more vague. *Discourse Processes, 49*, 523–538.
Levelt, W. J. M. (1983). Monitoring and Self-Repair in Speech. *Cognition, 14*(1), 41–104.
McQueen, J. M., & Huettig, F. (2012). Changing only the probability that spoken words will
  be distorted changes how they are recognized. *Journal of the Acoustical Society of America,
  131*(1), 509–517.
Niedzielski, N. (1999). The effect of social information on the perception of sociolinguistic vari-
  ables. *Journal of language and social psychology, 18*(1), 62–85.
Pickering, M. J., & Garrod, S. (2007). Do people use language production to make bpredictions
  during comprehension? *Trends in cognitive sciences, 11*(3), 105–110.
Sturt, P., Sanford, A. J., Stewart, A. J., & Dawydiak, E. (2004). Linguistic focus and good-
  enough representations: an application of the change-detection paradigm. *Psychonomic
  Bulletin & Review, 11*, 882–888.
Tanenhaus, M. K., Spivey-Knowlton, M. J., Eberhard, K. M., & Sedivy, J. E. (1995). Integration of
  visual and linguistic information in spoken language comprehension. *Science, 268*, 1632–1634.
Traxler, M. J., Williams, R. S., Blozis, S. A., & Morris, R. K. (2005). Working memory, animacy, and
  verb class in the processing of relative clauses. *Journal of Memory and Language, 53*, 204–224.
Uther, M., Knoll, M. A., & Burnham, D. (2007). Do you speak E-NG-LI-SH? A comparison of
  foreigner-and infant-directed speech. *Speech Communication, 49*(1), 2–7.
Van Berkum, J., van den Brink, D., Tesink, C. M., Kos, M., & Hagoort, P. (2008). The neural
  integration of speaker and message. *Journal of Cognitive Neuroscience, 20*, 580–591.
Veling, H., & van Knippenberg, A. (2004). Remembering can cause inhibition: Retrieval-induced
  inhibition as cue independent process. *Journal of Experimental Psychology. Learning,
  Memory, and Cognition, 30*, 315–318.

Chapter 12
Seeing and Believing: Social Influences on Language Processing

David W. Vinson, Rick Dale, Maryam Tabatabaeian
and Nicholas D. Duran

12.1 Introduction and Motivation

Most readers have likely experienced writing peacefully at a cafe, and being suddenly foisted into an uninvited conversation with a loose acquaintance, or even a stranger, who happens to be there. Approached while intimately nested within a paper or new analysis, some of us might try carefully to tailor our language to convince the interlocutor that we are not desperately trying to end the interaction so we can get back to our work. This subtle process is all but simple. A whole range of social factors from low-level visual processes such as observing the other's gaze, to higher-level processes such as knowledge of their belief states, unfolds simultaneously, and probably mostly implicitly. Put simply, language processing in these natural situations is undergirded by many sources of information: gaze, gesture, tone of voice, lexical to syntactic levels, topics of conversation, not-so-gently-executed dialogue moves and so on. This complex array of information *simultaneously* shapes our own language towards specific goals. These variables involved in language processing *in context* do not enjoy the benefits of laboratory distillation. They together incrementally guide how we process the dialogue and how we contribute to it, as we may nevertheless try to get out of it.

D.W. Vinson · R. Dale (✉) · M. Tabatabaeian
Cognitive and Information Sciences, University of California,
5200 N. Lake Rd, Merced, CA 95343, USA
e-mail: rdale@ucmerced.edu

D.W. Vinson
e-mail: dvinson@ucmerced.edu

N.D. Duran
Arizona State University, Tempe, USA

© Springer India 2015
R.K. Mishra et al. (eds.), *Attention and Vision
in Language Processing*, DOI 10.1007/978-81-322-2443-3_12

This example, and many other instances of language use in context, cast language as an active and social process, intimately involving both speaker and listener (Tanenhaus and Brown-Schmidt 2008). This may be obvious to many readers, yet much research on language processing focuses on phenomena closely related to what may be termed "monologue", such as decontextualized word recognition or sentence processing. Indeed, much of this research has investigated language production and comprehension independent of one another (Pickering and Garrod 2004). From this standpoint, language happens *to* the individual at a single moment and not *between* two or more individuals over time (see Kreysa and Pickering 2011 for review). Alternatively, the past decade or two has revealed a rapidly growing trend to shift the field's focus to mechanisms involved in what might be the most basic and natural form of communication: dialogue (Clark 1992, 1996; Garrod and Pickering 2004). As Clark (1996) and colleagues have famously argued, well before this recent trend began, instances of language behaviour are difficult to explain or understand without making reference to participants in the dynamic, incremental process of dialogue. This resurgent trend looks to dialogue with an eye to understanding the *mechanisms and processes* that underlie it. The work of Clark (1996) and others certainly formed part of the bedrock of this endeavour, primarily the manner in which coordination shapes everything from lexical choice (Brennan and Clark 1996) to the organisation of overt behaviours during interaction (Clark 2005). Yet, despite this intensive work, there still remain a number of important questions about the mechanisms driving dialogue (Garrod and Pickering 2004).

Our aim is to survey this trend by looking to *social factors*, such as social gaze, and how they influence language processing in context. One impactful and inherently social process is gaze following, or attending to the spatial location visually attended to by another (Friesen and Kingstone 1998). Specifically, observing another's gaze, under the right conditions, can affect the development of common ground (Bard et al. 2007): the mutually understood and shared content between interlocutors (Clark and Marshall 1981). Yet, as in our natural language situation described above, gaze following—and visual attention in general—operate alongside a range of other cognitive processes that also influence language comprehension. Other higher-level social processes naturally bear influence. For example, Brown-Schmidt and colleagues (2009b, 2011) found that taking another's perspective impacts the ability to disambiguate linguistic referents from their visual counterparts. Although observing another's gaze and understanding another's point of view seem like disparate processes, the language processing system has the potential to be influenced by both while comprehending in context. At the same time, effective social interaction can rely heavily on visual processes. Consider even the relatively lower-level process of phoneme perception, which can be highly affected by visual content. The McGurk effect demonstrates this powerfully (McGurk and MacDonald 1976; see also Johnson et al. 1999). Low-level processes such as gaze and gaze tracking, and higher-level processes such as knowledge and beliefs about another while taking their perspective, are not independent of each other; they mutually constrain each other during unfolding dialogue (see Brown-Schmidt and Hanna 2011 for review).

The above studies provide a brief introduction to the primary themes of this chapter: How do low- and high-level social processes impact language processing, and what role does vision play? First, we will review studies geared towards understanding how low-level social processes, such as observing another's gaze, impact language comprehension (Sect. 12.2). We then address higher-level social contexts where interlocutors must become highly attuned to the knowledge shared by their conversation partners (Sect. 12.3). This will be followed by a discussion of how many levels of processing work together during language usage in social context, using conversational deception as a case study (Sect. 12.4). We end by drawing on a dynamic approach to these processes, describing human interaction as a multilayered complex system that establishes particular strategies of operating (Dale et al. 2013; Fusaroli et al. 2013). By using this theoretical framework, we describe the future directions for mechanistic exploration (Sect. 12.5). As we argue below, the influence of such social factors is pervasive. Low-level and high-level processes, from seeing what another sees, to knowing what another knows, can sharply influence language comprehension. We begin with the importance of the eyes for language processing in context.

12.2 Seeing, and Seeing Seeing

Successful communication is sometimes mediated by the observation of another's gaze (Hanna and Brennan 2007) and by where their gaze is fixated (Gallup et al. 2012). Gaze behaviour has become a key variable in studies geared towards understanding the role of social factors in language comprehension. Readers of this volume are no doubt aware of these paradigms, many of which use eye-tracking technologies to capture gaze behaviour. Its use in research on language processing is now rather pervasive, including research on linguistically-mediated visual attention (Huettig et al. 2012), visual-world effects in language processing (Tanenhaus et al. 1995; Farmer et al. in press), disambiguation (Eberhard et al. 1995; Allopenna et al. 1998), knowledge states of an interaction partner (Brennan et al. 2010; Brown-Schmidt 2009a) and even the appearance or apparent goals of one's interlocutors (Laidlaw et al. 2011)—among many other linguistic variables (see Kreysa and Pickering 2011 for review). This massive array of findings shows that visual attention is crucial to multiple levels of language processing. At one level, the same phrase may result in entirely different gaze fixations dependent on access to specific visual content (Tanenhaus et al. 1995; cf. Cooper 1974). At the word level, gaze reveals when, in an auditory sentence stimulus, competition between potential referents occurs and when that ambiguity is resolved (Eberhard et al. 1995). Several of the chapters of this volume review this important research, revealing the intrinsic role visual attention plays in language processing. This opens up language comprehension to a battery of possible influences, the existence of which may only be possible through vision.[1] In our review here, we focus on the impact of these findings in the contexts of natural language usage, such as dialogue.

Consider, for example, the coupling between eye-movement patterns during interaction. Research on interaction has shown that successful communication is associated with the coupling of both posture (Shockley et al. 2003) and eye movements (Richardson and Dale 2005). For example, Richardson and Dale (2005) had a speaker view a grid of images depicting characters of a popular television series (e.g., *Friends*). Recording both speech and eye movements of the speaker, they were asked to explain the relationships between the characters. Separate participants were asked to listen to one speaker's recording while also viewing the same series of images. Importantly, listeners were not given access to the speaker's eye movements. Yet, eye movements of both speaker and listener were highly coupled. More importantly, listeners whose gaze pattern was more tightly coupled, closer in time to the gaze pattern of the speaker, performed better on a comprehension test. A follow-up experiment showed that when visual attention was drawn towards the image a speaker was addressing in real time, by flashing the corresponding image, faster responses were given on a comprehension test. In a following study, Richardson et al. (2007) showed synchronous gaze coupling to occur in real-time interactions, especially if dyads shared the same common ground about their topic of conversation.

These studies suggest the coupling between gaze patterns may draw interlocutors towards useful visual information, influencing dialogue more broadly. One may argue, however, that this research simply reveals how conversational structure constrains visual attention, but not as compellingly how visual attention feeds back and can influence language processing. Strong evidence for this may come from research on language acquisition, in word learning, where studies have shown the observation of another's gaze increases later comprehension. Yu et al. (2005) had English-speaking individuals listen to a story told in Mandarin Chinese depicting a child's picture book. Participants followed along with the corresponding images while some others were presented with an additional crosshair indicating the speaker's gaze fixations. Participants who observed the crosshair performed better on a Mandarin Chinese comprehension test. This shows more

---

[1]A reviewer of this chapter suggested that we consider the possibility that vision presents some unique sources of information not present in other modalities. This would certainly be a controversial thesis, though there is inarguably a unique benefit to visual attention and gaze that other modalities may not have. For example, gaze may reveal the knowledge of a task partner that may only be made explicit or implicit through an overt linguistic act such as a reference (Yu et al. 2005). Gaze fixations to objects or their presence in a visual array serves as potentially "cheap but efficient" information about the task and a task partner's knowledge (Bard 2007; Brown-Schmidt 2009b). These properties may indeed give vision some unique characteristics relative to other modalities—they may have lower thresholds to achieving the shared knowledge than (say) overt speech or gesture.

directly how low-level social factors such as gaze following can directly affect comprehension. Importantly, exact timing of the occurrence of speech and eye movements was not as important as the *coupling* between speech and eye movements. As long as both auditory and visual content were experienced as coupled—manipulated via lag between speech sounds and oculomotor movements—greater comprehension occurred (Yu et al. 2005). If substantially displaced, however, gaze had no impact. Therefore, attending to the corresponding visual information while engaged in conversation may be important for effective comprehension. Accurate comprehension is highly influenced by one's own visual attention and observation of another's gaze fixations. Further, visual and auditory coupling in the process of connecting visual referents with acoustic signals may also be crucial (with children, see examples in Yu and Smith 2012).

Perhaps when considering the pervasive influence of social variables in basic cognitive processing, these results should *not* come as a surprise. It is possible that attending to the spatial region attended to by another may be a reflexive process (Friesen and Kingstone 1998; Shepherd 2010; Kuhn and Kingstone 2009). For example, Friesen and Kingstone (1998) found that reaction times decreased in response to objects presented on the screen when a cartoon face in the centre of the screen gazed towards the region where the object was to appear. Further, reaction times did not decrease when cues were presented by non-social images (e.g., a garbled face stimulus). Gaze following is inherently social and impacts visual attention more so than other types of content that might occur simultaneously within our visual field. Gaze following can be used to orient our attention towards potentially relevant information while avoiding potentially irrelevant information (Gallup et al. 2012). Importantly, what captures visual attention may be the result of our social context. This means that the shared knowledge between two or more people, common ground (Clark and Marshall 1981), may be established more implicitly, emerging out of constraints imposed by one's social context and less by the active process of explicitly deciding what information will be shared.

This process of quick integration of another's gaze may indeed help in dialogue. Gaze following can be used to disambiguate visual referents within established common ground well before clarifying linguistic information is presented. Hanna and Brennan (2007) seated participants at a table across from one another. Each half of the table contained the same objects. Though aware of having the same objects, participants unable to view the other's objects were given access to their partner's eyes. On critical trials, one participant directed the other to pick up an object similar to another object (e.g., a blue circle with five dots opposed to a blue circle with six dots). On these trials, participants used the gaze of the director to disambiguate the correct referent well before linguistic disambiguation occurred. Using the director's gaze to locate the proper referent occurred even when the order of the director's display did not match the actor's display. Clearly social information acquired through vision is used to predict what actions should be taken before clarifying linguistic information is presented. Indeed, knowing the proper referents allows participants to act in accordance with a shared common ground and even predict what linguistic information will be presented next.

Despite these intriguing results, gaze is not a social factor that is without constraint from factors such as cognitive cost. If the conditions are not right, specifically when following another's gaze is not of benefit to completing an established goal, gaze following may not occur. According to Bard et al. (2007) one assumption made by most researchers is that common ground is established only when interlocutors are able to "[model] another's knowledge while maintaining his or her own" (p. 617). Alternatively, establishing common ground may be mediated by the goals of specific individuals especially when time may *not* permit one to model another's knowledge. In one experiment, Bard and colleagues had participants navigate a map while under a time constraint. Another participant provided instructions and feedback while a crosshair on a map supposedly indicated where, on a corresponding map, the instructing participant's gaze was located. The crosshair was manipulated at a crucial point to either "look" at a relevant or irrelevant landmark. Findings show participants remained unaffected by the supposed gaze of another, indicated by the position of the crosshair, when the crosshair landed on irrelevant stimuli. This suggests that modelling another's knowledge may be limited to only that which is relevant while under a time constraint. Furthermore, when under time pressure, integrating all possible knowledge of another into one's model is costly and simply not feasible.

This may seem to throw into question the *automatic* nature of gaze following, instead supporting the notion that high-level processes such as one's goals may mediate low-level social processes such as gaze following. More likely, social gaze and what it implies about an interaction partner are rarely independent of each other, and despite the seeming simplicity of the former, the latter can be considerably more complicated. So when gaze may reflect cognitively costly social modelling, it may simply not have the same quick effects as when it merely implies spatial orientation (Friesen and Kingstone 1998).

Throughout this section, we have reviewed studies showing the impact of basic, relatively lower-level, social content on language processing. These studies show that one interlocutor's access to the other's gaze influences task competency regardless of the roles played by each participant (Bard et al. 2007; Richardson et al. 2007). In some cases low-level social information can be "ignored" depending on associated information, such as relatively more complex information like goal-oriented behaviour. But results do suggest that lower-level processes such as observing another's gaze *can strongly influence* the structuring of higher-level goals such as decision-making (Friesen and Kingstone 1998), novel language comprehension (Yu et al. 2005), task performance (Brown-Schmidt 2009b), and their outcomes. In this sense, social content may be supplanted in place of more individual goals. Many of these goals are based on social content provided by one's visual context, and the belief about others' access to the same content within their own visual context. Throughout the next section we will emphasise the influence of social content as it permeates linguistic processing at the level of maintaining specific goals.

12.3 Vision and "Visual Belief"

The previous section addressed how linguistic processes are affected by lower-level social factors and how these factors are tightly coupled to visual processes. Yet these factors were shown to influence language only in specific contexts. When attending to the location of another's gaze, recognition of the appearance of objects in that location occurs sooner (Friesen and Kingstone 1998). However, these cues may be completely ignored when they serve no purpose of completing one's goals, or it is too cognitively costly (Bard et al. 2007). In fact, it could be argued that gaze following only occurs when it fits within the constraints of one's current goals. Other research on visual attention aims to uncover what and how much visual information goes unnoticed when nested within a goal-oriented context (see Simons and Chabris, 1999 for a first look into this literature). Here we review a few social contexts that show how lower-level visual factors are constrained and, in turn, linguistic processing.

There is always the risk of being misunderstood given the inherent ambiguity of language. Despite this risk, conversational partners are able to rapidly converge on a shared understanding, where changes in how sentences are structured and ideas expressed are seamlessly adapted in the fast moving context of conversation. To do so, people must be able to make predictions about what another is likely to understand given subtle sources of social information (cf. Pickering and Garrod 2013). One source that rapidly guides language processing is being aware of another's location in space. Simply knowing another's location has powerful effects of disambiguating referents in visual space. For instance, Hanna and Tanenhaus (2004) asked a speaker to read aloud instructions to a partner on how to prepare a cake, where sometimes the speaker asked for a package of cake mix. Crucially, one package of mix was within the speaker's reach while the other was not. By tracking eye movements of the addressee, gaze fixations of the addressee revealed they immediately considered the cake mix that was outside the speaker's reach. The addressee naturally considered the speaker to be asking for the package they could not reach on their own, showing no signs of referent competition. Gaze fixations reveal that linguistic processing is constrained by the possibilities for action implied by another's spatial location. Such consideration, based on visual cues of proximity and location, is but one example of how language use is employed against a backdrop of other knowledge, in this case of what others can see and do.

There are many other studies that attest to the complexity and pervasiveness of visual information in language processing, where simple visual cues provide the basis for assessment of another's knowledge or mental states. These include adjustments in linguistic processing based on whether one appears to be a child (Newman-Norlund et al. 2009), member of the same social category (Isaacs and Clark 1987), friend or stranger (Savitsky et al. 2011), or male or female (Senay and Keysar 2009). Moreover, adjustments are extended across a number of linguistic behaviours, from grammatical choice (Balcetis and Dale 2005), to pronunciation and prosody (Kraljic et al. 2008a, b), to spatial language (Galati et al. 2012; Schober 1993).

an entirely different beast when attempting to conceal valuable information in a high-risk interrogation.

Although the goals of conversational deception may vary, what is common throughout all contexts is that the high-level factors involved have a direct impact on the low-level behaviours that shape communication. In a study by De Paulo and Bell (1996), researchers examined how possessing knowledge about another's beliefs can lead to deception, which in turn, can alter various properties of language use. Participants were instructed to discuss their ideas about paintings that they had liked or disliked with people who sometimes introduced themselves as the artist and who also expressed various levels of investment with each painting (e.g., by stating, "This is one of my favorites", vs. "This is one that I did".). When investment by the artist was potentially high, but the participant did not particularly care for the work, participants were more likely to be dishonest. In doing so, they tended to delay or avoid clear answers, provide misleading information, and use language that exaggerated their liking for the painting. Thus, the participants here were able to rapidly adjust their linguistic and communicative behaviour based on inferences about another's beliefs.

The subtle social information that must be managed when lying to another can also be in the form of ongoing actions generated by the person being lied to. These actions are not independent of how the liar responds, but are very much shaped, intentionally or not, by the liar during the interaction. In the intentional case, Burgoon and colleagues (Burgoon et al. 1999) have shown that when deceivers interact with conversational partners who do not appear to be involved with the ongoing discourse, such as by avoiding eye contact, leaning backward, or turning their bodies to distance themselves, deceivers are more likely to engage in compensatory movement behaviours to increase their partner's involvement. These particular behaviours, such as increasing proximity and the number of gaze fixations on the other's face, are also accompanied by greater verbal involvement. Importantly, the non-verbal and verbal patterns expressed here are elicited by a situational context where there is a perceived need to mitigate suspicion, a belief brought about by visually attending to the low-level changes in the partner's behaviour. When situational factors change, such as when the threat of detection is less severe, deceivers may express distinct and opposite patterns of behaviour. For example, using eye-tracking techniques, Pak and Zhou (2013) have found that deceivers fixate the faces of interlocutors less often, and that averting gaze seems to increase in frequency during the deceptive act (cf. Vrij and Semin 1996).

The above studies also raise an interesting possibility that visual information may feedback into the dialogue structure itself. Along these lines, Doherty-Sneddon et al. (1997) found that co-presence (visibility through video) modulated the entire discourse structure of an interaction. So while visual attention to non-verbal behaviours both influences and is influenced by discourse, the deceptive case suggests that this may be a more complex functional relationship when processing the language and behaviour of one's interlocutor. The cues can sometimes compete, and give way to more or less effective social evaluations depending on how they are focused upon.

The consideration of social information in deceptive communication also extends beyond the deceiver to the recipient or observer of a lie. In a study conducted by Boltz et al. (2010), participants were instructed to listen to a conversation between a man and a woman whose speech rates and response latencies were varied as they answered a number of questions. Participants were then asked to guess who was lying and when. A correlation was found between responses labelled as lies and how long it took the man or woman to start answering each question. Participants associated short and on-time latencies with honesty and mostly took long latencies as a cue for deception. But the tendency to do so depended on the gender of the speaker and their perceived motivation to lie. When the content of a response made someone else appear more favourable, and was spoken by a female, participants were more likely to selectively overlook verbal cues of deception. On the other hand, when the content of a response made the speaker look more favourable, and was spoken by a male, the verbal cues were more strictly applied. These results suggest that generalisations based on speaker attributes can dramatically alter how language is processed when assessing deceptive intent.

The very complexity of this functional relationship—how high-level discourse demands and low-level perceptual and cognitive demands interrelate in natural language use—has not enjoyed as systematic a theoretical development as is greatly needed. One way of pursuing this systematic exploration, as we describe in our concluding section, is to treat the cognitive system as multiply constrained and adaptive, more like a complex web of interdependencies, rather than a system of many independent controllers or processes.

12.5 Self-organisation of Interaction

We have offered some discussion and review of how language comprehension is fundamentally shaped by social factors. We have focused in several places on the lower-level process of visual attention and gaze as both a social factor and cognitive process that shapes the comprehension of language. We have also shown that higher-level social factors, including the knowledge and beliefs about an interlocutor, sharply impact comprehension, including back onto the process of attention itself. The resulting view of the cognitive system is one of a complex, multilayered system that involves a variety of *interdependencies*—systems that interact actively during the process of language comprehension. It seems unlikely that there is a central computational executive which is simultaneously "computing the positions and velocities" of all of these bits and pieces of human interaction (Dale et al. 2013). Instead, there must be active flows of information continually and mutually interacting with one other.

In order to make tractable this abundance of multimodal and dynamic structures, it seems fruitful to consider a process of *self-organisation* as driving complex language processes such as comprehension in context. Self-organisation is based on the idea that a coherent performance, such as naturalistic language processing, is not "controlled centrally", but develops through a distributed process of mutual influence among the parts of a system. Such influence can cut across all levels. For example, if we learn a new fact about a conversation partner, it might shift our attention both in how we sample the visual array, but also in terms of what is to be said or interpreted. Here is where the concept of self-organisation becomes important: Two people interacting in a joint task come to form their behaviours through compensatory, complementary behaviours. These behaviours influence one another locally and incrementally, making the whole conversational performance itself a kind of self-organising "synergy" (Fusaroli et al. 2013). It is "self-organizing" in the sense that there is no one central system dictating how the interaction should unfold. Its fate is driven instead by the interdependencies among the parts as they function *together*.

Dale et al. (2013) discuss this problem as the "centipede's dilemma" of interaction research: Understanding how the various processes at play during language come to coordinate and work together. The famous children's poem by Craster has a toad ask a centipede, "Pray, which leg moves after which?" The centipede ponders this effortly, attempting awareness of this coordination, only to find that she disrupts her very ability to move. The same happens if we do this during conversation. The cognitive mechanisms involved in a conversational performance probably outnumber a centipede's legs, especially if we counted mechanisms unavailable to conscious report. So how do we coordinate everything? The standard approach of distilling channels and exploring its behaviour piece by piece may suffer the same consequence as the centipede. This is not to say such distillation is not required, as it probably is. It is to say that recourse to language in context, and exploring the interdependencies among many channels, should also be a central part of the explanatory agenda.

In this paper, we identified some "flows of information" across cognitive processes that provide clues. When *belief about the partner* is influenced by the context of conversation, this simple piece of information may serve to highlight or amplify particular expectations or processes (Brennan et al. 2010; Brown-Schmidt 2009a, b). This relatively high-level process "sets the stage" for particular organised patterns of attention and memory at a lower level. Surely constraints of accessibility and ease of processing will influence this at all levels (Shintel and Keysar 2009), but this is not to say that the *results* of social factors do not shift the overall strategic organisation of conversational performance at a longer timescale (Duran et al. 2011). The functional timescale of conversational performance is not on the scale of "immediate or initial access", as is sometimes implied by these minimalist theories. It is instead at the timescale of hundreds of milliseconds if not seconds. At this timescale we find language comprehension processes weaved together with larger-scale pragmatic interpretation, discourse structure, social expectations and belief, and so on. We cannot consider even the lower-level processes of attention as separate from these higher-level social factors.

But how do these lower-level processes constrain each other, and act together? Akin to the centipede's dilemma, rather than understanding the interaction "leg by leg by leg," we would suggest the idea of a "synergy" operating within and between people during coherent conversational performance. The behaviours that can mutually influence each other are quite numerous: turn-taking and rhythms, prosody or pauses, use of particular words or phrases, gesture and other bodily variables, facial expression, distribution of eye gaze, and so on. These flow into larger structures that are also numerous: adjacency pairs, topics of conversation and so on. Because these processes are often studied independently (or in small clusters), many theories tend to assume our cognitive system is composed of modules uniquely evolved or developed for each such process (Dale et al. 2013). But these can also be seen as an array of levels that are mutually constraining, and dynamically evolving, as two people come to form, in an important way, a "unit of analysis", and the interaction itself a stable, if temporary, synergy itself.

This is the notion of a synergy: a functional reduction of variability, where processes do not simply align, but can complement and compensate for each other. These different processes get coupled and constrained, moving the system into a lower-dimensional functional unit, and smaller number of stable categories—perhaps surprisingly simpler than what would be anticipated from the multidimensionality of the system itself (Shockley et al. 2009). For example, perhaps at the coarsest level of description in human interaction, one could see stable modes in the form of *arguing* (Paxton and Dale, 2013), or *flirting* (Grammer et al. 1998), or *joint decision-making* (Fusaroli and Tylén 2012), or *giving-directions* (Cassell et al. 2007). These have sometimes been referred to as "oral genres" (e.g., Busch 2007).

What is still lacking is a systematic agenda to uncover how these various processes work together to bring about *multimodal coordination* between two interacting people. We have argued in this chapter that visual attention is not independent of a range of other information sources. Social factors from gaze of another, or belief about another, can modulate the dynamics of one's attentional processes. So vision and attention are a key component, figuring into a heterogeneous assemblage of experimental techniques and observational analyses, and an associated array of diverse theoretical mechanisms that have yet to be integrated. But this array of mechanisms described above does not *merely* interact. They weave processes together into coherent interactive "structures". And it is a powerful force, much the way we experience that awkward cafe conversation that started this chapter. The great difficulty *many* of us seem to have with tailoring such short interactions is perhaps reflective of the rapid integration of diverse cognitive processes that underlie it.

References

Akmajian, A., Demers, R. A., & Harnish, R. M. (1987). *Linguistics: An introduction to language and communication* (2nd ed.). Cambridge, MA: MIT Press.

Allopenna, P. D., Magnuson, J. S., & Tanenhaus, M. K. (1998). Tracking the time course of spoken word recognition using eye movements: Evidence for continuous mapping models. *Journal of Memory and Language, 38*(4), 419–439.

Balcetis, E., & Dale, R. (2005). An exploration of social modulation of syntactic priming. In *Proceedings of the 27th Annual Meeting of the Cognitive Science Society* (pp. 184–189).

Bard, E. G., Anderson, A. H., Chen, Y., Nicholson, H. B., Havard, C., & Dalzel-Job, S. (2007). Let's you do that: Sharing the cognitive burdens of dialogue. *Journal of Memory and Language, 57*(4), 616–641.

Boltz, M. G., Dyer, R. L., & Miller, A. R. (2010). Jo are you lying to me? Temporal cues for deception. *Journal of Language and Social Psychology, 29*(4), 458–466.

Branigan, H., & Pearson, J. (2006). Alignment in human-computer interaction. In K. Fischer (Eds.), *How people talk to computers, robots, and other artificial communication partners*, (pp. 140–156).

Branigan, H. P., Pickering, M. J., Pearson, J., & McLean, J. F. (2010). Linguistic alignment between people and computers. *Journal of Pragmatics, 42*(9), 2355–2368.

Brennan, S. E., Galati, A., & Kuhlen, A. K. (2010). Two minds, one dialog: coordinating speaking and understanding. *Psychology of Learning and Motivation, 53*, 301–344.

Brennan, Susan E., & Clark, H. H. (1996). Conceptual pacts and lexical choice in conversation. *Journal of Experimental Psychology. Learning, Memory, and Cognition, 22*(6), 1482.

Brown-Schmidt, S. (2009a). Partner-specific interpretation of maintained referential precedents during interactive dialog. *Journal of Memory and Language, 61*(2), 171–190.

Brown-Schmidt, S. (2009b). The role of executive function in perspective taking during online language comprehension. *Psychonomic Bulletin & Review, 16*(5), 893–900.

Brown-Schmidt, S., & Hanna, J. E. (2011). Talking in another person's shoes: Incremental perspective-taking in language processing. *Dialog and Discourse, 2*, 11–33.

Buller, D. B., & Burgoon, J. K. (1996). Interpersonal deception theory. *Communication Theory, 6*, 203–242.

Burgoon, J. K. (2006). The dynamic nature of deceptive verbal communication. *Journal of Language and Social Psychology, 25*(1), 76–96.

Burgoon, J. K., Buller, D. B., White, C. H., Afifi, W., & Buslig, A. L. (1999). The role of conversational involvement in deceptive interpersonal interactions. *Personality and Social Psychology Bulletin, 25*(6), 669–686.

Busch, M. W. (2007). *Task-based pedagogical activities as oral genres: A systemic functional linguistic analysis*. ProQuest.

Cassell, J., Kopp, S., Tepper, P., Ferriman, K., & Striegnitz, K. (2007). Trading spaces: How humans and humanoids use speech and gesture to give directions. In T. Nishida (Ed.), *Conversational informatics* (pp. 133–160). New York: Wiley.

Clark, H. H. (n.d.), & C. P. Marshall. (1981). Definite reference and mutual knowledge. A. K. Joshi, B. L. Webber, & I. A. Sag (Eds.), *Elements of discourse understanding*. Cambridge: Cambridge University Press.

Clark, H H. (1992). *Arenas of language use*. Chicago: University of Chicago Press.

Clark, H. H. (1996). *Using language* (Vol. 4). Cambridge: Cambridge University Press.

Clark, H. H. (2005). Coordinating with each other in a material world. *Discourse studies, 7*(4–5), 507–525.

Cooper, R. M. (1974). The control of eye fixation by the meaning of spoken language: A new methodology for the real-time investigation of speech perception, memory, and language processing. *Cognitive Psychology, 6*(1), 84–107.

Dale, R., Fusaroli, R., Duran, N. D., & Richardson, D. C. (2013). The self-organization of human interaction. In B. Ross (Ed.), *Psychology of learning and motivation* (Vol. 59, pp. 43–95). Elsevier Inc: Academic Press.

De Paulo, B. M., & Bell, K. L. (1996). Truth and investment: Lies are told to those who care. *Journal of Personality and Social Psychology, 71*(4), 703.

Doherty-Sneddon, G., Anderson, A., O'Malley, C., Langton, S., Garrod, S., & Bruce, V. (1997). Face-to-face and video-mediated communication: A comparison of dialogue structure and task performance. *Journal of Experimental Psychology: Applied, 3*(2), 105–125. doi:10.1037/1076-898X.3.2.105.

Duran, N. D. & Dale, R. (2012). Increased vigilance in monitoring others' mental states during deception. In N. Miyake, D. Peebles, & R. P. Cooper (Eds.), *Proceedings of the 34th annual conference of the cognitive science society* (pp. 1518–1523). Austin: TX: Cognitive Science Society.

Duran, N. D., & Dale, R., Kello, C., Street, C. N. H., & Richardson, D. C. (2013). Exploring the movement dynamics of deception. Frontiers in Cognitive Science. Gilbert, D. T. (1991). How mental systems believe. *American Psychologist, 46*, 107–119.

Duran, N. D., Dale, R., & Kreuz, R. J. (2011). Listeners invest in an assumed other's perspective despite cognitive cost. *Cognition, 121*(1), 22–40.

Eberhard, K. M., Spivey-Knowlton, M. J., Sedivy, J. C., & Tanenhaus, M. K. (1995). Eye movements as a window into real-time spoken language comprehension in natural contexts. *Journal of Psycholinguistic Research, 24*(6), 409–436.

Farmer, T. A., Anderson, S. E., Freeman, J. B., & Dale, R. (in press). Coordinating motor actions and language. In P. Pyykkonen & M. Crocker (Eds.), *Visually situated language comprehension*. Amsterdam: John Benjamins.

Friesen, C. K., & Kingstone, A. (1998). The eyes have it! Reflexive orienting is triggered by nonpredictive gaze. *Psychonomic Bulletin & Review, 5*(3), 490–495.

Fusaroli, R., & Tylén, K. (2012). Carving language for social interaction: A dynamic approach. *Interaction studies, 13*, 103–123.

Fusaroli, R., Rączaszek-Leonardi, J., & Tylén, K. (2013). Dialog as interpersonal synergy. *New Ideas in Psychology, 32*, 1–11.

Galati, A., Michael, C., Mello, C., Greenauer, N. M., & Avraamides, M. N. (2012). The conversational partner's perspective affects spatial memory and descriptions. *Journal of Memory and Language*. Retrieved from http://www.sciencedirect.com/science/article/pii/S0749596X12001040.

Gallup, A. C., Hale, J. J., Sumpter, D. J., Garnier, S., Kacelnik, A., Krebs, J. R., & Couzin, I. D. (2012). Visual attention and the acquisition of information in human crowds. *Proceedings of the National Academy of Sciences, 109*(19), 7245–7250.

Garrod, S., & Pickering, M. J. (2004). Why is conversation so easy? *Trends in cognitive sciences, 8*(1), 8–11.

Grammer, K. (1990). Strangers meet: Laughter and nonverbal signs of interest in opposite-sex encounters. *Journal of Nonverbal Behavior, 14*(4), 209–236.

Grammer, K., Fink, B., & Renninger, L. (2002). Dynamic systems and inferential information processing in human communication. *Neuro Endocrinology Letters, 23*(Suppl 4), 15–22.

Grammer, K., Kruck, K. B., & Magnusson, M. S. (1998). The courtship dance: Patterns of nonverbal synchronization in opposite-sex encounters. *Journal of Nonverbal Behavior, 22*(1), 3–29.

Hanna, J. E., & Brennan, S. E. (2007). Speakers' eye gaze disambiguates referring expressions early during face-to-face conversation. *Journal of Memory and Language, 57*(4), 596–615.

Hanna, J. E., & Tanenhaus, M. K. (2004). Pragmatic effects on reference resolution in a collaborative task: Evidence from eye movements. *Cognitive Science, 28*(1), 105–115.

Hanna, J. E., Tanenhaus, M. K., & Trueswell, J. C. (2003). The effects of common ground and perspective on domains of referential interpretation. *Journal of Memory and Language, 49*(1), 43–61. doi:10.1016/S0749-596X(03)00022-6.

Horton, W. S., & Gerrig, R. J. (2005). The impact of memory demands on audience design during language production. *Cognition, 96*(2), 127–142.

Horton, W. S., & Slaten, D. G. (2012). Anticipating who will say what: The influence of speaker-specific memory associations on reference resolution. *Memory & Cognition, 40*(1), 113–126.

Huettig, F., Mishra, R. K., & Olivers, C. N. (2012). Mechanisms and representations of language-mediated visual attention. *Frontiers in Psychology, 2*, 394.

Isaacs, E. A., & Clark, H. H. (1987). References in conversation between experts and novices. *Journal of Experimental Psychology: General, 116*(1), 26–37.

Johnson, K., Strand, E. A., & D'Imperio, M. (1999). Auditory–visual integration of talker gender in vowel perception. *Journal of Phonetics, 27*(4), 359–384.

Keysar, B., Barr, D. J., & Horton, W. S. (1998). The egocentric basis of language use: Insights from a processing approach. *Current Directions in Psychological Sciences, 7*, 46–50.

Keysar, B., Lin, S., & Barr, D. J. (2003). Limits on theory of mind use in adults. *Cognition,* *89*(1), 25–41.

Kraljic, T., Brennan, S. E., & Samuel, A. G. (2008a). Accommodating variation: Dialects, idiolects, and speech processing. *Cognition, 107*(1), 54–81.

Kraljic, T., Samuel, A. G., & Brennan, S. E. (2008b). First impressions and last resorts how listeners adjust to speaker variability. *Psychological Science, 19*(4), 332–338.

Kreysa, H., & Pickering, M. J. (2011). Eye movements and dialogue. Retrieved from http://pub.uni-bielefeld.de/publication/2028210.

Kronmüller, E., & Barr, D. J. (2007). Perspective-free pragmatics: Broken precedents and the recovery-from-preemption hypothesis. *Journal of Memory and Language, 56*(3), 436–455.

Kuhn, G., & Kingstone, A. (2009). Look away! Eyes and arrows engage oculomotor responses automatically. *Attention Perception and Psychophysics, 71*, 314–327.

Laidlaw, K. E. W., Foulsham, T., Kuhn, G., & Kingstone, A. (2011). Potential social interactions are important to social attention. *Proceedings of the National Academy of Sciences, 108*(14), 5548–5553.

McGurk, H., & MacDonald, J. (1976). Hearing lips and seeing voices. Retrieved from http://www.nature.com/nature/journal/v264/n5588/abs/264746a0.html.

Nadig, A. S., & Sedivy, J. C. (2002). Evidence of perspective-taking constraints in children's online reference resolution. *Psychological Science, 13*(4), 329–336.

Newman-Norlund, S. E., Noordzij, M. L., Newman-Norlund, R. D., Volman, I. A., de Ruiter, J. P., Hagoort, P., & Toni, I. (2009). Recipient design in tacit communication. *Cognition, 111*(1), 46–54.

Pak, J., & Zhou, L. (2013). Eye gazing behaviors in online deception. *AMCIS 2013 Proceedings.* Retrieved from http://aisel.aisnet.org/amcis2013/ISSecurity/RoundTablePresentations/3.

Paxton, A., & Dale, R. (2013). Argument disrupts interpersonal synchrony. *Quarterly Journal of Experimental Psychology, 66* (11), 2092–2102.

Pickering, M. J., & Garrod, S. (2004). Toward a mechanistic psychology of dialogue. *Behavioral and Brain Sciences, 27*(2), 169–189.

Pickering, M. J., & Garrod, S. (2013). Forward models and their implications for production, comprehension, and dialogue. *Behavioral and Brain Sciences, 78*, 49–64.

Richardson, D. C., & Dale, R. (2005). Looking to understand: The coupling between speakers' and listeners' eye movements and its relationship to discourse comprehension. *Cognitive Science, 29*(6), 1045–1060.

Richardson, D. C., Dale, R., & Kirkham, N. Z. (2007). The art of conversation is coordination common ground and the coupling of eye movements during dialogue. *Psychological Science, 18*(5), 407–413.

Richardson, D. C., Dale, R., & Tomlinson, J. M. (2009). Conversation, gaze coordination, and beliefs about visual context. *Cognitive Science, 33*(8), 1468–1482.

Savitsky, K., Keysar, B., Epley, N., Carter, T., & Swanson, A. (2011). The closeness- communication bias: Increased egocentrism among friends versus strangers. *Journal of Experimental Social Psychology, 47*, 269–277.

Schober, M. F. (1993). Spatial perspective-taking in conversation. *Cognition, 47*(1), 1–24.

Senay, I., & Keysar, B. (2009). Keeping track of speaker's perspective: The role of social identity. *Discourse Processes, 46*(5), 401–425.

Shepherd, S. V. (2010). Following gaze: Gaze-following behavior as a window into social cognition. *Frontiers in Integrative Neuroscience, 4*. Retrieved from http://www.ncbi.nlm.nih.gov/pmc/articles/pmc2859805/.

Shintel, H., & Keysar, B. (2009). Less is more: A minimalist account of joint action in communication. *Topics in Cognitive Science, 35*(2), 281–322.

Shockley, K., Richardson, D. C., & Dale, R. (2009). Conversation and coordinative structures. *Topics in Cognitive Science, 1*(2), 305–319.

Shockley, Kevin, Santana, M.-V., & Fowler, C. A. (2003). Mutual interpersonal postural constraints are involved in cooperative conversation. *Journal of Experimental Psychology:
Human Perception and Performance, 29*(2), 326.

Simons, D. J., & Chabris, C. F. (1999). Gorillas in our midst: Sustained inattentional blindness
for dynamic events. *Perception, 28*(9), 1059–1074.

Tanenhaus, M. K., & Brown-Schmidt, S. (2008). Language processing in the natural world.
Philosophical Transactions of the Royal Society B: Biological Sciences, 363(1493), 1105.

Tanenhaus, M. K., Spivey-Knowlton, M. J., Eberhard, K. M., & Sedivy, J. C. (1995). Integration
of visual and linguistic information in spoken language comprehension. *Science, 268*(5217),
1632–1634.

Vrij, A., & Semin, G. R. (1996). Lie experts' beliefs about nonverbal indicators of deception.
Journal of Nonverbal Behavior, 20(1), 65–80.

White, C., & Burgoon, J. (2006). Adaptation and communicative design. *Human Communication
Research, 27*(1), 9–37.

Yu, C., Ballard, D. H., & Aslin, R. N. (2005). The role of embodied intention in early lexical
acquisition. *Cognitive Science, 29*(6), 961–1005.

Yu, C., & Smith, L. B. (2012). Embodied attention and word learning by toddlers. *Cognition,
125*(2), 244–262. doi:10.1016/j.cognition.2012.06.016.